IET HEALTHCARE TECHNOLOGIES SERIES 16

EEG Signal Processing

Other volumes in this series:

EEG Signal Processing

Feature extraction, selection and classification methods

Edited by
Wai Yie Leong

The Institution of Engineering and Technology

Published by The Institution of Engineering and Technology, London, United Kingdom

The Institution of Engineering and Technology is registered as a Charity in England & Wales (no. 211014) and Scotland (no. SC038698).

First published 2019

The Institution of Engineering and Technology
Michael Faraday House
Six Hills Way, Stevenage
Herts, SG1 2AY, United Kingdom

www.theiet.org

British Library Cataloguing in Publication Data
A catalogue record for this product is available from the British Library

ISBN 978-1-78561-370-8 (hardback)
ISBN 978-1-78561-371-5 (PDF)

Typeset in India by MPS Limited
Printed in the UK by CPI Group (UK) Ltd, Croydon

Contents

Foreword

A Brain Computer Interface (BCI) system monitors the brain activity and translates features related to the user's intent or feeling, into device commands. The electro-encephalography (EEG) is the most common method in order to record the brain activity in BCI systems. It is a non-invasive method that requires relatively simple and inexpensive equipment, and it is easier to use than other methods. Nevertheless, EEG-based BCIs provide modest speed and accuracy so it is necessary to use multichannel systems and proper signal processing methods. EEG signal processing is divided into several stages: feature extraction, selection and classification.

Feature extraction methods obtain specific information from EEG signals. These features can be useful in order to discriminate among different mental tasks. Then, using selection methods, a subgroup of the most relevant features for classification is chosen, namely

- Spectral features achieved from Fourier transform.
- Blind source separation
- Optimisation approach
- Autoregressive models
- Nonlinear methods
- Genetic algorithms
- Unsupervised learning

Feature classification methods allow from the selected features, to determine what class is the most probable for a specific sample. To that purpose, the aims of the book is to focus on Feature extraction methods to obtain specific information from EEG signals. These features can be useful in order to discriminate among different mental tasks. This book emphasizes strategies, case studies and clinical practices. Advanced Signal Processing methods will also be discussed in this title.

Ir Prof Wai Yie Leong

Chapter 1

EEG extraction for meditation

Lewis Tee[1] and Wai Yie Leong[1]

1.1 Introduction

Meditation, in recent years, is receiving renewed interest by researchers [1–6]. Meditation is a practice with long traditions in human history. Despite the long standing in history, research regarding meditation was not well concluded in literature for the past several decades [7]. The neurophysiological process of meditation and long-term impact is also not well known [8].

Numerous benefits have been associated with meditation [2,4,9,10]; however, proposals of meditation as a beneficial practice were met with skepticism due to the lack of rigor and quality in measurements found in early studies [8,11]. Until the framework of meditation is well established, it would be a challenge to present the effects of meditation in an irrevocable manner. The author is in the opinion that measures of meditation must be more thoroughly explored and established before the effects (beneficial or otherwise) of meditation could be effectively examined.

In this study, the focus is placed on measures of brain activities that are associated with meditation. With the intention that a physiological common ground that is universal across differing meditative activities could be found here.

Electroencephalogram (EEG) is the selected method of measurement. EEG measurement produces a time series signal that represents the neural activity of the brain. It holds the advantage of being a painless, noninvasive, relatively quick, and economical procedure. Electrodes are placed on the scalp of the subject, with no pre-procedure requirements (i.e., fasting), nor post procedural side effects (i.e., nausea, surgical wounds).

The EEG device records a subject's brain electrical activity, and the resulting data can be applied to study meditation activities [7,12]. A review is performed upon existing methods used for EEG signal processing. This chapter examined EEG signal processing steps that are commonly applied, namely data preparation and feature extraction.

EEG signal, as a common among biomedical signal, is often noisy, contaminated, with data in high-dimensional space [13]. Effective signal processing is used to identify and extract features that are relevant to the object of study that may

[1]Faculty of Engineering and Information Technology, MAHSA University, Malaysia

otherwise be hidden [14–16]. Computer assisted signal processing can offer expedited extraction and classification of data, improved accuracy, and reliability while reducing strenuous human workload and related human errors.

The author acknowledges that researches have previously attempted to streamline meditation, and have proposed to classify a broad range of practice into two archetypes: Focused Attention (FA) meditation and Open Monitoring (OM) meditation [8]. This difference is defined by the method taken in achieving meditation. Both methods call for a comfortable and relaxed physical and mental state. FA has the practitioner placing attention upon an object (breathing, visualization, etc.), while OM has the practitioner opening to allow a variety of thoughts to freely flow through the mind while being attached to none of the thoughts that arise. Both methods achieve a common goal, where the practitioner's mind is no longer focused upon logical thought processes.

For the purpose of discussion in this chapter, a simple, generic definition of meditation is offered—A voluntary mental exercise that disengages the mind from logical thought process, giving rise to mental relaxation and peaceful emotions.

1.2 EEG signal processing

The term electroencephalogram (EEG) has been coined by Hans Berger, a German psychiatrist, in 1924 denoting the recording of brain waves [17]. Brain waves [15] are not actual waves emitted by the brain, but are signals produced by measuring the voltage differences across two points of the scalp. It is however named as such due to the rhythmic sinusoidal wave forms that appear on the measured signal. Brainwaves appear to reflect some of the functional states of the brain, and by using signal decomposition and analysis techniques, it is possible to extract and classify EEG features that are associated to event-related potentials, specific brain functions, or physical conditions.

The Nyquist principle (which states that the sampling rate of the signal must exceed twice the maximum frequency to be detected) is a basic criterion that must be met in order to avoid signal aliasing or undetectable interference. When the Nyquist criterion is not met, two sine waves of different frequency can have identical sampled data if one or both waves have a frequency that is more than half the sampling frequency, shown as follows. Equation (1.1) shows the Fourier transform of the original signal $x(t)$, giving $X(f)$:

$$X(f) = \int_{-\infty}^{\infty} x(t)e^{-i2\pi ft} \, dt \qquad (1.1)$$

The Poisson summation of the above is shown in (1.2):

$$X_s(f) = \sum_{k=-\infty}^{\infty} X(f - kf_s) \qquad (1.2)$$

where the X_s of sine waves with $f > \frac{f_s}{2}$ could not be distinguished from the lower frequency component. Modern EEG measurement devices sample signals at a rate of at least 128 Hz, or 250 Hz/256 Hz, up to over 1000 Hz. As most EEG signal of interest lies between 0.5 Hz and 30 Hz range, these signals lie well within the measurement range of standard EEG measurement devices. There also exists evidence of Gamma waves (30–100 Hz) observed in the human brain. Gamma waves of interest are currently observed in the regions of 30–50 Hz, which are again well within the measurement range of modern EEG devices.

1.2.1 Data collection

Modern EEG procedure is typically noninvasive. The EEG consists of at least two, usually more, low-impedance gold-plated electrodes that are placed on the subjects' scalp using conductive adhesive paste [18]. One electrode is placed on the reference point, the ear mastoid bone, and the rest placed across points of interest.

Due to the fact that each individual brain neuron produces only a very small electrical current, a change in voltage is measureable only when a large group of neurons fire simultaneously [19]. The electromotive force (EMF) of this signal (activation of a group of neurons) must then propagate from the cerebral cortex through layers of meninges, scalp, and scalp tissue, before the magnetic component of the EMF is detected by the EEG electrode. Due to this fact, the spatial resolution of EEG is poor and electrodes placed next to each other would detect virtually no differences. As such, an international standard 10–20 electrode placement system [20] was adopted by the International Federation in Electroencephalography and Clinical Neurophysiology in 1958 to indicate formal EEG measurement spots that have proven to be fruitful in past research (shown in Figure 1.1).

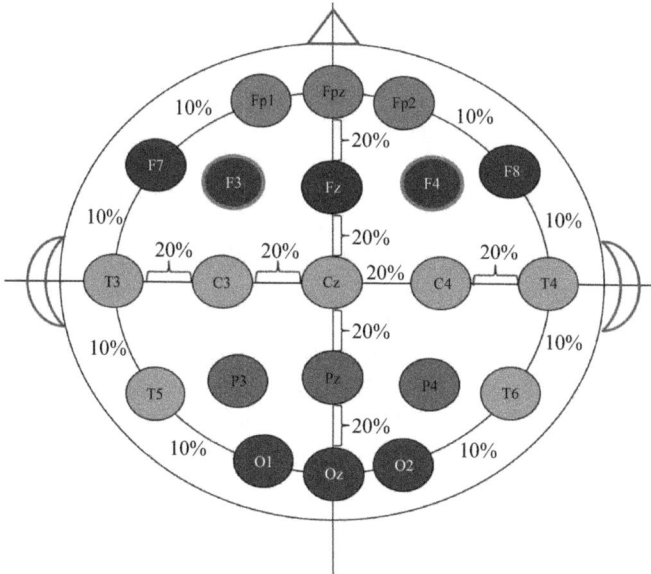

Figure 1.1   The top view of patient's scalp overlaid with the 10–20 standard electrode placement map

1.2.2   Data preparation

Data preparation generally serves the purpose of removing signal contamination and delivers cleaned data for the next stage, feature extraction.

Brainwaves are continuous signals that reflect a person's brain activity. In a typical EEG measurement process, a common reference is selected at an arbitrary location, usually at the mastoid behind the ears. The source signal is the measured potential difference between two points located on the person's scalp, one being the site of interest and the other the reference point. An EEG recording is a digital signal sampled (at regular interval) from the source signal. Raw EEG data at first glance look like noise. That is because raw EEG data comprises five signal sources [15]:

1. Targeted biosignal of brain
2. Non-targeted physiological signal of other sources (e.g., ECG, EOG, and EMG)
3. Scalp—Electrode interface interference (e.g., sweat artifact)
4. Power grid interference (50 Hz/60 Hz)
5. Other noises (e.g., body movement, breathing, footsteps)

Only the brain signal is desirable; the other signals would be considered as contamination, or artifacts, and needed to be removed or reduced prior to subsequent data extraction and analysis [21] (to be discussed in Section 2.3).

1.2.3   Filters

In addition to the commonly performed linear detrending and mean subtraction, filtering is a corner stone in removing signal contamination.

An anti-aliasing low-pass filter applied at the input of the EEG recording device filters out signals at frequencies higher than half the sampling rate. This removes anti-aliasing created by signals with frequencies beyond the EEG recording device's measurement capability according to the Nyquist Criterion discussed previously.

High-pass filter [22] removes low-frequency (cut off at 0.5 Hz) contamination from body movement, electrode drift, sweat artifact, which appears as a gentle slope as the conductivity at the tissue–electrode interface slowly changes due to the change in ionic composition caused by sweating.

A notch filter [22] centered at 50 Hz or 60 Hz is typically applied to remove power grid interference.

Application of frequency filters requires the interference signal and target signal to occupy difference frequency range. However, in practice, there are certain interferences that occupy the same frequency space as the target signal. One example is when the study involves investigation of slow sleep wave (i.e., 0.5–4 Hz), where over filtration using a low-frequency filter may result in potential data loss.

It is advisable to take precautionary steps, such as minimizing body movement, regulating ambient temperature to reduce sweating, maintaining good electrode contact, with the intent to minimize the need to filter the signal.

Furthermore, along with EEG, there exist at the same time within the subject's body at least three other types of bio-electrical signal, namely ECG, EOG, and

EMG. These signals are typically not bounded within a particular frequency band and require other processing technique, such as ICA, discussed in Section 2.2.3.

Artifacts from eye blinks are one of the most influential contaminations in EEG signals [23] and must be removed from the signal. Several techniques have been proposed to detect eye blink artifacts, such as threshold amplitude [24]. This method is easy to apply, but presents several drawbacks [25], i.e., (1) low accuracy leading to over rejection of data segments, (2) unable to adapt to variable duration of the eye blink, and (3) unable to detect partial artifact in a segmented epoch if the artifact peak was not present (thus not meeting the amplitude threshold). Independent Component Analysis, discussed in Section 2.2.3, is another method to remove eye blink artifacts. Chang *et al.* [25] has proposed single channel ruled based eye blink detection with adaptive eye blink duration algorithm.

1.2.4 Principal component analysis

Depending on the data, some EEG Signal can be considered high dimensional data, and analysis of such raw signal requires complex computational processes. Such data may be subjected to dimension reduction process (e.g., principal component analysis (PCA)), where the most relevant data are extracted and reconstructed as Feature Vectors for subsequent processing or classification stages [26].

PCA is a statistical technique often used in facial recognition and bioengineering processing application and has been successfully applied in EEG signal processing as well [27–30]. It is a technique used for extracting significant pattern from high-dimensional data.

PCA is an orthogonal linear transformation that projects the original data onto a new coordinate system, where the projected data are expressed with the greatest variance along the first principal component, the second greatest variance along the second principal component, and so forth, with the first loading vector having to satisfy (1.3).

$$
\begin{aligned}
v_{(1)} &= \arg\max_{\|v\|=1}\left\{\|Xv\|^2\right\} \\
&= \arg\max_{\{v\}=1} v^T X^T X v \\
&= \arg\max\left\{\frac{v^T X^T X v}{v^T v}\right\}
\end{aligned}
\tag{1.3}
$$

and subsequent loading vector $v_{(k)}$ that expresses the greatest variance of the projected data with (1.4).

$$
v_{(k)} = \arg\max_{\|v\|=1}\left\{\|\hat{X}_k v\|^2\right\} = \arg\max\left\{\frac{v^T \hat{X}_k^T \hat{X}_k v}{v^T v}\right\}
\tag{1.4}
$$

Finally, the decomposition of $\mathbf{X}$ is given as $\mathbf{T} = \mathbf{XV}$, where $\mathbf{X}$ is an n-by-p data matrix, with n number of rows, which correspond to the number of observations (in this case, EEG channels), and p number of columns, which correspond to the number of variables (data sequence). $\mathbf{V}$ (the coefficient matrix) is a p-by-p matrix, with each column containing the coefficients of one principal component in descending order of component variance, also referred to as eigenvectors of $\mathbf{X}^T\mathbf{X}$, which is proportional to the covariance matrix of the dataset $\mathbf{X}$.

Feature Vectors can be formed from a selected set of eigenvectors (typically the more significant components) for the purpose of dimension reduction. By projecting the original dataset $\mathbf{X}$ with p number of variables onto a new space (with the same number of p variables) that is uncorrelated through the transformation of $\mathbf{T} = \mathbf{XV}$. Components with lesser significance can be removed by truncating the transformation using $\mathbf{T_L} = \mathbf{XV_L}$, where L is an integer of the first L loading vectors and the resulting matrix $\mathbf{T_L}$ is now an n-by-L matrix having only L columns.

1.2.5   Independent component analysis

Because EEG recording easily reflects signal from sources within and without the brain, the contaminated signal can be corrected with the application of independent component analysis (ICA) [21]. EEG recording can be seen as data that are generated by the mixing of several different sources of brain activity, from different parts of the brain, as well as other biomedical sources (muscular movement signal, ECG, etc.). By applying ICA to the resulting mixed signal, independent components can be extracted to either reveal hidden data or be removed if deemed as artifacts.

For the sake of computational simplicity and feasibility, multivariate data, such as EEG or other biomedical signals, are often assumed to have Gaussian distribution and are linear representations of statistically independent signal sources. ICA algorithm isolates statistically independent sources, termed Independent Components, which are then viewed as linear combinations of the source signal. Artifact independent component can be identified and removed, resulting in a signal that is free from the specific artifact. This method of artifact removal has presented success in the removal of eye blink artifact and muscle movement artifact [31–34].

ICA [35] in general, has a requirement that the recorded signals are assumed independent sources, given by (1.5) and (1.6), where in the recorded signals x, there are n number of linear combination of n independent components, denoted by s_1, $s_2, \ldots, s_n$.

$$x_j = a_{j1}s_1 + a_{j2}s_2 + \cdots + a_{jn}s_n \tag{1.5}$$

$$x = \sum_{k=1}^{n} a_k s_k \tag{1.6}$$

In (1.5), a_{jn} is an unknown parameter that is dependent on the distance and attenuation between the source and the recorder. In order to solve this set of equations, with a_{jn} being unknown, it is necessary to assume $s_1, s_2, \ldots, s_n$ are statistically independent, and derive the estimates of a_{jn} based on statistical properties of s_n, possible under the condition $j \geq n$.

For the purpose of computational convenience, (1.6) is rewritten in matrix form, shown in (1.7) with $\mathbf{x}$ being a vector of mixed (observed) data, $\mathbf{s}$ a random vector representing the (latent) source, and **A** a matrix containing unknown variables a_{jn}.

$$\mathbf{x} = \mathbf{As} \qquad (1.7)$$

ICA operations also assume **A** to be a square matrix, and components of **s** are statistically independent as mentioned above. By estimating the matrix **A**, and computing it's inverse, **V**, we have

$$\mathbf{s} = \mathbf{Vx} \qquad (1.8)$$

where **V** is a linear transformation of **x**, which produces maximum independence in the components of **s**.

Generally speaking, ICA requires as many recording of mixed signals, **x**, as there are latent source, *s*. In EEG, *s* multichannel recording would be required. Studies have achieved ICA source separation using single channel data, however there are additional conditions, such as having stationary signal with sources that are disjointed in the frequency domain [36], or working in combination with another decomposition method, e.g., EMD [37].

Other methods of decomposing the signal such as Wavelet and Empirical Mode Decomposition, and isolating the specific wavelet decomposition/IMFs of said ocular artifacts for removal has been met with success as well [27].

1.2.6 Segmentation and manual artifact deletion

EEG signal is non-stationary in nature. Figure 1.2 shows a raw EEG signal where the subject's mental state changed from the first state (0–34 s) to a second state (49–78 s), with interferences generated by movement, which happened in between the shift. A baseline drift can also be seen in the second state after the 49 s mark. Segmentation can be applied to ease the processing of this signal. In Figure 1.3, two 8-s segments were extracted from each state, and filtered through a 1 Hz high-pass Butterworth filter.

Interferences seen in Figure 1.2 were non-rhythmic (not of a specific frequency band nor conform to an identifiable pattern), or simply exceeded the dynamic range of the amplifier and appeared as a signal with its peak cut off. These interferences

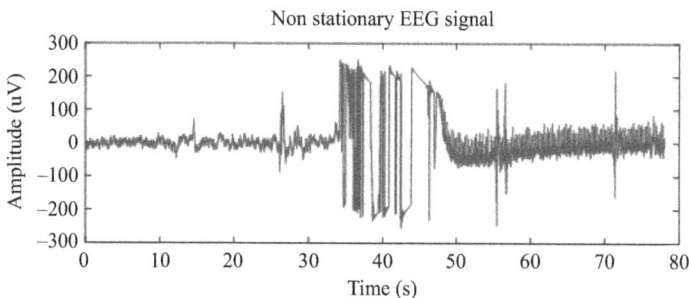

Figure 1.2 *Raw signal, naturally non-stationary with movement artifact between 35 and 48 s mark and baseline drift after the 49 s mark*

are difficult to remove by use of filters or algorithms because they do not consist of regular patterns. Artifacts not removed by filters or algorithms are manually rejected at this stage. Manual deletion is a straight forward approach and commonly practiced [38] as a last resort strategy to visually inspect and manually delete segments of contaminated data. This approach can be a tedious task, and subject to human error.

Segmentation is an advantageous processing step to create a quasi-stationary state, seen in Figure 1.3 for further processing steps that require a signal to be stationary.

Length of segments vary, and the precision in deciding the exact length does not result in any overly significant impact. There exist certain determining criteria

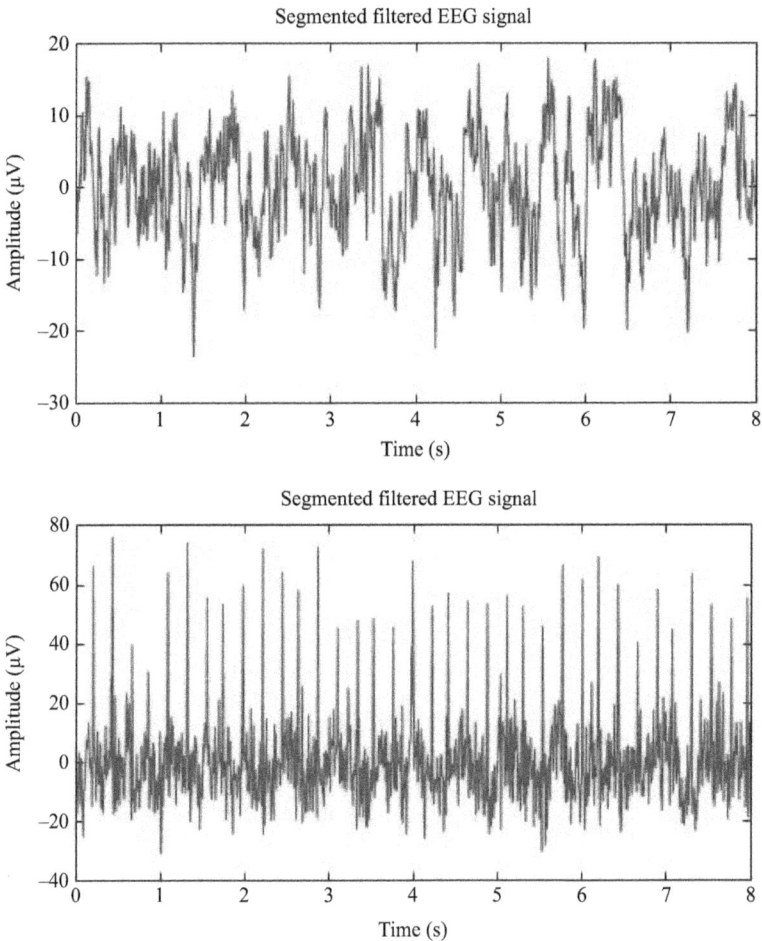

Figure 1.3   High-pass filtered, artifact-free, quasi-stationary segments (top) and extracted from raw signal (bottom)

for segment length, such that each segment must exceed at least one cycle of the target signal frequency. Shorter segments are lighter on computational load and provide a quasi-stationary signal. Longer segments, while benefiting data hungry algorithms, may be non-stationary.

Adaptive segmentation is a viable option to obtain optimum presentation of stationary signal. In adaptive segmentation, each segment is not uniform in length. The criteria for adaptive segmentation are often described by the longest artifact-free segment possible while remaining a stationary signal. Adaptive segmentation offers the best of both worlds at the expense of computational load. However, it may adversely contribute to signal processing time as it requires relatively more complex processing stage. This needs to be taken into consideration for processes with time-sensitive results (e.g., real-time measurement).

1.3   Feature extraction

Feature extraction is the stage where specific data are extracted from the vast amount of available data for the next processing step—classification.

Feature extraction attempts to convert the original complicated or even dimensionally sparse signal to a simpler set of data or to create a new set of data (feature vectors) while retaining significant representation of the original signal. This process, when done successfully, reduces the computational and time resources required to parse through the original signal to achieve the desired data classification [39].

Pattern detection and recognition are limited by signal features, contaminations, EEG recording device constraints, and subject dependent issue [26]. To overcome some of these limitations, research and development in feature extraction techniques are required.

A study can, and usually does, utilize more than one extracted feature set to complement one another for higher accuracy in the classification stage.

1.3.1   Review of some feature extraction methods

Over the last two decades, many researches have addressed automatic EEG signal processing, most, if not all, methods generally fall into one of the four following methods [40]: (1) time domain analysis, (2) frequency domain analysis, (3) time–frequency analysis, and (4) nonlinear/complexity analysis.

1.3.1.1   Time domain analysis
Instantaneous statistics
These are data calculated from statistical metrics such as mean, median, minimal/maximal amplitude, range, standard deviation, and higher order statistics such as skewness and kurtosis. While these may be considered as fundamental data, with an appropriate approach, they can yield valuable information as demonstrated by Wallant *et al.* [39], where maximal amplitude and standard deviation was successfully applied to the automatic detection of bad and noisy EEG channels.

Amplitude mean

Signal mean subtraction is commonly performed to study signal distribution. However, doing so may prove to overlook information embedded within the signal mean. It can be seen in the following result: in Figure 1.4, the amplitude mean of the EEG signals representing two different mental activities performed by subjects are significantly different. The amplitude mean of meditation, a relaxing mental exercise, is shown to be much lower, average by one order of magnitude, when compared to the signal amplitude mean measured during post-meditation. Detailed data are tabulated in Appendix A.

A classification accuracy of 84.06% was achieved in this study using 5.25E-3 as the cut-off level for a yes–no classifier for meditation.

Hjorth parameters

The Hjorth parameters are also indicators in the time domain that is applicable as EEG feature [41–43]. Hjorth parameters consist of Activity, Mobility, and Complexity, described as follows:

$$\text{Activity} = \text{var}(x(t)) \tag{1.9}$$

$$\text{Mobility} = \sqrt{\frac{\text{Activity}(x'(t))}{\text{Activity}(x(t))}} \tag{1.10}$$

$$\text{Complexity} = \frac{\text{Mobility}(x'(t))}{\text{Mobility}(x(t))} \tag{1.11}$$

The Activity (1.9), Mobility (1.10), and Complexity (1.11) of the time domain signal $x(t)$ are also the zero-order moment (signal power), second-order moment

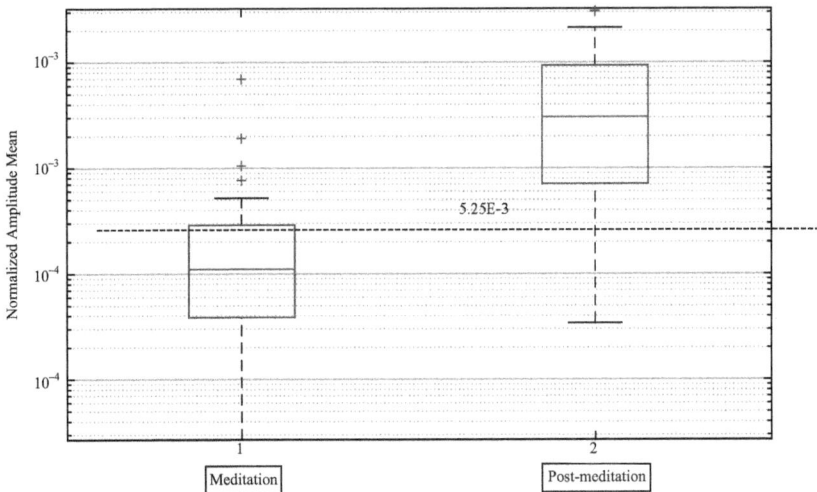

Figure 1.4   *Normalized amplitude mean of meditation signal versus post-meditation signal from nine subjects*

(mean frequency), and fourth-order moment (change in frequency), respectively, of the power density spectrum. While the Hjorth parameters appear to give us information pertaining to the frequency domain, it offers signal feature extraction in the time domain, and potentially skipped some of the complexities that are usually associated with frequency domain operators such as fast Fourier transform (FFT), short-time Fourier transform (STFT), or wavelets, which are discussed in Section 1.3.1.2.

1.3.1.2   Frequency domain analysis

The frequency domain presents data across the frequency domain instead of time and is often used for feature extraction.

Power spectral density

Power spectral density (PSD) is a very common feature extracted from EEG. Fast Fourier transform is applied to the autocorrelation data of the time domain signal, which converts the data into the frequency domain, and subsequently plotted as PSD. PSD in μV^2/Hz displays how the power of a time domain signal $x(t)$ is distributed in terms of frequency.

The truncated Fourier transform $\hat{x}_T(\omega)$, where the signal is integrated over a finite period between time 0 and T, is written as

$$\hat{x}_T(\omega) = \frac{1}{\sqrt{T}} \int_0^T x(t)e^{-i\omega t}dt \tag{1.12}$$

and the power spectral density $S_{xx}(\omega)$ is computed as

$$S_{xx}(\omega) = E\left[|\hat{x}_T(\omega)|^2\right] \tag{1.13}$$

where E is the expected value. However, as EEG data are a discrete signal instead of a continuous signal, the PSD, $\bar{S}_{xx}(\omega)$, is obtained using summation over N samples instead of integration over T period, where $\Delta t = \frac{T}{N}$, and denoted as

$$\bar{S}_{xx}(\omega) = \frac{(\Delta t)^2}{T} \left| \sum_{n=1}^{N} x_n e^{-i\omega n} \right|^2 \tag{1.14}$$

Analyzing the PSD of a signal can quickly reveal essential characteristic of a signal in the frequency domain, and serves as an important foundation for signal processing. Upon transformation, a signal is decomposed into multiple individual sinusoidal waves and segregated into discrete frequencies. As a widely accepted common practice, waves with frequencies 0.5–4 Hz are labeled as Delta Waves, 4–7 Hz are labeled as Theta Waves, 7–14 Hz as Alpha Waves, 11–1 Hz as Sigma Waves (less prominently used), 14–30 Hz as Beta Waves, and beyond 30 Hz as Gamma Waves, shown in Figure 1.5.

Studies using EEG PSD [38] demonstrated capability in detecting differences in grammar processing (grammatical vs ungrammatical). Wallant *et al.* [39] suggested that PSD can be obtained and individual band power be compared among different bands of choice, malleable according to the design of experiment. The application of

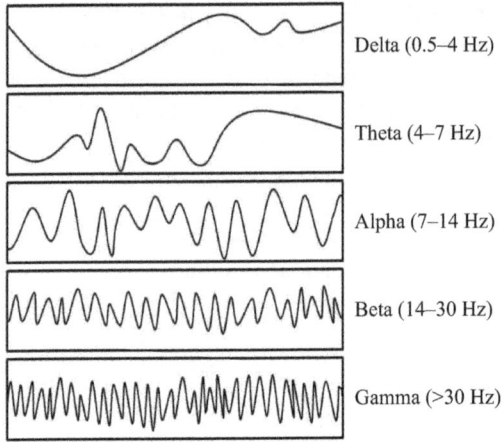

Figure 1.5   Representation of time series brain wave signals and respective frequency bands

logarithmic compression to band power calculation is an extension to PSD that is often considered and has been shown to enhance PSD evaluation [44–47].

However, Fourier analysis presents certain shortcomings, primarily because basic Fourier processes assume the signal to be stationary, which means that the frequency of the signal does not change with time. The FFT presents the frequency component of the signal under the assumption that it is present at all times, as FFT cannot report when a particular frequency component is present. The short-time Fourier transform discussed in the following section was developed in response to this issue.

1.3.1.3   Time–frequency extraction methods

Time–frequency analysis incorporates both time and frequency information of the signal. Classical time–frequency methods such as STFT and spectrogram plots localized segments of frequency data as a function of time.

Short-time Fourier transform

STFT approach takes a signal and cuts it into segments of identical length. Fourier transform is applied to each segment, and the resulting frequency domain data are plotted against the temporal axis of the original signal. Having some data overlap in the individual segments is common. The STFT provides frequency and phase information of the local segment, and when plotted against time, a change in local spectra is obtained.

STFT retains the limitation of Fourier transform, where the signal is assumed to be stationary within the segmented window. With a predefined window length, time and frequency resolutions are fixed, and as such a certain degree of compromise between these two parameters must be determined and accepted. It would be helpful to decide beforehand if the feature of interest lies within the lower or higher frequency band, and determine the optimum time window width, generally termed narrowband (good time resolution) or wideband (good frequency resolution) to extract the target data.

STFT, $X(\tau, \omega)$, of the original signal $x(t)$ is written as

$$X(\tau, \omega) = \int_{-\infty}^{\infty} x(t)w(t - \tau)e^{-i\omega t}dt \tag{1.15}$$

where the window function $w(t)$ is typically a Gaussian window. However, as EEG data are typically discrete time data, $x(n)$, the discrete time STFT, is written as

$$X(m, \omega) = \sum_{-\infty}^{\infty} x(n)w(n - m)e^{-i\omega n} \tag{1.16}$$

with $w(n)$ as the window.

Due to the simple, unvarying window function, the computational time required from STFT is shorter compared to the continuous wavelet transform and was deemed more appropriate in time-sensitive, real-time application [48].

Spectrogram

By taking the magnitude squared of the resulting data from the STFT process discussed above, gives the following spectrogram:

$$\text{spectrogram}(\tau, \omega) = |X(\tau, \omega)|^2 \tag{1.17}$$

The spectrogram is a graphical display of the frequency response over time and provides an intuitive way to interpret the time-frequency information compared to deciphering raw STFT data [38].

Time–frequency decomposition methods offer both time and frequency components information. Different methods present these information in different ways. The temporal versus frequency resolution compromised in STFT analysis inevitably lead to the development of other more adaptive methods that can provide good time resolution for high-frequency components and good frequency resolution for low-frequency components. Two frequently used methods with adaptive time–frequency resolution, the Wavelet Transform and Hillbert–Huang Transform, are discussed in Sections 1.3.1.3.3 and 2.3.2.3.

Wavelet Transform

The Wavelet Transform can be seen as an expansion to the STFT; while this is not strictly true, the Wavelet Transform does offer information similar to the STFT. Due to the fact that EEG is a non-stationary signal, a time-varying spectral estimation technique such as wavelet has proven to be popular feature extraction methods [44,49–52].

However, the Wavelet Transform offers certain advantage over the STFT, as Wavelet Transform decomposes a time series signal and expresses it as a series of wavelets using varying window sizes. Long windows are used to obtain good

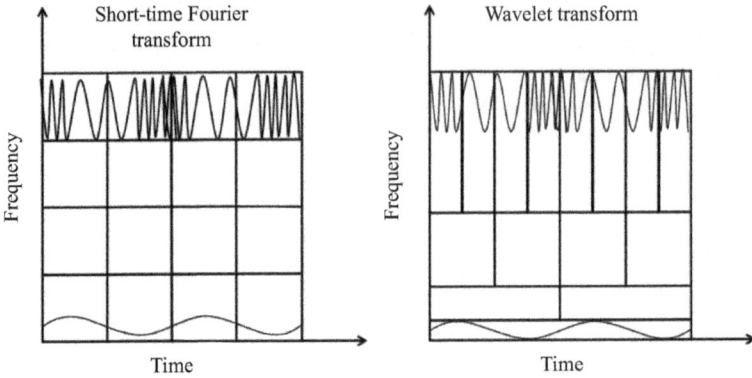

Figure 1.6   Comparison of time and frequency resolution capabilities between STFT and WT

frequency resolution at low frequencies and short windows are used to obtain good time resolution when capturing high-frequency components.

Figure 1.6 compares the time and frequency resolution of STFT versus Wavelet. As can be seen in the figure, STFT struggles to estimate the frequency of low-frequency components with a fixed time window that is too short. Subsequently, STFT could not separate the time in which two different higher frequency components occur because the fixed window is too long. When we look at the wavelet transform, the mother wavelet is dilated to completely capture the entire cycle of the low-frequency component and compressed to separate the time in which the higher frequency components occur. Generally speaking, the smaller a window, the better the time resolution, the poorer the frequency resolution, and vice versa. However, wavelet is able to offer good time resolution for higher frequency component while maintaining good frequency resolution (due to components being in high frequency). In the same way, wavelet offers good frequency resolution for low-frequency component while maintaining good time resolution for the same reasoning.

The mathematical model of the Continuous Wavelet Transform is written as

$$CWT(\tau, s) = \frac{1}{\sqrt{|s|}} \int_{-\infty}^{\infty} x(t) \cdot \psi * \left(\frac{t - \tau}{s}\right) dt \tag{1.18}$$

where $\psi(t)$ is the mother wavelet, a window of finite length; τ is the translation (location of window); and s is the dilation, a scaling factor. All windows used are a compressed or dilated version of the mother wavelet.

Continuous Wavelet Transform, however, does pose as a complex calculation challenge as the τ and s constantly change. To facilitate calculation, the wavelet transform is often performed in a discrete form.

The recorded signal $x[n]$ is decomposed through a series of filters seen in Figure 1.7. The mother wavelet, $g[n]$, is a high-pass filter, which decomposes the signal and outputs detail coefficients, with D_1 being the Level 1 coefficient, D_2

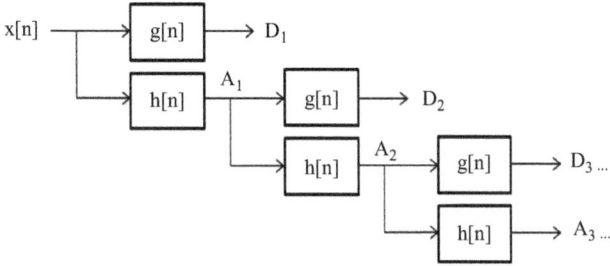

Figure 1.7   Discrete Wavelet Transform filter banks

being the Level 2 coefficient, and so forth. At the same time, the signal $x[n]$ is passed through a low-pass filter with an impulse response $h[n]$ written as

$$y[n] = \sum_{k=-\infty}^{\infty} x[k]h[n-k] \tag{1.19}$$

and $h[n]$ is a quadrature mirror filter of $g[n]$, with the relationship between these two filters written through their respective z-transform as

$$G(z) = zH(-z^{-1}) \tag{1.20}$$

The low-pass filter, $h[n]$, outputs an approximation of the signal that becomes the input for the next decomposition stage. At each stage, half of the signal is removed, and the signal is down sampled by 2. Each decomposition stage (output from the low-pass filter) halves the time resolution and doubles the frequency resolution. At the following stage, the result is given by

$$y[n] = \sum_{k=-\infty}^{\infty} x[k]h[2n-k] \tag{1.21}$$

Following this decomposition process, the input signal $x[n]$ must be a multiple of 2^n, where n is the number of decomposed levels. If $n = 6$ (i.e., 6 levels of decomposition), given $2^6 = 64$, then the data sequence to be decomposed must have at least 64 data, or multiples of 64. However, keep in mind that in order to satisfy the Nyquist criterion, the minimum number to samples must at least double 2^n as shown in Figure 1.8.

1.3.1.4 Nonlinear analysis

While STFT and wavelet transform are commonly applied to process EEG signal, both are linear processes. EEG is often assumed to be linear and stationary (achieved through segmentation), in order for the signal to be decomposed and evaluated using certain techniques that assume linearity, or even stationarity.

However, EEG signal changes accordingly to the functional state of the brain, and the signal source is a complex biological organ. Therefore, it is reasonable to regard EEG as a non-stationary, nonlinear signal. In this section, we discuss decomposition methods that take the nonlinear nature of EEG into consideration.

| Original signal x[n] 128 samples 0–64 Hz | | Wavelet decomposition | | | | |

A6	D6	D5	D4	D3	D2	D1
2 samples	2 samples	4 samples	8 samples	16 samples	32 samples	64 samples
0–1 Hz	1–2 Hz	2–4 Hz	4–8 Hz	8–16 Hz	16–32 Hz	32–64 Hz

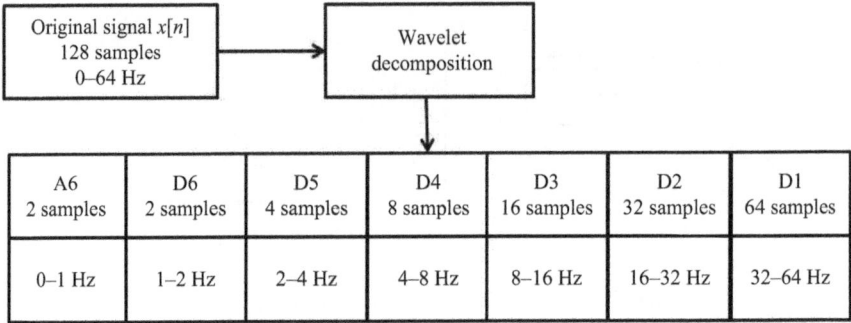

Figure 1.8   Analysis for selection of wavelet decomposition level for selected signal sampled at 128 Hz

Hillbert–Huang Transform

Empirical mode decomposition (EMD) [53–55] method is capable of decomposing nonlinear data into multiple IMF (Intrinsic mode functions) and is an adaptive process without the limitation of a predefined basis function or segment length compromise [56].

IMFs are sifted by first identifying local extrema in the signal $x(t)$. An upper envelope is created by connecting all local maxima using a cubic spline line, and a lower envelope is created by connecting all local minima using the same method. Mean of the upper and lower envelope is denoted as m_1.

The proto-IMF component, denoted as h_1, is shown in (1.22).

$$h_1 = x(t) - m_1 \tag{1.22}$$

To calculate the first IMF component, the same process of creating upper and lower envelopes for h_1 is performed, giving m_{11} as the mean of h_1's envelopes. h_{11} is the first IMF (where $k = 1$) derived in (1.23)

$$h_{1(k)} = h_{1(k-1)} - m_{1(k)} \tag{1.23}$$

All IMFs must satisfy these conditions: (1) Difference in the number of zero crossings and the number of extrema is 1 or less. (2) The mean value between the local maxima and local minima is 0 [40]. The decomposition of signal $x(t)$ can then be expressed as

$$x(t) = \sum_{k=1}^{K} imf_k(t) + r_k(t) \tag{1.24}$$

with K IMFs and $r_k(t)$ is the residue that is a monotonic function.

Data from the IMFs extracted from EEG signal provide local amplitude and frequency information, and based on this, weighted frequencies data can be obtained via the Hilbert Transform forming the Hilbert Spectral Analysis.

Higher order spectral analysis

Higher order spectral analysis (HOSA) is a natural extension of the power spectral analysis. The second moment is written as

$$\sigma^2(t_1) = E(x(t)x(t+t_1))\qquad(1.25)$$

The power spectrum, the Fourier transform of the second moment, is a representation of a Gaussian process and assumes signal linearity. The third moment is written as

$$\gamma(t_1, t_2) = E(x(t)x(t+t_1)x(t+t_2))\qquad(1.26)$$

Bispectrum, the Fourier transform of the third moment, examines the relationship of the sine waves at two frequencies, f_1 and f_2, and as well as the $f_1 + f_2$ frequency. The mathematical model is written as

$$B(f_1, f_2) = |X(f_1) \cdot X(f_2) \cdot X * (f_1 + f_2)|\qquad(1.27)$$

where X is the Fourier transform coefficient at the respective frequencies of f_1 and f_2, and $X*$ is the complex conjugate of X. For a signal that is likely to be nonlinear, bispectrum can provide additional information such as phase coupling between the frequency components, while suppressing Gaussian noise [57].

There is a drawback in HOSA, where good estimations require a large number of data. One recommendation suggests using N^2 number of samples [58,59], where N is the number of data points in the FFT calculations.

Fractal dimension

Fractal dimension measures the complexity of the signal [60–63]. Complexity measurement is sensitive to noise and faces the challenge of limited data availability. FD measures self-similarities, which is often seen in systems of nature. The brain, which is a biological organ, too displays self-similarities on temporal and spatial scales [64]. According to Zappasodi *et al.* [64], a single channel EEG has an FD range in between one and two. FD was observed to decrease in association to Beta decrease and Alpha increase in stroke patient during recovery periods. Zappasodi *et al.* suggested FD is capable of capturing the loss of complexity that reflects system dysfunction due to damage, revealing a structure–function correlation observable using FD measurement.

1.3.1.5 Multi-channel EEG analysis

Finally, it ought to be reminded that EEG signal recorded from the brain is not a standalone single signal by itself. Each signal is reflecting a group of neurons, and it is highly likely that groups of neurons in the brain are interlinked, and the activation of neurons at one location is correlated to the activation of other neuron groups. When more than one EEG signal is measured, it is advantageous to place the electrodes at strategic locations, where these signals can then be studied together using cross-correlation or coherence (akin to cross-correlation in the frequency domain) analysis.

Cross-correlation

To begin with data in the time domain, the cross-covariance of two signals, $x(t)$ and $y(t)$, is given by

$$\gamma_{XY}(\tau) = E[(X_t - \mu_X)(Y_{t+\tau} - \mu_Y)] \tag{1.28}$$

and the cross-correlation is the cross-covariance divided by the standard deviation of $x(t)$ and $y(t)$, respectively

$$\rho_{XY}(\tau) = \frac{E[(X_t - \mu_X)(Y_{t+\tau} - \mu_Y)]}{\sigma_X \sigma_Y} \tag{1.29}$$

where μ_X and μ_Y are the mean of $x(t)$ and $y(t)$, respectively. The mean and standard deviation are constant under the assumption that $x(t)$ and $y(t)$ are stationary. As such, the results of cross-covariance and cross-correlation are independent of t.

Spectral coherence

Moving into the frequency domain, the Cross Spectral Density, or Cross-Spectrum, is the Fourier transform of γ_{xy}, where $\gamma_{xy}(\tau)$ is the Cross-Covariance. Cross-Spectrum G_{xy} is written as

$$G_{xy}(f) = \sum_{\tau=0}^{\infty} \gamma_{xy}(\tau) e^{-2\pi i \tau f} \tag{1.30}$$

which gives a complex result of real and imaginary parts

$$G_{xy}(f) = A_{xy}(f) + i\psi_{xy}(f) \tag{1.31}$$

The spectral coherence, $C_{xy}(f)$, in turn expresses the spectrum in dimensionless units by taking the magnitude square, written as

$$C_{xy}(f) = \frac{|G_{xy}(f)|^2}{G_{xx}(f)G_{yy}(f)} \tag{1.32}$$

Multi-signal analysis immediately gives a different perspective of the source we are analyzing. Varying degrees of cross-correlation or coherency in multi-channel EEG data imply that activity in different parts of the brain function in relation with each other. However, due to the nature of EEG measurement, which measures the EMF detected on the scalp after propagating through layers of tissue and bones (as discussed in Section 2.1), there is the possibility that high correlation/coherence between two channels are due to a common source.

1.4   Conclusion

In this chapter, several different feature extraction methods were discussed. Time series signal often has self-defining, signature patterns embedded within. Each feature extraction method aims to recover some of these valuable patterns in their unique algorithm. Depending on the nature of the signal, differences in some features are likely to be more prominent than others. The act of selecting the appropriate extraction method that reveals significant features is an art in itself.

The evolution of feature extraction was also discussed. Many feature extraction methods prove to be very promising in their strength, yet some methods hold certain limitation. Handicapped methods evolve, as can been seen in the development of STFT and Spectrogram from the Fourier transform, and subsequently the "spiritual succession" of STFT by the Wavelet Transform.

EEG features function like a set of Global Positioning Satellites (GPS) [65–72]. For GPS, in order for a location to be triangulated, at least three GPS satellite signals must be received, and more satellite signals are required for increased precision. Likewise, data of one extracted EEG feature by itself may provide certain valuable information, two or more features are usually used in conjunction to reliably interpret and predict the functional states of the brain.

Appendix A

Participant ID	Meditation		Post-meditation	
	Data point	Signal mean	Data point	Signal mean
#1	F3	0.000365	F3	0.02984
	F3	0.000572	F3	N/A
	F4	0.002141	F4	0.008256
	F4	0.002678	F4	0.002068
#2	F3	0.000645	F3	0.1506
	F3	0.01052	F3	0.03092
	F4	0.001784	F4	0.09326
	F4	0.003978	F4	0.08784
#3	F3	0.002511	F3	0.01091
	F3	0.000371	F3	0.000381
	F4	0.00016	F4	0.05905
	F4	0.00029	F4	0.008816
#4	F3	0.003186	F3	0.3031
	F3	0.001095	F3	0.128
	F4	0.00308	F4	0.2141
	F4	0.000027	F4	0.09768
#5	F3	0.00761	F3	0.03266
	F3	0.06929	F3	0.02466
	F4	0.000833	F4	0.1083
	F4	0.005201	F4	0.05943
#6	F3	0.000838	F3	0.09266
	F3	0.000636	F3	0.1078
	F4	0.000402	F4	0.01077
	F4	0.001122	F4	0.006005
#7	F3	0.000507	F3	0.002291
	F3	0.001892	F3	0.002663
	F4	0.001525	F4	0.005343
	F4	0.001492	F4	0.002817

(Continues)

(*Continued*)

Participant ID	Meditation		Post-meditation	
	Data point	Signal mean	Data point	Signal mean
#8	F3	0.000155	F3	0.001714
	F3	0.001927	F3	0.000343
	F4	8.55E-05	F4	N/A
	F4	0.000172	F4	N/A
#9	F3	0.003905	F3	0.091
	F3	0.000183	F3	0.0237
	F4	0.01917	F4	0.3073
	F4	0.000755	F4	0.01675

References

[1]   A. Lutz, A. P. Jha, J. D. Dunne, and C. D. Saron, "Investigating the phenomenological matrix of mindfulness-related practices from a neurocognitive perspective," *Am. Psychol.*, vol. 70, no. 7, pp. 632–658, 2015.

[2]   S. Dimidjian and Z. V. Segal, "Prospects for a clinical science of mindfulness-based intervention," *Am. Psychol.*, vol. 70, no. 7, pp. 593–620, 2015.

[3]   A. Kruis, H. A. Slagter, D. R. W. Bachhuber, R. J. Davidson, and A. Lutz, "Effects of meditation practice on spontaneous eyeblink rate," *Psychophysiology*, vol. 53, no. 5, pp. 749–758, 2016.

[4]   M. A. Rosenkranz, A. Lutz, D. M. Perlman, *et al.* "Reduced stress and inflammatory responsiveness in experienced meditators compared to a matched healthy control group," *Psychoneuroendocrinology*, vol. 68, pp. 117–125, 2016.

[5]   J. Wielgosz, B. S. Schuyler, A. Lutz, and R. J. Davidson, "Long-term mindfulness training is associated with reliable differences in resting respiration rate," *Scientific Reports*, vol. 6, 27533, 2016.

[6]   D. Dentico, F. Ferrarelli, B. A. Riedner, *et al.*, "Short Meditation Trainings Enhance Non-REM Sleep Low-Frequency Oscillations," *PLoS One*, vol. 11, no. 2, pp. 1–18, 2016.

[7]   B. R. Cahn and J. Polich, "Meditation states and traits: EEG, ERP, and neuroimaging studies.," *Psychol. Bull.*, vol. 132, no. 2, pp. 180–211, 2006.

[8]   A. Lutz, H. a. Slagter, J. D. Dunne, and R. J. Davidson, "Attention regulation and monitoring in meditation," *Trends Cogn. Sci.*, vol. 12, no. 4, pp. 163–169, 2008.

[9]   T. W. Kjaer, C. Bertelsen, P. Piccini, D. Brooks, J. Alving, and H. C. Lou, "Increased dopamine tone during meditation-induced change of consciousness," *Cogn. Brain Res.*, vol. 13, no. 2, pp. 255–259, 2002.

[10] K. Rubia, "The neurobiology of meditation and its clinical effectiveness in psychiatric disorders," *Biol. Psychol.*, vol. 82, no. 1, pp. 1–11, 2009.

[11] P. Sedlmeier, J. Eberth, M. Schwarz, *et al.*, "The psychological effects of meditation: A meta-analysis," *Psychol. Bull.*, vol. 138, no. 6, pp. 1139–1171, 2012.

[12] T. Takahashi, T. Murata, T. Hamada, *et al.*, "Changes in EEG and autonomic nervous activity during meditation and their association with personality traits," *Int. J. Psychophysiol.*, vol. 55, no. 2, pp. 199–207, 2005.

[13] F. Lotte, M. Congedo, L. Anatole, F. Lotte, M. Congedo, and L. Anatole, "A review of classification algorithms for EEG-based brain – computer interfaces. To cite this version: A review of classification algorithms for EEG-based brain-computer interfaces," *J. Neural. Eng.*, vol. 4, pp. 24, 2007.

[14] I. J. Rampil, "A primer for EEG signal processing in anesthesia," *Anesthesiology*, vol. 89, no. 10, pp. 980–1002, 1998.

[15] M. Teplan, "Fundamentals of EEG measurement," *Meas. Sci. Rev.*, vol. 2, pp. 1–11, 2002.

[16] F. Lotte, "A tutorial on EEG signal processing techniques for mental state recognition in brain-computer interfaces," *Brain-Computer Music Interfacing*, 2014.

[17] T. F. Collura, "History and evolution of electroencephalographic instruments and techniques.," *J. Clin. Neurophysiol.*, vol. 10. pp. 476–504, 1993.

[18] G. Ungless, *The Activewave User Guide.* Cambridgeshire, UK: CamNTech Ltd., 2014.

[19] A. J. Rowan and E. Tolunsky, *Primer of EEG.* Philadelphia: Butterworth Heinemann, 2003.

[20] H. H. Jasper, "The ten-twenty electrode system of the International Federation," *Electroencephalogr. Clin. Neurophysiol.*, vol. 10, no. 2, pp. 371–375, 1958.

[21] M. Chaumon, D. V. M. Bishop, and N. A. Busch, "A practical guide to the selection of independent components of the electroencephalogram for artifact correction," *J. Neurosci. Methods*, vol. 250, pp. 47–63, 2015.

[22] L.-C. Teofilo, *Fundamentals of Sleep Technology.* Philadelphia, PA: Lippincott Williams & Wilkins, 2012.

[23] D. Hagemann and E. Naumann, "The effects of ocular artifacts on (lateralized) broadband power in the EEG," *Clin. Neurophysiol.*, vol. 112, no. 2, pp. 215–231, 2001.

[24] H. Nolan, R. Whelan, and R. B. Reilly, "FASTER: Fully automated statistical thresholding for EEG artifact rejection," *J. Neurosci. Methods*, vol. 192, no. 1, pp. 152–162, 2010.

[25] W.-D. Chang, H.-S. Cha, K. Kim, and C.-H. Im, "Detection of eye blink artifacts from single prefrontal channel electroencephalogram," *Comput. Methods Programs Biomed.*, vol. 124, pp. 19–30, 2015.

[26] J. Atkinson and D. Campos, "Improving BCI-based emotion recognition by combining EEG feature selection and kernel classifiers," *Expert Syst. Appl.*, vol. 47, pp. 35–41, 2016.

[27] R. Patel, S. Sengottuvel, M. P. Janawadkar, K. Gireesan, T. S. Radhakrishnan, and N. Mariyappa, "Ocular artifact suppression from EEG using

ensemble empirical mode decomposition with principal component analysis," *Comput. Electr. Eng.*, vol. 54, pp. 78–86, 2016.

[28]   I. Nejadgholi and M. Bolic, "A comparative study of PCA, SIMCA and Cole model for classification of bioimpedance spectroscopy measurements," *Comput. Biol. Med.*, vol. 63, pp. 42–51, 2015.

[29]   A. a. Putilov, "Principal component analysis of the EEG spectrum can provide yes-or-no criteria for demarcation of boundaries between NREM sleep stages," *Sleep Sci.*, vol. 8, no. 1, pp. 16–23, 2015.

[30]   F. M. De Blasio, R. J. Barry, E. M. Bernat, and G. Z. Steiner, "Time-frequency PCA of event-related EEG changes in the orienting reflex," *Int. J. Psychophysiol.*, vol. 94, no. 2, pp. 169–170, 2014.

[31]   D. Mantini, M. G. Perrucci, S. Cugini, A. Ferretti, G. L. Romani, and C. Del Gratta, "Complete artifact removal for EEG recorded during continuous fMRI using independent component analysis," *Neuroimage*, vol. 34, no. 2, pp. 598–607, 2007.

[32]   B. W. Mcmenamin, A. J. Shackman, L. L. Greischar, and R. J. Davidson, "Electromyogenic Artifacts and Electroencephalographic Inferences Revisited," *Neuroimage*, vol. 1, no. 54, pp. 4–9, 2011.

[33]   A. Delorme, T. Sejnowski, and S. Makeig, "Enhanced detection of artifacts in EEG data using higher-order statistics and independent component analysis," *Neuroimage*, vol. 34, no. 4, pp. 1443–1449, 2007.

[34]   B. W. Mcmenamin, A. J. Shackman, J. S. Maxwell, *et al.*, "Validation of ICA-based myogenic artifact correction for scalp and source-localized EEG," *Neuroimage*, vol. 49, no. 3, pp. 1–34, 2010.

[35]   A. Hyvärinen and E. Oja, "Independent component analysis: algorithms and applications," *Neural Netw.*, vol. 13, no. 4–5, pp. 411–430, 2000.

[36]   M. E. Davies and C. J. James, "Source separation using single channel ICA," *Signal Process.*, vol. 87, no. 8, pp. 1819–1832, 2007.

[37]   B. Mijović, M. De Vos, I. Gligorijević, J. Taelman, and S. Van Huffel, "Source separation from single-channel recordings by combining empirical-mode decomposition and independent component analysis," *IEEE Trans. Biomed. Eng.*, vol. 57, no. 9, pp. 2188–2196, 2010.

[38]   J. M. Schneider, A. D. Abel, D. A. Ogiela, A. E. Middleton, and M. J. Maguire, "Developmental differences in beta and theta power during sentence processing," *Dev. Cogn. Neurosci.*, vol. 19, pp. 19–30, 2016.

[39]   D. C. t Wallant, V. Muto, G. Gaggioni, *et al.*, "Automatic artifacts and arousals detection in whole-night sleep EEG recordings," *J. Neurosci. Methods*, vol. 258, pp. 124–133, 2016.

[40]   R. Djemili, H. Bourouba, and M. C. Amara Korba, "Application of empirical mode decomposition and artificial neural network for the classification of normal and epileptic EEG signals," *Biocybern. Biomed. Eng.*, vol. 36, no. 1, pp. 285–291, 2015.

[41]   S.-H. Oh, Y.-R. Lee, and H.-N. Kim, "A novel EEG feature extraction method using Hjorth parameter," *Int. J. Electron. Electr. Eng.*, vol. 2, no. 2, pp. 106–110, 2014.

[42] C. Vidaurre, N. Krämer, B. Blankertz, and A. Schlögl, "Time domain parameters as a feature for EEG-based brain-computer interfaces," *Neural Netw.*, vol. 22, no. 9, pp. 1313–1319, 2009.

[43] R. M. Mehmood and H. J. Lee, "EEG based emotion recognition from human brain using Hjorth parameters and SVM," *Int. J. Bio-Science Bio-Technology*, vol. 7, no. 3, pp. 23–32, 2015.

[44] T. H. Aspiras and V. K. Asari, "Log power representation of EEG spectral bands for the recognition of emotional states of mind," in Information, Communications and Signal Processing (ICICS) 2011 8th International Conference, 2011, pp. 1–5.

[45] C. Brunner, M. Billinger, C. Vidaurre, and C. Neuper, "A comparison of univariate, vector, bilinear autoregressive, and band power features for brain-computer interfaces," *Med. Biol. Eng. Comput.*, vol. 49, no. 11, pp. 1337–1346, 2011.

[46] A. Delorme and S. Makeig, "EEGLAB: An open source toolbox for analysis of single-trial EEG dynamics including independent component analysis," *J. Neurosci. Methods*, vol. 134, no. 1, pp. 9–21, 2004.

[47] W. Klimesch, M. Doppelmayr, H. Wimmer, *et al.*, "Alpha and beta band power changes in normal and dyslexic children," *Clin. Neurophysiol.*, vol. 112, no. 7, pp. 1186–1195, 2001.

[48] M. Kemal Kıymık, G. İnan, A. Dizibüyük, and A. Mehmet, "Comparison of STFT and wavelet transform methods in determining epileptic seizure activity in EEG signals for real-time application," *Comput. Biol. Med.*, vol. 35, no. 7, pp. 603–616, 2005.

[49] J. Rafiee, M. A. Rafiee, N. Prause, and M. P. Schoen, "Wavelet basis functions in biomedical signal processing," *Expert Syst. Appl.*, vol. 38, no. 5, pp. 6190–6201, 2011.

[50] V. Tarantino, P. Bisiacchi, and G. Sparacino, "A wavelet methodology for EEG time-frequency analysis in a time discrimination task," *Int. J. Bioelectromagn.*, vol. 11, no. 4, pp. 185–188, 2009.

[51] A. Procházka, J. Kukal, and O. Vyšata, "Wavelet transform use for feature extraction and EEG signal segments classification," *2008 3rd Int. Symp. Commun. Control. Signal Process. ISCCSP 2008*, pp. 719–722, 2008.

[52] O. A. Rosso, M. T. Martin, A. Figliola, K. Keller, and A. Plastino, "EEG analysis using wavelet-based information tools," *J. Neurosci. Methods*, vol. 153, no. 2, pp. 163–182, 2006.

[53] K. Al-subari, S. Al-baddai, A. M. Tomé, and G. Volberg, "Analysis of EEG data collected during a contour integration task," *PLoS One*, pp. 1–27, 2015.

[54] J. R. Huang, S. Z. Fan, M. F. Abbod, K. K. Jen, J. F. Wu, and J. S. Shieh, "Application of multivariate empirical mode decomposition and sample entropy in EEG signals via artificial neural networks for interpreting depth of anesthesia," *Entropy*, vol. 15, no. 9, pp. 3325–3339, 2013.

[55] N. E. Huang and Z. Wu, "a review on Hilbert-Huang Transform: Method and its applications," vol. 46, no. 2007, pp. 1–23, 2008.

[56] Q. Liu, Y. F. Chen, S. Z. Fan, M. F. Abbod, and J. S. Shieh, "A comparison of five different algorithms for EEG signal analysis in artifacts rejection for monitoring depth of anesthesia," *Biomed. Signal Process. Control*, vol. 25, pp. 24–34, 2016.

[57] A. Goshvarpour, A. Goshvarpour, S. Rahati, and V. Saadatian, "Bispectrum estimation of electroencephalogram signals during meditation," *Iran. J. Psychiatry Behav. Sci.*, vol. 6, no. 2, pp. 48–54, 2012.

[58] J. W. A. Fackrell, P. R. White, J. K. Hammond, R. J. Pinnington, and A. T. Parsons, "The interpretation of the bispectra of vibration signals—," *Mech. Syst. Signal Process.*, vol. 9, no. 3, pp. 257–266, 1995.

[59] J. Fackrell, P. R. White, J. K. Hammond, R. J. Pinnington, and A. T. Parsons, "The interpretation of the bispectra of vibration signals—II. Experimental results and applications," *Mech. Syst. Signal Process.*, vol. 9, no. 3, pp. 267–274, 1995.

[60] H. Azami, H. Hassanpour, J. Escudero, and S. Sanei, "An intelligent approach for variable size segmentation of non-stationary signals," *J. Adv. Res.*, vol. 6, no. 5, pp. 687–698, 2015.

[61] T. Bojić, A. Vuckovic, and A. Kalauzi, "Modeling EEG fractal dimension changes in wake and drowsy states in humans–a preliminary study," *J. Theor. Biol.*, vol. 262, no. 2, pp. 214–222, 2010.

[62] L. Zhang, A. Butler, C. Sun, V. Sahgal, G. Wittenberg, and G. Yue, "Fractal dimension assessment of brain white matter structural complexity post stroke in relation to upper-extremity motor function," *Brain Res.*, vol. 1228, pp. 229–240, 2008.

[63] R. D. King, B. Brown, M. Hwang, T. Jeon, and A. George, "Fractal dimension analysis of the cortical ribbon in mild Alzheimer's disease," *Neuroimage*, vol. 53, no. 2, pp. 471–479, 2010.

[64] F. Zappasodi, E. Olejarczyk, L. Marzetti, G. Assenza, V. Pizzella, and F. Tecchio, "Fractal dimension of EEG activity senses neuronal impairment in acute stroke," *PLoS One*, vol. 9, no. 6, pp. 1–8, 2014.

[65] A. Accardo, M. Affinito, M. Carrozzi, and F. Bouquet, "Use of the FD for the analysis of EEG time series," *Biol. Cybern.*, vol. 77, no. 5, pp. 339–350, 1997.

[66] W. Y. Leong and R. S. Tung, *Sleep Disorder Recognition System*, Paperback, Lap Lambert Academic Publishing AG & Co Kg, 2013, ISBN 3659311219.

[67] W. Z. Chee and W. Y. Leong, *Remote Upper Limb Tracking System*, Lap Lambert Academic Publishing AG & Co Kg, 2012, ISBN 13: 9783845405179.

[68] W. Y. Leong and C. R. Andrew Ng, "Left-handedness detection," *Int. J. Smart Sensing Intell. Syst.*, vol. 7, no. 2, 2014.

[69] W. Y. Leong and C. M. Than, "Features of sleep apnea recognition and analysis," *Int. J. Smart Sensing Intell. Syst.*, vol. 7, no. 2, 2014.

[70] W. Y. Leong, "Implementing blind source separation in signal processing and telecommunications," The University of Queensland, PhD Thesis, 2006.

[71] D. Tan and W. Y. Leong, "Sleep disorder detection and identification," *Procedia Eng.*, vol. 41, pp. 289–295, 2012.

[72] W. Y. Leong, "Hidden defects diagnosis using parameter optimization," *Appl. Mech. Mater.* (ISSN: 1660-9336), 2012.

Chapter 2

EEG in auditory selective attention

Yin Fen Low[1], Daniel J. Strauss[2], and Yun-Huoy Choo[3]

Following modern terminology, attention is a decision process; the systematic admission of information into consciousness. It is viewed as the process of selecting some of the many confronted inputs. In theory, the selection can be random. However, humans are able to perform a nonrandom selection. For instance, drivers in a junction with traffic lights are able to focus on the lights rather than on other stimuli present in the scene. The mechanism in charge of the selection is termed "selective attention". Generally, selective attention may be defined as a process by which the perception of certain stimuli in the environment is enhanced relative to other concurrent stimuli of lesser immediate priority. A classical auditory example of this phenomenon is the well-known cocktail party effect, wherein a person can selectively listen to one particular speaker, while ignoring several other simultaneous conversations or background noise and thus enabling us to talk in a noisy place [1]. With the advances of neuroimaging technologies and signal processing methods, we have started to understand the neural correlates of selective attention through identifying and quantifying it using electroencephalographic (EEG) activities.

EEG recordings can noninvasively track with high temporal resolution the brain activity associated with different types of stimulus events. By analyzing changes in the event-related potentials (ERPs) as a function of the direction of attention, one can make inferences about the timing, level of processing, and anatomical location of stimulus selection processes in the brain [2]. The scalp electrical potentials that produce EEG are thought to be generated by the extracellular ionic currents caused by dendritic electrical activity (i.e., excitatory and inhibitory postsynaptic potentials EPSP/IPSP) [3]. So, what we see in the human EEG is the synchronous excitatory and/or inhibitory input into a large population of nerve cells. With EEG, it is possible to get a glimpse of neural activity from the whole

[1]Machine Learning and Signal Processing Research Group (MLSP), Centre for Telecommunication Research & Innovation (CeTRI), Fakulti Kejuruteraan Elektronik & Kejuruteraan Komputer (FKEKK), Universiti Teknikal Malaysia Melaka (UTeM), Malaysia

[2]Faculty of Medicine, Systems Neuroscience and Neurotechnology Unit, Saarland University, Homburg, Germany

[3]Computational Intelligence and Technologies (CIT) Research Group, Faculty of Information and Communication Technology, Universiti Teknikal Malaysia Melaka, Malaysia

cortex. This makes EEG a very potent tool to study the interaction between brain areas and different cortical networks.

This chapter highlights the use of the EEG in the neural correlates of auditory selective attention studies, where an objective quantification measure of the EEG synchrony is introduced to analyze the N1–P2 wave of auditory late responses (ALRs). Studies were carried out with normal hearing subjects as well as tinnitus patients.

2.1   Pioneer studies on neural correlates of auditory selective attention

The well-studied human auditory ERP components are N1, a negative component at around 100 ms (thus, also called N100) and P2, subsequent positive wave peak at 160–200 ms (also called P200). Figure 2.1 shows the N1 and P2 waves. The neural activity reflected in this wave is presumably associated with the auditory cortex [4,5]. In an early study of selective attention by Spong *et al.* [6], the N1 and P2 waves are considerably larger when the sound is to be attended than when it is to be ignored. In an intermodal attention task, the click-evoked N1–P2 response is significantly larger when the subject is attending to the click comparing to reading [7]. In a dichotic listening experiment (analog of *cocktail party effect*) where subjects attended selectively to tones in one ear and ignored tones of a different frequency in the other ear, the stimuli delivered to the attended ear elicited considerably larger N1 than the responses elicited by the same stimuli to the same ear when unattended [8]. In light of the rather early onset latency of the attention-related negativity (60–70 ms post-stimulus), Hillyard *et al.* [8] proposed that the N1 effect might reflect an early stimulus selection process of the sort hypothesized by [9,10], and other, variously termed "stimulus set," "filtering," "attenuation," "channel selection," or "input selection" (Figure 2.1).

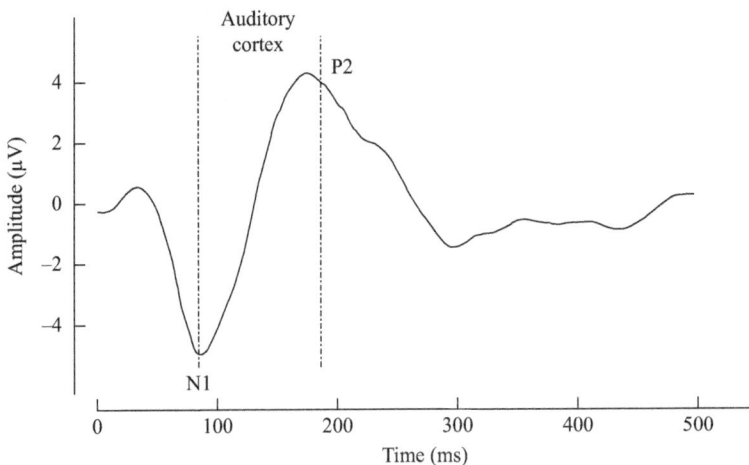

Figure 2.1   Auditory late response: N1 and P2 waves are anatomically associated with the auditory cortex

In some other studies, the N1 effect was found to be more pronounced when multiple channels of stimuli were presented [11], when inter-stimulus intervals (ISIs) were reduced [12], when increasing stimulus intensity [13–15], and when the tones were fainter or masked with noise [16]. Hillyard and Picton [17] proposed that the increase in task difficulty brought by these manipulations requires the subject to commit more of his/her processing resources to the attended channel, thus leaving fewer resources to process the irrelevant channels and increasing the selectivity of processing. The relative amplitudes of N1 waves elicited by stimuli in different channels depended upon whether attention was focused upon a single channel, or divided among two or more channels; this further suggests that this ERP was a sign of the allocation of attentional resources or capacity among the competing inputs [18,19].

2.2   Single sweep ALRs and wavelet-phase stability (WPS)

The investigation of the neural correlates of selective attention has been focused mainly on the average of the N1 and/or P2 components of ALRs. Typically, a large number of ALR sweeps is used in identifying neural correlates of auditory selective attention due to a poor signal-to-noise ratio (SNR). For example, in studies that were conducted by the groups of Picton [7,8,15,20,21], Näätänen [22,23], and Woldorff [24–26], as well as other recent studies, e.g., [27–29], the number of sweeps that has been used is typically more than 100. Some studies even analyzed more than 1,000 sweeps. This has led to a lengthy EEG recording and processing time. Also, subjects are easily exhausted during the task performing.

Another pertinent problem of the ensemble averaging method is that the method does not offer a view into dynamics of sweep sequences. This is because some important information contained in the single sweep sequences, such as the evolution of sweeps sequences, i.e., phase jitters and local amplitude fluctuations, are not reflected in the averaged signal [30,31]. Consequently, neural correlates of neurophysiological processes might not be obtained from the averaged signal. In order to tackle these obstacles, an analysis of single sweeps is suggested.

Recently, time-scale coherence measures based on the complex wavelet transform (CWT) have been introduced, which take the non-stationary nature of evoked potentials into account, in contrast to conventional coherence based on the frequency information alone [32]. This wavelet coherence increases with the correlation of the envelopes between two signals as well as if their phases show smaller variations in time [32]. In contrast to the analysis of averaged potentials, the amplitude information of single sweep ERP turned out to be fragile in some cases [30]. Large amplitude fluctuations can easily be introduced by slight accidental changes in measurement setup over time. Since the signals exhibit a high degree of variance from one sweep to another, even robust amplitude-independent synchronization measures, such as the time-scale entropy [33], can hardly be applied to assess their synchronization stability.

To be independent of amplitude fluctuations, one can focus on the wavelet phase coherence exclusively [32]. The wavelet phase coherence defined in [32] is mainly applied to measure the degree of phase locking of two signals in time, e.g., obtained from two different sites. Although such large-scale measures of cortical potentials based on synchronization provide no direct link between effects at the scale of neurons, recent multiscale models of ERPs [34] representing corticotha-lamic loops may also justify their use [35].

Note that the estimation of the phase relation from experimental data represents an inverse problem in a mathematical sense. This class of inverse problem has been thoroughly investigated in nonlinear dynamics, in particular, for weakly coupled self-sustained chaotic oscillators [36]. Meanwhile, the role of phase locking in modern biosignal processing in a more general sense as presented here can be found in [37].

The importance of the phase in signals has been emphasized by Oppenheim and Lim [38,39] using the Fourier representation. Numerical experiments have been used to illustrate the similarity between a signal and its only phase-reserved reconstruction. More recently, the significance of phases in the continuous wavelet representation of analytic signals has also been shown [40]. Besides that, a statistical interpretation of the usefulness of phase information in signal and image reconstructions is given in [41]. Particularly, authors in [41] have demonstrated that a random distortion of the phases can dramatically distort the reconstructed signal, while a random distortion of the magnitudes will not. Results from these studies reveal that the phase of a signal contains much more important information compared to the amplitude, as a signal can be reconstructed without suffering from a significant degradation of the quality by solely using the phase information.

Generally, the extraction of the EEG phase can be done via two closely related approaches: (i) the Hilbert transform (or analytic signal approach) and (ii) the wavelet transform. As pointed out by most of the studies, the performance of both these methods is comparable [42–45]. However, the Hilbert phase and Hilbert amplitude have direct physical meaning only for narrow band signals [46,47]. Meanwhile, the wavelet transform can be thought as equivalent to band-pass filtering of the signal, which makes the pre-filtering unnecessary. As a result, a measure called the WPS has been proposed to quantify neural correlates of selective auditory attention that are reflected in the ALR single sweeps.

Let us consider $\psi_{s,\tau}(\cdot) = |s|^{-1/2}\psi((\cdot - \tau)/s)$, where $\psi \in L^2(\mathbb{R})$ is the wavelet satisfying the admissibility criterion,

$$0 < C_\psi = \int_{\mathbb{R}} \frac{|\mathcal{F}(\omega)|^2}{|\omega|}d\omega < \infty, \tag{2.1}$$

where C_ψ denotes the admissibility constant, $\mathcal{F}(\omega)$ is the Fourier transform of the wavelet ψ, and $s, \tau \in \mathbb{R}$, $s \neq 0$. The wavelet transform:

$$\mathcal{W}_\psi : L^2(\mathbb{R}) \to L^2\left(\mathbb{R}^2, \frac{dsd\tau}{s^2}\right) \tag{2.2}$$

of a signal $f \in L^2(\mathbb{R})$ with respect to the wavelet ψ is given by the inner L^2-product:

$$(\mathcal{W}_\psi f)(s,\tau) = \langle f, \psi_{s,\tau} \rangle_{L^2} = \int_{\mathbb{R}} f(t)\psi^*_{s,\tau}(t)dt, \tag{2.3}$$

where the asterisk denotes complex conjugation. From the equation, we can see that the wavelet transform expands functions in terms of wavelets $\psi_{s,\tau}(\cdot)$, which are generated in the form of translations (time-shift) and dilations (scales) of a fixed function called the *mother wavelet* ψ. Obviously, it is different from the Fourier transforms in which the expansion of functions is in terms of trigonometric polynomials. Wavelets are characterized by a fast decay or compact support, i.e., they are essentially limited to a finite interval. The wavelets obtained in this way have distinct properties. They are relatively localized in time and frequency, permitting a closer connection between the function being represented and their coefficients. For a larger scale, the transform yields a global view of the signal with a high sensitivity for low-frequency components, while for a smaller scale, the transform provides information about short high-frequency components of the signal. In general, one can choose any type of wavelet to use, see [48] for more details and an introduction to wavelets. Note that the scale s can always be associated with a pseudo-frequency F_a in Hz by:

$$F_a = \frac{F_\psi}{s\Delta}. \tag{2.4}$$

Here Δ is the sampling period and F_ψ is the center frequency of the wavelet.

For the determination of the phase stability, we need an adaptation of the derived phase locking measure between two signals to our problem. The phase stability of a sequence $F = \{f_n \in L^2(\mathbb{R}): n = 1, \cdots, N\}$ of N sweeps, $\Gamma_{s,\tau}(F)$ is defined as:

$$\Gamma_{s,\tau}(F) = \frac{1}{N} \left| \sum_{n=1}^{N} e^{i\arg((\mathcal{W}_\psi f_n)(s,\tau))} \right|. \tag{2.5}$$

Equation (2.5) yields a value in the range of 0 and 1. We have a perfect phase stability for a particular s and τ for $\Gamma_{s,\tau}(F) = 1$ and a decreasing stability for smaller values due to phase jittering. The performance of the proposed WPS used as an objective evaluation of the large-scale neural correlates of auditory selective attention has been studied thoroughly in [49]. The result showed that the measure allows a reliable discrimination of the attentional conditions compared to the widely used wavelet coherence and correlation coefficient methods. Interestingly, it is found that the number of response sweeps that are needed to perform the differentiation is largely reduced by using the proposed measure as a synchronization measure.

2.3   WPS and the neural correlates of selective attention

The proposed stability measure had been further investigated in a study on the normal healthy subjects as well as chronic tinnitus patients who underwent compact music therapy with attention task. The aim is to affirm that the measure is linked to attention. Thus, it can be used as an objective measure of large-scale neural correlates of attention.

2.3.1   Study on the normal healthy subjects

The subjects were ten student volunteers (aged 26.7 ± 2.5, 4 females) with normal hearing (thresholds ≤ 15 dB HL in the standard frequencies of the audiogram) recruited from Saarland University. The parameters of the stimuli are shown in Table 2.1. Before the recording started, every subject underwent training sessions in order to make sure that they understood the nature of the task and to ensure that they were familiar with the task in the experiment. Later, the randomized stimulation (i.e., tones with three different frequencies were presented in random order and random ISI) was delivered to the right ear of the subject. Meanwhile, the left ear was presented with relaxing music which served as a distractor. The whole experiment needed about 20 min to complete. Subjects were required to pay their attention to the stimulus and detect the target tones by pushing a button during the first 10 min of the experiment (termed as the "attended condition"). The target tones appear as about 30% of the stimuli. A sign was given to the subject after 10 min, and the subjects were instructed to ignore the tone stimuli (the so-called "unattended condition"). All experiments were conducted in a sound-attenuated room with subjects' eyes closed lying comfortably on a bed. Electrodes impedances were kept below 5 kΩ in all measurements (filter: 1–30 Hz, sampling frequency: 512 Hz). An artifact filter was used to remove responses that exceeded 50 μV.

Single sweeps of a particular subject in both attended and unattended conditions are plotted in Figure 2.2. Prominent traces of negative amplitude around 80 ms (the N1 wave) and positive amplitude around 160 ms (the P2 wave) are clearly shown in the attended condition when the subject was required to detect the target tones. Since the subject ignored the presented tones during the unattended condition, attention modulated components in ALRs (such as the N1 wave and the P2 wave) are less synchronized with the incoming stimuli, thus demonstrating larger phase fluctuation effects than the attended condition.

Figure 2.3 shows the phase stability of a subject for both conditions at three different stimuli tones with $s = 40$ as an example. Note that the scale can always be associated with a pseudo frequency as described in Equation 2.4. For this scale (i.e., about 6.4 Hz), the temporal resolution is rather satisfactory and the differences in this

Table 2.1   Parameters of stimuli used in the study

Parameter	Remark
Stimulus type	Pure tones (1 kHz, 1.3 kHz, and 1.6 kHz)
Stimulus duration	40 ms
Stimulus rise/fall time	5 ms/5 ms
Stimulus plateau	30 ms
ISI	1–2 s (random)
Stimulus intensity	80 dB HL
Electrode placement	Vertex (ref); forehead (ground); channels 1 and 2 (right and left mastoid)

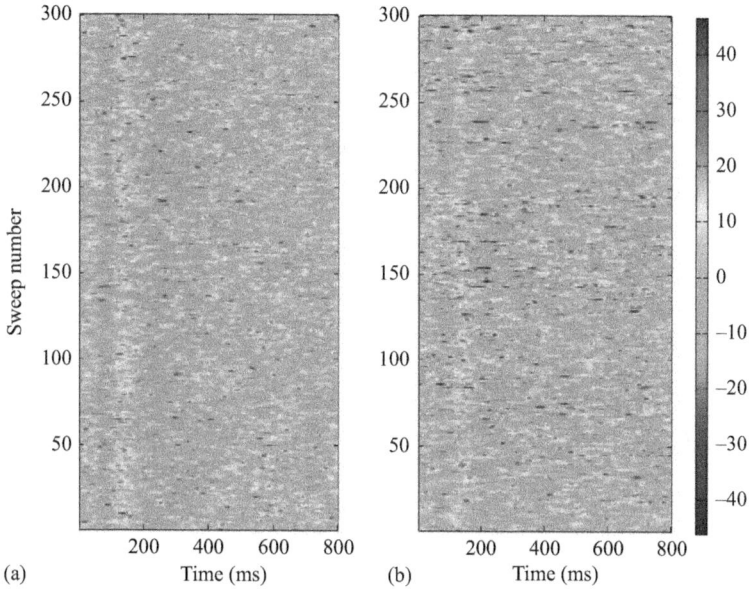

Figure 2.2 Single sweep plots of a particular subject in (a) attended and (b) unattended conditions

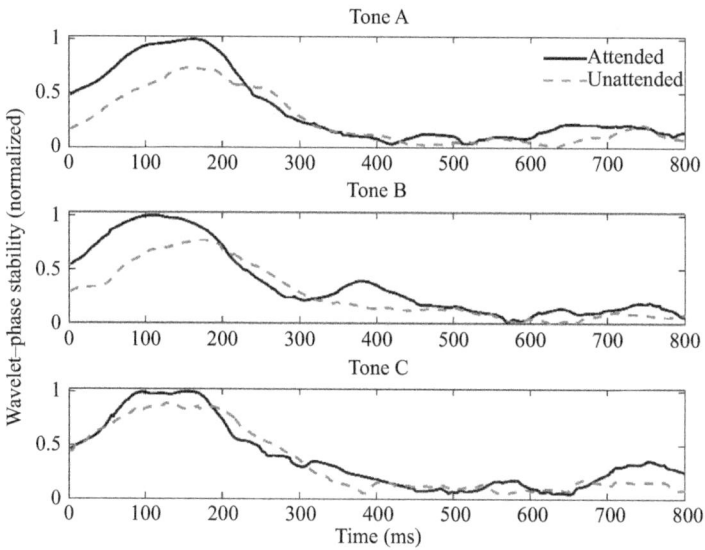

Figure 2.3 The WPS (s = 40) of a subject for three different tones in areas of both the conditions

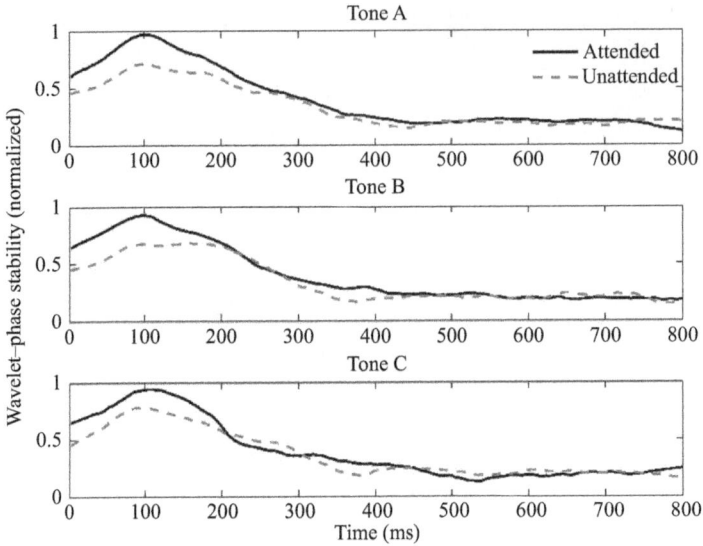

Figure 2.4   The normalized grand averaged difference of the WPS (s = 40) for all the tones in both the conditions

frequency band are also clearly noticeable. The fourth-derivative of the complex Gaussian function (the wavelet) and a total of 150 sweeps of each condition are in all analyses. It is observed that, the difference in the stimulus pitch results in distinct phase stability value. As shown in the figure, the phase stability of the attended condition is always larger than the unattended condition at the N1 wave for all tones. Meanwhile, the grand averaged differences of the phase stability for attended and unattended conditions were evaluated and the results are depicted in Figure 2.4. The major and significant differences (Wilcoxon test, $p < 0.05$) of the phase stability are associated with the time interval between 70 and 130 ms where the N1 wave is located.

2.3.2   Study on tinnitus patients (pre- and post-music therapy)

A total of ten patients who suffered from chronic tonal tinnitus and had no record of neurological or audiological pathology other than the tinnitus and potentially a tinnitus-related hearing impairment participated in the study (averaged age of 54.5 ± 7.5, one female). However, one male patient left the treatment on his personal request. Therefore, only data from nine patients is showed here. Data measurements were performed along with the assistance of a psychologist on duty at the Deutsches Zentrum für Musiktherapieforschung (Viktor Dulger Institut) DZM e. V., Heidelberg, Germany before and after the therapy (5 days separated). The experiment parameters, procedures, electrode placement, and data processing followed the details in Section 2.3.1.

Figure 2.5 presents the normalized grand average of the WPS in attended and unattended conditions for all tones before and after the therapy. Note that the

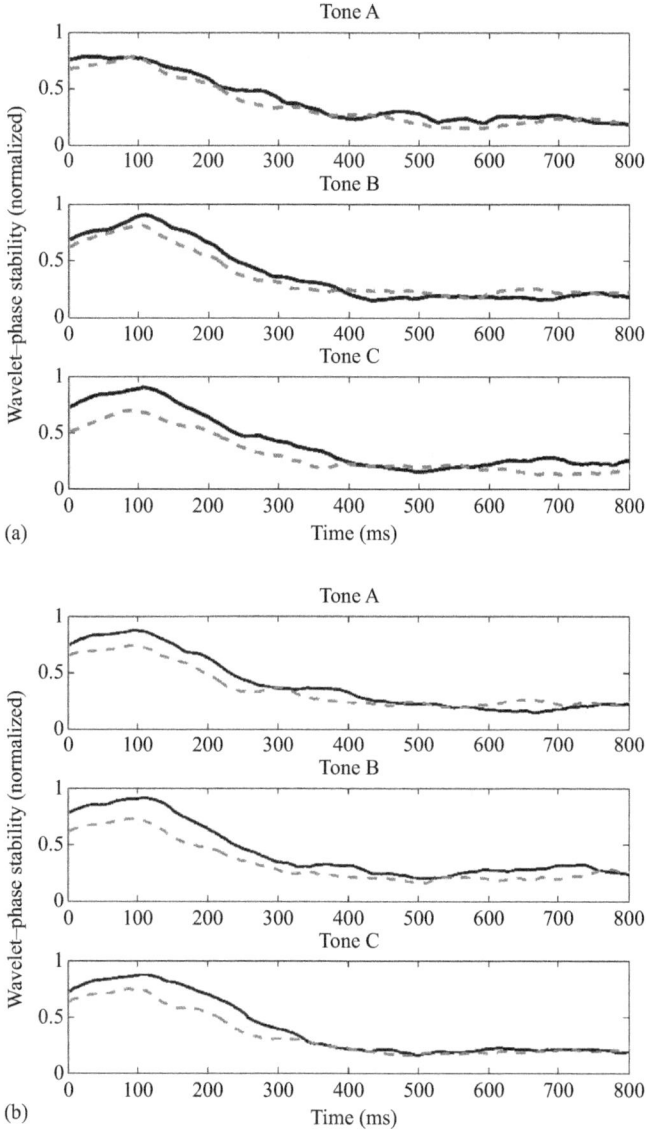

Figure 2.5   The normalized grand average of the WPS for all tones (a) before and
            (b) after the therapy (s = 40 as example)

wavelet transform for scale $s = 40$ was shown in the figure. Visually, a major difference was found at the time interval of the N1 wave in all tones. However, this
difference did not reach the significance level (Wilcoxon test, $p < 0.2$) before the
therapy. In contrast, there is a significant difference (Wilcoxon test, $p < 0.05$) in
the target tones after the therapy.

In addition, one can evaluate the therapeutic effect based on tinnitus questionnaires (TQ). This evaluation gives a lower score for decreasing in tinnitus
impact from the therapy. Therefore, it is useful to investigate the relationship
between our measure and the TQ scores of patients. Figure 2.6 depicts a summary
of the normalized mean phase stability at the N1 wave (80–130 ms) for all patients
before and after the therapy for the target tones, while Table 2.2 presents the list of

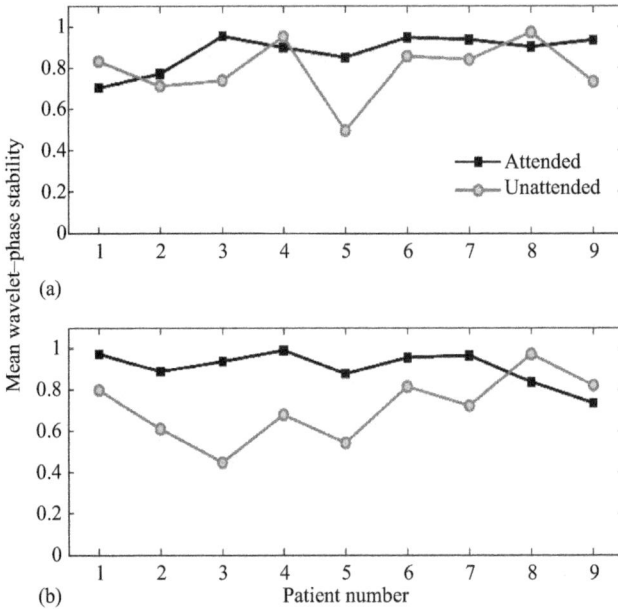

*Figure 2.6   An overview of the normalized mean phase stability of the target tones
at the N1 wave (80–130 ms) for all patients (a) before and (b) after the
therapy*

*Table 2.2   TQ scores of patients before and after
the therapy*

Patient number	Before the therapy	After the therapy
1	52	35
2	35	22
3	31	21
4	32	22
5	70	54
6	34	18
7	31	14
8	50	42
9	55	53

TQ scores of patients before and after the therapy. As shown here, the TQ scores decreased after the therapy (from 43.2 ± 13.2 to 31.2 ± 14.4) which is correlated with our finding, except for two patients (numbers 8 and 9).

2.3.3 Study on tinnitus decompensated patients

A total of 29 tinnitus patients participated in the study. They were separated into a group of compensated patients (tinnitus of degree 1 and 2, 18 patients) and decompensated patients (tinnitus of degree 3 and 4, 11 patients) by the 4 degree tinnitus differentiation scheme in [50] which is a German version of the questionnaire by Hallam. There was no significant difference (Wilcoxon test was applied) between the age and gender distribution among the group of compensated and decompensated patients. Also, there was no significant difference between the groups regarding tinnitus pitch which ranged between 125 and 10 kHz. Also, with respect to the auditory threshold between 125 and 10 kHz, there was no significant difference between the groups at any measured frequency. Only patients with a chronical tinnitus participated in the study. There was a significant difference between the groups regarding the time since the tinnitus appeared. In the decompensated group, the tinnitus emerged in average 4 years earlier.

ALRs were obtained using a commercially available device (Evostar, Pilot-Blankenfelde, Berlin, Germany) in a sound-proof chamber. In each measurement, tone bursts were presented with a stimulation rate of 1 burst per 2.5 s at 80 dB hearing level. The burst had a constant frequency of 1 kHz in all patients. All the patients in this study had tinnitus pitches at least 1 kHz away from the signal frequency of 1 kHz. In this way, we made sure that the tinnitus signal and the stimulus do not coincide in frequency. For patients with a one-sided tinnitus, the contralateral ear to the tinnitus was stimulated according to [51].

Regarding the instructions to the patients, we followed Walpurger *et al.* [52] in their habituation experiments, i.e., the patients were asked to lie comfortably, relax, and think about something nice. The patients were monitored during the experiment. None of the included patients were sleeping during the experiment. Artifacts were excluded from the analysis by the internal artifact filter of the system. Single sweeps were recorded using electrodes placed at the left and right mastoid, the vertex, and the upper forehead. Electrode impedances were below 5 kΩ in all measurements (filter: 0.3–30 Hz, sampling frequency: 500 Hz).

The motivation for the current study is provided by a tinnitus model of adaptive resonance as described in the following section. This model is based on the Jastreboff tinnitus model [53] combined with the adaptive resonance theory (ART) of cognitive sensory processing, see [54] and references therein.

2.3.3.1 The role of attention in the tinnitus decompensation

Tinnitus is a conscious sensation of sound experienced in the absence of acoustic stimulation. Chronic tinnitus is experienced by a majority of the population over the age of 40 [55–59]. Tinnitus perceptions are heterogeneous in their pathogenesis, characteristics, and impact for a patient's life. Although some patients, the compensated patients, can cope well with their tinnitus, decompensated patients suffer from severe psychosocial complications, making tinnitus even a contributing factor to suicide [60].

Typically, tinnitus is associated with at least some extent of hearing loss, usually in the high-frequency domain, and reorganization of activity throughout the processing hierarchy of the auditory system [59,61,62]. In animal studies, cochlear lesions change synaptic excitability in the auditory brainstem, cochlear nucleus [63], and in the auditory cortex [64] where they lead to increased spontaneous activity and synchronization of single units [65,66]. Moreover, changes of the evoked response amplitude were observed in the cochlear nerve [67,68], in the auditory midbrain (inferior colliculus) [67–70], and in the auditory cortex [67,70–72]. The presence of tinnitus was verified in behavioral studies using the same kinds of lesions [73–75].

In humans with tinnitus, increments of evoked signal amplitude were reported for several components of the acoustically evoked signal, the middle latency response (MLR) [76], the steady-state response (SSR) [77,78], and the N1 wave in late ALR [79] and are supposed to express cortical functional reorganization [80]. Neuroimaging studies using PET [81], fMRI [82], and repetitive transcranial magnetic stimulation (rTMS) [83] consistent with EEG and magnetoencephalogram (MEG) studies report subcortical and cortical tinnitus-related changes in activation and excitability. Volumetric studies suggest that there may be structural correlates of these functional changes [84,85].

It is widely accepted that the subjective distress due to tinnitus is mainly determined by non-auditory [86,87] with central mechanisms related to attention playing a key role [88–90]. Tinnitus-related increments in the amplitude of auditory-evoked signals were interpreted to reflect the deterioration of inhibition and upregulation of gain for input-deprived frequency bands in the afferent auditory pathway including auditory cortex [59,91]. Interestingly, similar amplitude increments of evoked potential components were reported in healthy subjects as an effect of attention MLR [92,93], SSR [94], and N1 [8,95], suggesting that the amplitude enhancements of the evoked responses in tinnitus could reflect attention toward the tinnitus percept. This assumption is also supported by the work of others [52,89,96].

2.3.3.2   The oscillatory tinnitus model

A mathematical framework of the cognitive tinnitus processing may be provided by ART of Grossberg (e.g., see [97] and references therein), in which top–down projections are the key mechanism for solving the stability–plasticity dilemma. ART is a representative theory of a fundamental paradigm shift in cognitive neuroscience, see [98] for a review. Whereas classical theories of sensory processing consider the brain as a passive and stimulus-driven bottom–up or feedforward hierarchically organized neural architecture, bidirectional theories such as ART claim that sensory processing is a highly active process with strong top–down interactions. Many cognitive models based on ART have been suggested so far [97] and recently ART has also been adapted to the auditory system for auditory scene analysis and source segregation [99]. The common mechanism of all these models is that sensory stimuli activate top–down expectations whose signals are matched against the bottom–up data. Top–down expectations originating from learning processes focus the attention on information which matches to them.

In this way, these expectations synchronize, amplify, and modify the activity of cells within the attentional focus and suppress the activity of others. When linking ART to the Jastreboff tinnitus model, a similar mechanism of subcortical and cortico-cortical top–down interactions can be expected if the attentional focus, e.g., driven by negative associations, is on the signal tinnitus as in decompensated tinnitus patients. Neurobiological evidence of such attention–synchronization mechanism was found in the visual system in [100] where the synchronity of neural groups in the visual cortex is strongly influenced by attention.

Consequently, to sum up, according to ART, it can be expected that there is a predominate processing of the tinnitus signal in decompensated patients, regarding expectation and attention. Other signals are suppressed and lead to less synchronized responses in the auditory cortex due to cortico-cortical top–down projections. Thus, neural correlates of these top–down projections might be reflected in the synchronization stability of single sweep sequences of ALRs. The combined model is illustrated in Figure 2.7.

In Figure 2.8, the averaged WPS is shown for the group of compensated and decompensated tinnitus patients ($s = 40$). The significant differences of the phase stability are associated with the interval between 100 and 200 ms where the N1 and the P2 waves are located.

Due to the subjective evaluation, a rather strong overlap between tinnitus patients of degree 2 and 3 is expected. Therefore, for the following experiments in

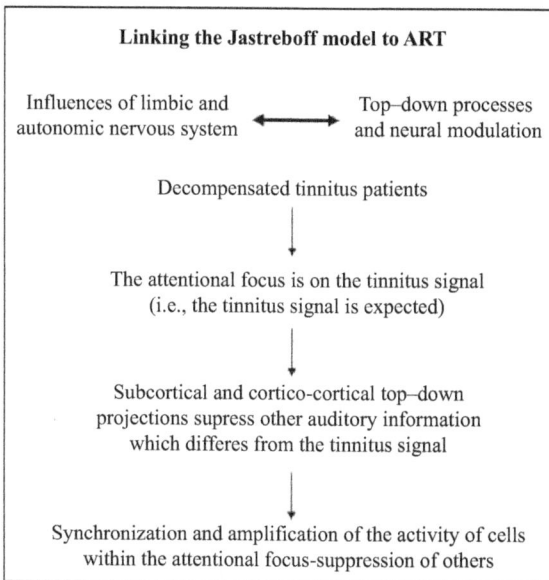

Figure 2.7 Oscillatory tinnitus model

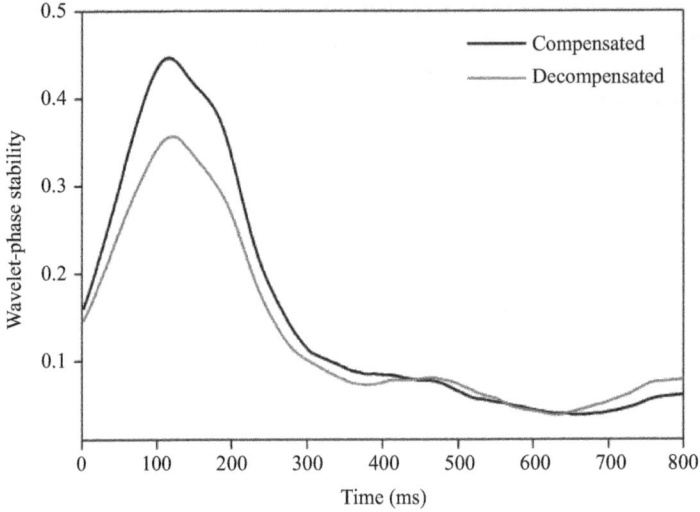

Figure 2.8   The averaged difference of the WPS for s = 40

which we analyze the evolution of the phase stability over the sweep sequence, we focus our interest in patients with tinnitus of degree 1 (T1 group) and 4 (T4 group), i.e., the most compensated and decompensated ones. As an example for a T1 and T4 patient, we have shown the quantity $e^{i\arg((\mathcal{W}_\psi f_n)(s,\tau))}$ $(n = 1, \ldots, N)$ in line for $s = 40$ and $\tau = 100$. In this figure, a complex number (with absolute value of 1) associated with a sweep $n + 1$ is "attached" (linearly translated with conserved absolute value and phase) to the complex number associated with sweep n (each circle represents one sweep) in Figure 2.9. It is obvious to see that the sum of the individual sweeps for the T1 patient would result in a much larger value as for the decompensated T4 patient which is the fundamental concept of our approach.

Figure 2.10 shows the phase difference between consecutive pairs of sweeps, of a total of 1,000 sweeps, averaged for the T1 and T4 group. A slight decrease of the phase stability between consecutive pairs of sweeps for the compensated patients (T1) is noticeable in this figure. However, it is worth to emphasize that this measure allows just for a comparison of neighboring sweeps with the inclusion of a far-field coherence, i.e., over many sweeps.

As mentioned earlier, it is impossible to analyze the amplitude of individual potentials in single sweeps. However, using a time-scale maximal value detection algorithm [101], we tried to estimate the amplitude of consecutive packages of ten averaged sweeps for patients with tinnitus of degree 1 and degree 4, i.e., the most compensated and decompensated patients as shown in Figure 2.11. Since it is difficult to draw a conclusion from the highly fluctuating curves, a smoothed version as bold line is also plotted. A rather slight habituation in the T1 group as reflected in the decreasing negative amplitude is noticeable.

In order to validate our approach, we shattered our data segments in groups composed of various criteria. The following three experiments have been

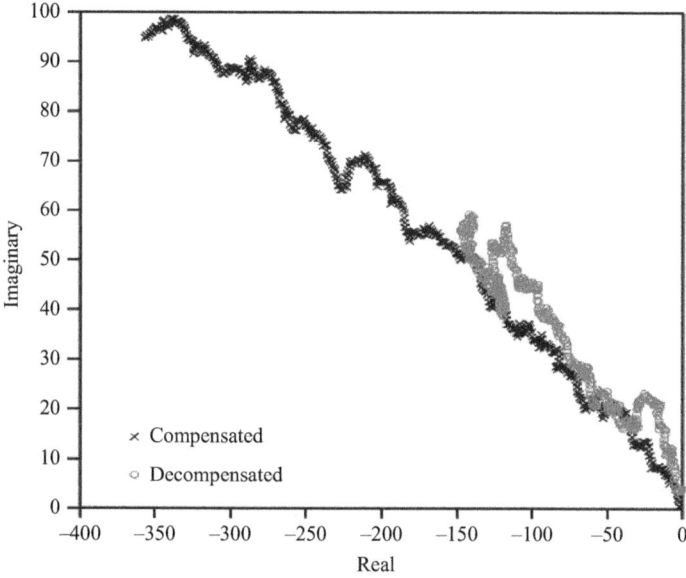

Figure 2.9   The evolution of ALR sweeps in the complex plane for a T1 and T4 patient (for s = 40 and τ = 100)

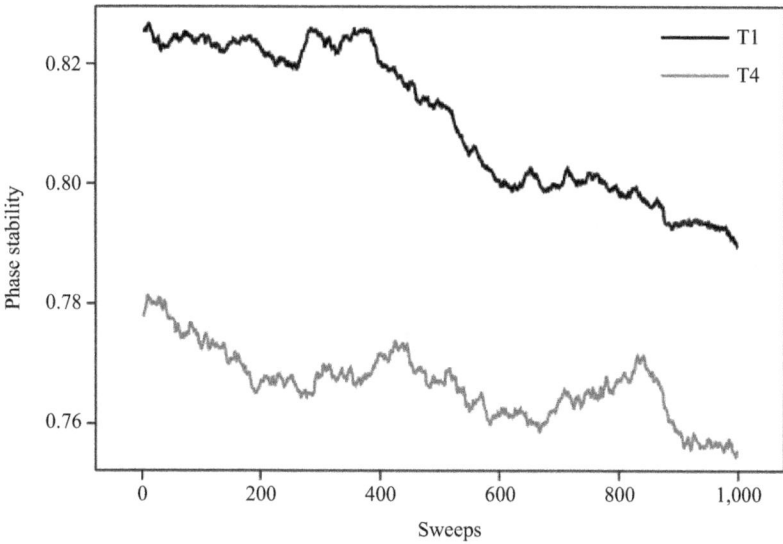

Figure 2.10   The consecutive difference of the phase from one sweep (m) to its neighboring sweep (m + 1) for tinnitus patients of degree 1 (T1) and degree 4 (T4) (smoothed)

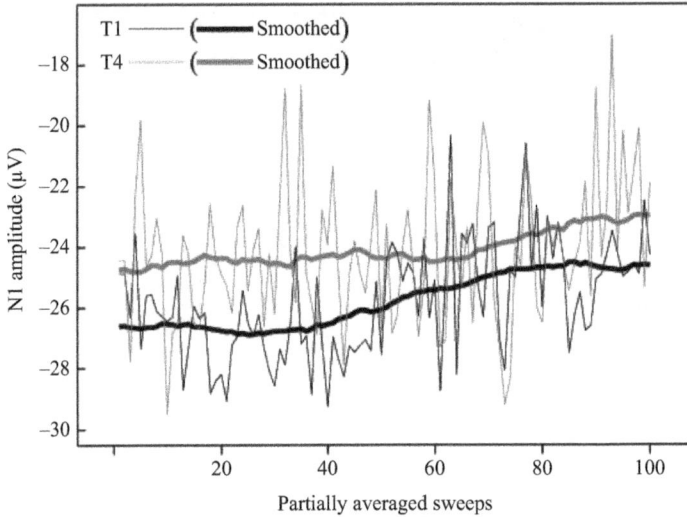

*Figure 2.11   The mean N1 amplitude for all patients with tinnitus degree 1 (T1)
and degree 4 (T4) for consecutive partially averaged (ten
consecutive) sweeps of a total of 1,000 sweeps*

implemented in order to investigate whether there are other factors which may
separate our data segments and patients, respectively.

(a) *Experiment 1*: We used a random perturbation of the data segments such that
we generated two random groups with the same number of patients similar to
the compensated and decompensated group. We repeated this experiment four
times, i.e., we generated four different sets of randomly composed groups. In
all these experiments, there was no significant difference between the groups,
showing that an accidental composition of the patient groups cannot reproduce our result for the group of compensated and decompensated patients.

(b) *Experiment 2*: Due to the well-known problem of a hearing loss in tinnitus
patients, we tried to get a rather homogeneous group of patients regarding the
hearing loss. However, the following experiments may help to exclude significant influences of the hearing capabilities of our patients/ears on our
results.

Experiment 2 (i): We separated the data segments into a group of ears with an
average hearing loss of less or equal 15 dB (30 ears) and more than 15 dB (28
ears). There was no significant difference between the groups, showing that
hearing loss is not able to shatter our data segments and the group of ears/
patients, respectively.

Experiment 2 (ii): In an additional experiment, we removed data segments of
ears with an increased hearing loss (more than 20 dB) at a stimulus frequency
of 1 kHz. This yielded data segments of five ears (mean: 34 dB, SD: 11.4 dB)
which we removed from our original set of data segments analyzed in the

paper. Removing those data segments did not change our results significantly regarding the group separation of compensated and decompensated tinnitus patients. Consequently, it can be concluded that an increased hearing loss (with the bounds defined by our group of patients) does not allow a group separation using our analysis scheme, showing that an influence of hearing losses can be excluded in our study.

(c)   *Experiment 3*: We also generated two different groups of patients according to their degree of depression with a shattering threshold of 18 points at the Beck depression scale. There was no significant difference between the group with increased degree of depression (>18 points, 6 patients) and the remaining group (≤18 points, 23 patients).

In summary, besides the tinnitus compensation and decompensation, we found no separation criteria for the patient population that results in significant differences.

2.4   Remarks

A novel approach to the objective quantification of large-scale neural correlates of selective attention using the WPS of ALR sequences has been presented. Particularly, the extracted measure is able to differentiate the attended and unattended conditions. This finding confirms that the phase stability of ALRs is linked to attention in which higher attention level that is locked to the stimulus produces a larger phase synchronization stability and vice versa. Interestingly, there is also an enlargement of the N1 wave in the attended condition compared to the unattended condition. This outcome is in line with ERP-based studies of auditory attention that have been reported so far.

The WPS is a time-scale measure which is exclusively based on the phase information of single sweeps as suggested. It is important to note that this measure is not applied as direct time locking measure since the responses in both groups are stimulus locked. We evaluated the quality and stability of the response over the stimulus sequences in terms of time-resolved phase information.

This measure is independent from the fragile amplitude information. Although there is no 1:1 map between the applied large-scale measure and the small-scale neuronal group synchronization, recent multiscale models of ERPs representing corticothalamic loops may also justify the use of this large-scale measure [34]. Especially, the large-scale neural models developed [35]; [102,103] are able to reproduce our experimental results of neural correlates of auditory selective attention and habituation reflected in single sweeps by means of phase stability.

Due to the analysis of single sweeps, the presented approach provides a direct or real-time monitoring which has great potential to be used in therapeutic neurofeedback-based control systems. An initial attempt in developing such a possible therapy has already been conducted in [104] and the results are motivating. Particularly, the system requires only a minimum training for solving the task; subjects learned quickly and established the capability to control and regulate their attention effectively.

The proposed approach was also applied to quantify neural correlates of auditory selective attention in the tinnitus decompensation. In particular, the neural correlates related to attention on an auditory stimulus and the tinnitus signal, respectively, that reflected in ALRs were studied. The WPS measure provides a reliable discrimination between compensated and decompensated tinnitus patients groups. More importantly, the result obtained allows an interpretation which is based on a model linking ART to the Jastreboff tinnitus model.

The role of passive attention in the tinnitus decompensation has been examined in [105] subjectively. These authors found evidence for an attentional focus on the tinnitus ear in subjects with an unilateral tinnitus. They assumed a passive attention bias which results from listening to the continuous endogenously generated sound. The authors of [105] also pointed out that if selective attention is increased by the tinnitus, an automatic attentional bias might be assumed. This is also supported by a study of Goodwin and Johnson [106]. These authors proposed that for the tinnitus signal, a particular process is involved which is related to the enhancement of a tinnitus-like signal in the periphery. This is of course in accordance with the adaptive resonance model as discussed before. Primitive mechanisms introducing an attentional bias to streams from the exogeneous system, which are in later processing stages picked up by the endogenous system, are also in conformity to other modern models of auditory selective attention, e.g., see the model of Wrigley and Brown [107] which is based on auditory scene segregation by Bregman [108].

Since decompensated tinnitus patients pay too much attention to the tinnitus signal [53,109], the signal tinnitus is expected by higher auditory areas in these patients, employing ART terms, and thus matches to the top–down projections which synchronize the cells within the focus of attention to this particular signal. The activity of other cells is suppressed such that these patients can hardly synchronize to other signals such as the tone bursts applied in this study. These patients cannot habituate to the stimuli. In this sense, our findings are in accordance to [52] where decompensated tinnitus patients showed a less distinct habituation of the N1–P2 wave amplitude differences compared to compensated tinnitus patients using averaged ALR trials.

In the study of the tinnitus patients with compact music therapy, significant differences in all tones in terms of the phase stability after the therapy is found compared to before the therapy. The finding can be interpreted in such a way that these tinnitus patients suffer from the inability to habituate toward the tinnitus tone and to divert their attention to other acoustic stimuli. It is suggested that the tinnitus tone is always in the focus of attention. Based on the idea of tinnitus generation by top–down processes, the influence of two different pathways in the tinnitus generation was speculated. On one hand, we expect a corticofugal amplification by focusing the attentional resources to the tinnitus auditory stream, due to its high subjective importance [110]. On the other hand, we assume a malfunctioning of attentional guidance, i.e., the inability to habituate due to simultaneous activations of cortical regions of emotional processing, for example, the amygdala. These activations give a higher weight to the tinnitus signal so that preventing it from habituation as it is "assumed" to be important [111]. After the therapy, the cognitive attentional processing in patients has increased greatly through the training approach which emphasizes on self-effective control mechanism. In other words, the direct effect of such training is that patients are able to guide their attention abilities effectively.

2.5 Conclusion

The neural correlates of auditory selective attention that reflected in the EEG can be objectively quantified by using the proposed measure, i.e., the WPS. It is a time-scale measure constructed from the CWT that focus on the phase information of the EEG signal. It has been reinforced and confirmed that it is linked to attention in the studies with healthy and tinnitus subjects, as a synchronization measure. In particular, the WPS of ALRs allows for a reliable discrimination of the attentional conditions compared to the widely used wavelet coherence and correlation coefficient methods. The number of response sweeps that are needed to perform the differentiation is largely reduced by using the proposed measure especially for the target tones. In addition, with the analysis of single sweeps, our approach provides a real-time monitoring of the attentional levels. Thus, the approach can be directly adapted in medical applications. For example, the approach will benefit in clinical diagnosis and treatment for tinnitus patients as well as other attentional-related disorders. It is noted that the proposed approach has to be carefully evaluated by conducting more clinically oriented studies. Apart from this, the approach is also useful in developing non-medical brain–computer interface (BCI) applications that are based on human attention (or intention).

References

[1] Cherry, E. C. (1953). Some experiments on the recognition of speech, with one and two ears. *J Acoust Soc Amer*, 25:975–979.

[2] Woldorff, M. (1999). *Auditory Attention*. The MIT Encyclopedia of the Cognitive Science, MIT Press, Cambridge, MA.

[3] Buzsaki, G. (2006). *Rhythms of the Brain*. Oxford University Press, New York, USA.

[4] Hall, J. W. (1992). *Handbook of Auditory Evoked Responses*. Allyn and Bacon, Needham Heights, MA.

[5] Verkindt, C., Bertrand, O., Perrin, F., Echallier, J. F., and Pernier, J. (1995). Tonotopic organization of the human auditory cortex: N100 multiple dipole analysis. *Electroencephalogr Clin Neurophysiol*, 96:143–156.

[6] Spong, P., Haider, M., and Lindsley, D. (1965). Selective attentiveness and cortical evoked responses to visual and auditory stimuli. *Science*, 148:395–397.

[7] Picton, T. W., Hillyard, S. A., Galambos, R., and Schiff, M. (1971). Human auditory attention: a central or peripheral process. *Science*, 173:351–353.

[8] Hillyard, S. A., Hink, R. F., Schwent, V. L., and Picton, T. W. (1973). Electrical signs of selective attention in the human brain. *Science*, 182:177–180.

[9]   Broadbent, D. (1970). *Stimulus Set and Response Set: Two Kinds of Selective Attention*. Appleton-Century-Crofts, New York.

[10]   Treisman, A. (1969). Strategies and models of selective attention. *Psych Review*, 76:282–299.

[11]   Schwent, V. and Hillyard, S. A. (1975). Auditory evoked potentials and multi-channel selective attention. *Electroencephalogr Clin Neurophysiol*, 38:131–138.

[12]   Schwent, V., Hillyard, S., and Galambos, R. (1976). Selective attention and the auditory vertex potential. I: effects of stimulus delivery rate. *Electroencephalogr Clin Neurophysiol*, 40:604–614.

[13]   Knight, R., Hillyard, S., Woods, D., and Neville, H. (1981). The effects of frontal cortex lesions on event-related potentials during auditory selective attention. *Electroencephalogr Clin Neurophysiol*, 28:571–582.

[14]   Ritter, W., Simson, R., and Vaughan, H. (1988). Effects on the amount of stimulus information processed on negative event-related potentials. *Electroencephalogr Clin Neurophysiol*, 28:244–258.

[15]   Hillyard, S. (1981). Selective auditory attention and early event-related potentials: a rejoinder. *Canad J Psychol*, 35:159–174.

[16]   Schwent, V., Hillyard, S. A., and Galambos, R. (1976). Selective attention and the auditory vertex potential. II: effects of signal intensity and masking noise. *Electroencephalogr Clin Neurophysiol*, 40:615–622.

[17]   Hillyard, S. A. and Picton, T. W. (1979). Event-related brain potentials and selective information processing in man. *Progress Clin Neurophysiol*, 6:1–50.

[18]   Hink, R., Van Voorhis, S., Hillyard, S., and Smith, T. (1977). The division of attention and the human auditory evoked potential. *Neuropsychologia*, 15:597–605.

[19]   Parasuraman, R. (1978). Auditory evoked potentials and divided attention. *Psychophysiology*, 15:460–465.

[20]   Keating, L. W. and Ruhm, H. B. (1971). Some observations on the effects of attention to stimuli on the amplitude of the acoustically evoked response. *Audiology*, 10:177–184.

[21]   Hillyard, S., Simpson, G., Woods, D., VanVoorhis, S., and Munte, T. (1984). *Event-Related Brain Potentials and Selective Attention to Different Modalities*. Cortical Integration, New York.

[22]   Näätänen, R., Gaillard, A. W. K., and Mäntysalo, S. (1978). Early selective auditory attention effect on evoked responses reinterpreted. *Acta Psychol*, 42:313–329.

[23]   Näätänen, R. and Michie, P. (1979). Early selective attention effects on the evoked potential. A critical review and reinterpretation. *Biol Psychol*, 8:81–136.

[24]   Woldorff, M., Hansen, J. C., and Hillyard, S. A. (1987). Evidence for effects of selective attention in the mid-latency range of the human auditory event–related potential. *Curr Trend Event-Related Pot Res*, 40:146–154.

[25]   Woldorff, M., Hackley, S., and Hillyard, S. (1991). The effects of channel-selective attention on the mismatch negativity wave elicited by deviant tones. *Psychophysiology*, 28:30–42.

[26]   Woldorff, M. (1995). Selective listening at fast stimulus rates: so much to hear, so little time. *Perspect. Event-Related Pot Res.*, 44:32–51.

[27]   Coch, D., Sanders, L. D., and Neville, H. J. (2005). An event-related study of selective auditory attention in children and adults. *J Cogn Neurosci*, 17:605–622.

[28]   Luo, Y.-J. and Wei, J.-H. (1999). Cross-modal selective attention to visual and auditory stimuli modulates endogenous ERP components. *Brain Res*, 842:30–38.

[29]   Neelon, M. F., Williams, J., and Garell, P. C. (2006). The effects of auditory attention measured from human electrocorticograms. *Clin Neurophysiol*, 117:504–521.

[30]   Kolev, A. and Yordanova, J. (1997). Analysis of phase-locking is informative for studying event-related potentials. *Biol Cybern*, 76:229–235.

[31]   Strauss, D. J., Delb, W., Plinkert, P. K., and Schmidt, H. (2004). Fast detection of wave V in ABRs using a smart single sweep analysis system. In *Proceedings of the 26th International Conference of the IEEE Engineering in Medicine and Biology Society*, pp. 458–461, San Francisco, USA.

[32]   Lachaux, J.-P., Rodriguez, E., Martinerie, J., and Varela, F. J. (1999). Measuring the phase synchrony in brain signals. *Hum Brain Map*, 8:194–208.

[33]   Strauss, D. J., Delb, W., and Plinkert, P. K. (2004). Objective detection of the central auditory processing disorder: a new machine learning approach. *IEEE Trans Biomed Eng*, 51:1147–1155.

[34]   Robinson, P. A., Rennie, C. J., Rowe, D. L., O'Connor, S. C., and Gordon, E. (2005). Multiscale brain modelling. *Phil Trans Royal Soc London*, B360:1043–1050.

[35]   Low, Y. F., Trenado, C., Delb, W., D'Amelio, R., and Strauss, D. J. (2006). Large-scale inverse and forward modeling of adaptive resonance in the tinnitus decompensation. In *28th International Conference of the IEEE Engineering in Medicine and Biological Society*, pp. 2585–2588, New York City, USA.

[36]   Rosenblum, M., Pikovsky, A., Kurths, J., Schäfer, C., and Tass, P. A. (2001). Phase synchronization: from theory to data analysis (Chapter 9). In Hoff, A. J., editor, *Handbook of Biological Physics*, pp. 279–321, Elsevier B.V., Amsterdam, Netherlands.

[37]   Rosenblum, M., Pikovsky, A., and Kurths, J. (2004). Synchronization approach to analysis of biological system. *Fluctuation Noise Lett*, 1:L53–L62.

[38]   Oppenheim, A. V. and Lim, J. S. (1981). The importance of phase in signals. *Proc IEEE*, 69(5):529–541.

[39]   Hayes, M. H., Lim, J. S., and Oppenheim, A. V. (1980). Signal reconstruction from the phase or magnitude. *IEEE Trans Acoust, Speech, Sig Processing*, 28:672–680.

[40]   Grossmann, A., Kronland-Martinet, R., and Morlet, J. (1987). Reading and understanding continuous wavelet transforms. In *Wavelets. Time–Frequency Methods and Phase Space, Proceedings of the International Conference*, Marseille, France.

[41] Ni, X. and Huo, X. (2007). Statistical interpretation of the importance of phase information in signal and image reconstruction. *Stat Probab Lett.*, 77:447–454.

[42] Bruns, A. (2004). Fourier, Hilbert, and wavelet based signal analysis: are they really different approaches? *J Neurosci Method*, 137:321–332.

[43] Kijewski-Correa, T. and Kareem, A. (2006). Efficacy of Hilbert and wavelet transforms for time–frequency analysis. *J Engin Mech*, 132(10):1037–1049.

[44] Quian Quiroga, R., Kraskov, A., and Grassberger, P. (2002). Performance of different synchronization measures in real data: a case study on electroencephalographic signals. *Am Phys Soc*, 65:0419031–14.

[45] Quyen, M. L., Foucher, J., Lachaux, J.-P. *et al.*, (2001). Comparison of Hilbert transform and wavelet methods for the analysis of neural synchrony. *J Neurosci Method*, 111:83–98.

[46] Boashash, B. (1992). Estimating and interpreting the instantaneous frequency of a signal-part 1: fundamentals. *Proc IEEE*, 80(4):83–95.

[47] Bedrosian, E. (1962). *A Product Theorem for Hilbert Transforms.* Memorandum, United States Air Force Project RAND, Santa Monica, CA..

[48] Louis, A. K., Maass, P., and Rieder, A. (1997). *Wavelets: Theory and Application.* John Wiley & Sons, Baffins Lane, Chichester, West Sussex.

[49] Low, Y. F. and Strauss, D. J. (2011). A performance study of the wavelet-phase stability (WPS) in auditory selective attention. *Brain Res Bull*, 86(1–2), 110–117. doi:10.1016/j.brainresbull.2011.06.012.

[50] Goebel, W. and Hiller, W. (1998). Tinnitus–Fragebogen (TF). *Ein Instrument zur Erfassung von Belastung und Schweregrad bei Tinnitus.* Hofgrefe, Göttingen, Germany.

[51] Lockwood, A. H., Salvi, R. J., Coad, M. L., Towsley, M. L., Wack, D. S., and Murphy, B. W. (1998). The functional neuroanatomy of tinnitus: evidence for limbic system links and neural plasticity. *Neurology*, 50:114–120.

[52] Walpurger, V., Herbing-Lennartz, G., Denecke, H., and Pietrowsky, R. (2003). Habituation deficits in auditory event-related potentials in tinnitus complainers. *Hear Res*, 181:57–64.

[53] Jastreboff, P. J. (1990). Phantom auditory perception (tinnitus): mechanism of generation and perception. *Neurosci Res*, 8:221–254.

[54] Grossberg, S. (2005). Linking attention to learning, expectation, competition, and consciousness (Chapter 107). In Itti, L. and Tsotsos, J., editors, *Neurobiology of Attention*, pp. 652–662, Elsevier, Inc., Philadelphia, USA.

[55] Evered, D. and G., L. (1981). Tinnitus. viii. In *Ciba Pharmaceutical Co. Medical Education Administration*, p. 325, Summit, NJ.

[56] Hazell, J. (1990). Tinnitus and disability with ageing: adaptation and management. *Acta Otolaryngol Suppl*, 476:202–208.

[57] Feldmann, H. (1992). Tinnitus. *Dtsch Med Wochenschr*, 117:480.

[58] Baguley, D. M. (2002). Mechanisms of tinnitus. *Br Med Bull*, 63:195–212.

[59] Eggermont, J. J. and Roberts, L. E. (2004). The neuroscience of tinnitus. *Trends Neurosci*, 27:676–682.

[60]   Delb, W., D'Amelio, R., Schonecke, O., and Iro, H. (1999). Are there psychological or audiological parameters determining the tinnitus impact. In Hazell, J. W. P., editor, *Proceedings of the 6th Tinnitus Seminar*, pp. 446–451, Cambridge, UK, Oxford University Press.

[61]   Henry, J. A., Meikle, M., and Gilbert, A. (1999). Audiometric correlates of tinnitus pitch: insights from the tinnitus data registry. In *Proceedings of the Sixth International Tinnitus Seminar*, pp. 51–57.

[62]   Mahlke, C. and Wallhäusser-Franke, E. (2004). Evidence for tinnitus-related plasticity in the auditory and limbic system, demonstrated by arg3.1 and c-fos immunocytochemistry. *Hear Res*, 195(1–2):17–34.

[63]   Francis, H. W. and Manis, P. B. (2000). Effects of deafferentation on the electrophysiology of ventral cochlear nucleus neurons. *Hear Res*, 149: 91–105.

[64]   Kotak, V. C., Fujisawa, S., Lee, F. A., Karthikeyan, O., Aoki, C., and Sanes, D. H. (2005). Hearing loss raises excitability in the auditory cortex. *J Neurosci*, 25:3908–3918.

[65]   Norena, A. J. and Eggermont, J. J. (2003). Changes in spontaneous neural activity immediately after an acoustic trauma: implications for neural correlates of tinnitus. *Hear Res*, 183:137–153.

[66]   Seki, S. and Eggermont, J. J. (2003). Changes in spontaneous firing rate and neural synchrony in cat primary auditory cortex after localized tone–induced hearing loss. *Hear Res*, 180(1–2):28–38.

[67]   Qiu, C., Salvi, R., Ding, D., and Burkard, R. (2000). Inner hair cell loss leads to enhanced response amplitudes in auditory cortex of unanesthetized chinchillas: evidence for increased system gain. *Hear Res*, 139:153–171.

[68]   Wang, J., Ding, D., and Salvi, R. J. (2002). Functional reorganization in chinchilla inferior colliculus associated with chronic and acute cochlear damage. *Hear Res*, 168:238–249.

[69]   Salvi, R. J., Saunders, S. S., Gratton, M. A., Arehole, S., and Powers, N. (1990). Enhanced evoked response amplitudes in the inferior colliculus of the chinchilla following acoustic trauma. *Hear Res*, 50:245–257.

[70]   Sun, W., Lu, J., Stolzberg, D., Gray, L., Deng, A., Lobarinas, E., and Salvi, R. J. (2009). Salicylate increases the gain of the central auditory system. *Neuroscience*, 159(1):325–334.

[71]   Yang, G., Lobarinas, E., Zhang, L., Turner, J., Stolzberg, D., Salvi, R., and Sun, W. (2007). Salicylate induced tinnitus: Behavioral measures and neural activity in auditory cortex of awake rats. *Hear Res*, 226:244–253.

[72]   Syka, J. and Rybalko, N. (2000). Threshold shifts and enhancement of cortical evoked responses after noise exposure in rats. *Hear Res*, 139:59–68.

[73]   Bauer, C. A., Brozoski, T. J., Rojas, R., Boley, J., and Wyder, M. (1999). A behavioural model of chronic tinnitus in rats. *Otolaryngol – Head Neck Surg*, 121(4):457–462.

[74]   Jastreboff, P. J., Brennan, J. F., and Sasaki, C. T. (1988). An animal model for tinnitus. *Laryngoscope*, 98:280–286.

[75] Kaltenbach, J. A., Zacharek, M. A., Zhang, J., and Frederick, S. (2004). Activity in the dorsal cochlear nucleus of hamsters previously tested for tinnitus following intense tone exposure. *Neurosci Lett*, 355:121–125.

[76] Gerken, G. M., Hesse, P. S., and Wiorkowski, J. J. (2001). Auditory evoked responses in control subjects and in patients with problem-tinnitus. *Hear Res*, 157:52–64.

[77] Diesch, E., Andermann, M., Flor, H., and Rupp, A. (2010b). Interaction among the components of multiple auditory steady-state responses: enhancement in tinnitus patients, inhibition in controls. *Neuroscience*, 167(2):540–553.

[78] Wienbruch, C., Paul, I., Weisz, N., Elbert, T., and Roberts, L. E. (2006). Frequency organization of the 40 Hz auditory steady-state response in normal hearing and in tinnitus. *NeuroImage*, 33:180–194.

[79] Kadner, A., Viirre, E., Wester, D. C. *et al.* (2002). Lateral inhibition in the auditory cortex: an EEG index of tinnitus? *Neuroreport*, 13:443–446.

[80] Wienbruch, C., Paul, I., Weisz, N., Elbert, T., and Roberts, L. E. (2006). Frequency organization of the 40 Hz auditory steady-state response in normal hearing and in tinnitus. *NeuroImage*, 33:180–194.

[81] Langguth, B., Eichhammer, P., Kreutzer, A. *et al.* (2006). The impact of auditory cortex activity on characterizing and treating patients with chronic tinnitus – first results from a PET study. *Acta Otolaryngol Suppl*, 556:84–88.

[82] Smits, M., Kovacs, S., De Ridder, D., Peeters, R. R., van Hecke, P., and Sunaert, S. (2007). Lateralization of functional magnetic resonance imaging (fMRI) activation in the auditory pathway of patients with lateralized tinnitus. *Neuroradiology*, 49(8):669–679.

[83] Kleinjung, T., Vielsmeier, V., Landgrebe, M., Hajak, G., and Langguth, B. (2008). Transcranial magnetic stimulation: a new diagnostic and therapeutic tool for tinnitus patients. *Int Tinnitus J*, 14:112–118.

[84] Schneider, P., Andermann, M., Wengenroth, M. *et al.* (2009). Reduced volume of heschl's gyrus in tinnitus. *NeuroImage*, 45(3):927–939.

[85] Landgrebe, M., Langguth, B., Rosengarth, K., Braun, S., Koch, A., and Kleinjung, T. (2009). Structural brain changes in tinnitus: grey matter decrease in auditory and non-auditory brain areas. *NeuroImage*, 46(1):213–218.

[86] Jastreboff, P. J. (1990). Phantom auditory perception (tinnitus): mechanism of generation and perception. *Neurosci Res*, 8:221–254.

[87] Zenner, H. P., Pfister, M., and Birbaumer, N. (2006). Tinnitus sensitization: sensory and psychophysiological aspects of a new pathway of acquired centralization of chronic tinnitus. *Otol Neurotol*, 8:1054–1063.

[88] Jacobson, G., Calder, J., Newman, C., Peterson, E., Wharton, J., and Ahmad, B. (1996). Electrophysiological indices of selective auditory attention in subjects with and without tinnitus. *Hear Res*, 97:66–74.

[89] Strauss, D. J., Delb, W., D'Amelio, R., Low, Y. F., and Falkai, P. (2008). Objective quantification of the tinnitus decompensation by synchronization measures of auditory evoked single sweeps. *IEEE Trans Neural Syst Rehabil Eng*, 16(1):74–81.

[90]   Trenado, C., Haab, L., Reith, W., and Strauss, D. J. (2009). Biocybernetics of attention in the tinnitus decompensation: an integrative multiscale modeling approach. *J Neurosci Methods*, 178:237–47.

[91]   Diesch, E., Andermann, M., Flor, H., and Rupp, A. (2010b). Interaction among the components of multiple auditory steady-state responses: enhancement in tinnitus patients, inhibition in controls. *Neuroscience*, 167(2):540–553.

[92]   Poghosyan, V. and Ioannides, A. A. (2008). Attention modulates earliest responses in the primary auditory and visual cortices. *Neuron*, 58:802–813.

[93]   Woldorff, M. and Hillyard, S. (1990). Attentional influence on the mismatch negativity. *Behav Brain Sci*, 13:261–262.

[94]   Müller, N., Schlee, W., Hartmann, T., Lorenz, I., and Weisz, N. (2009). Top–down modulation of the auditory steady-state response in a task-switch paradigm. *Front Hum Neurosci*, 3. 10.3389/neuro.09.001.2009.

[95]   Arthur, D. L., Lewis, P. S., Medvick, P. A., and Flynn, E. R. (2000). A neuromagnetic study of selective auditory attention. *Electroencephalogr Clin Neurophysiol*, 78:348–360.

[96]   Delb, W., Strauss, D. J., Low, Y. F. *et al.* (2008). Alterations in event related potentials (ERP) associated with tinnitus distress and attention. *Appl Psychophysiol Biofeedback*, 33:211–221.

[97]   Grossberg, S. (2005). Linking attention to learning, expectation, competition, and consciousness. In Itti, L. and Tsotsos, J., editors, *Neurobiology of Attention*, pp. 652–662.

[98]   Engel, A. K., Fries, P., and Singer, W. (2001). Dynamic predictions: oscillations and synchrony in top-down processing. *Nature Rev Neurosci*, 2:704–718.

[99]   Grossberg, S., Govindarajan, K. K., Wyse, L. L., and Cohen, M. A. (2004). ARTSTREAM: a neural network model of auditory scene analysis and source segregation. *Neural Networks*, 17:511–536.

[100] Fries, P., Reynolds, J. H., Rorie, A. E., and Desimone, R. (2001). Modulation of oscillatory neural synchronization by selective visual attention. *Science*, 23:1560–1563.

[101] Strauss, D. J., Delb, W., and Plinkert, P. K. (2004a). Analysis and detection of binaural interaction in auditory brainstem responses by time–scale representations. *Comput Biol Med.*, 24:461–477.

[102] Trenado, C., Haab, L., Reith, W., and Strauss, D. J. (2009a). Biocybernetics of attention in the tinnitus decompensation: an integrative multiscale modeling approach. *J Neurosci Methods*, 178:237–247.

[103] Trenado, C., Haab, L., and Strauss, D. J. (2009b). Corticothalamic feedback dynamics for neural correlates of auditory selective attention. *IEEE Trans Neural Syst Rehabil Eng*, 17:46–52.

[104] Busse, M., Low, Y. F., Corona-Strauss, F. I., Delb, W., and Strauss, D. J. (2008). Neurofeedback by neural correlates of auditory selective attention as possible application for tinnitus therapies. In *Conference Proceedings of the IEEE Engineering in Medcine and Biology Society*, pp. 5136–5139.

[105] Cuny, C., Norena, A., El Massioui, F., and Chéry-Croze (2004). Reduced attention shift in response to auditory changes in subjects with tinnitus. *Audiol Neuro Otol*, 9:294–302.

[106] Goodwin, P. E. and Johnson, R. M. (1980). A comparison of reaction times to tinnitus and non-tinnitus frequencies. *Ear Hear*, 1:148–155.

[107] Wrigley, S. N. and Brown, G. J. (2004). A computational model of auditory selective attention. *IEEE Trans Neural Networks*, 15:1151–1163.

[108] Bregman, A. S. (1999). *Auditory Scene Analysis*. MIT Press, Cambridge, MA.

[109] Hallam, R. S., Jakes, S. C., and Hinchcliffe, R. (1988). Cognitive variables in tinnitus annoyance. *Br J Clin Psychol*, 31:613–621.

[110] Suga, N., Xiao, Z., Ma, X., and Ji, W. (2002). Plasticity and corticofugal modulation for hearing in adult animals. *Neuron*, 36:9–18.

[111] Haab, L., Wallhäusser-Franke, E., Trenado, C., and Strauss, D. J. (2009). Modeling limbic influences on habituation deficits in chronic tinnitus aurium. In *Conference Proceedings of the IEEE Engineering in Medcine and Biology Society*, pp. 4234–4237, Minneapolis, Minnesota, USA.

Chapter 3

Investigating EEG signal detection, feature optimisation, and extraction method for sleep apnea

Leong Wai Yie[1]

To detect the sleep apnea electroencephalogram (EEG) signal, several feature extraction and optimisation methods were investigated in this chapter. The sleep apnea signals were acquired in this experiment. This chapter researched on the abnormalities in EEG for those who suffered from sleep apnea. The statistical correlation measurement of the EEG brain signals was analysed mainly to identify the abnormalities and specific features of patients who suffered from sleep apnea. The features and characteristics of the EEG signals were measured using the fundamental section of the Hilbert–Huang Transform (HHT) decomposition method to breakdown EEG sleep apnea data into finite and smaller components. Based on this research, the fundamental Empirical Mode Decomposition (EMD), Bivariate decomposition and white noise-based Ensemble EMD (EEMD) to the targeted EEG data method were investigated to obtain instantaneous frequency data. All these three methods were used to analyse the extracted sleep apnea EEG signals and features. Based on the analysis, using EMD in feature extraction, the abnormalities could be detected. The feature extraction performance would have greatly been significantly enhanced when the EEG samples used were lower. Based on our observation, the abnormalities and signal segmentations shown in the Event-Related Potential and intrinsic that has illustrated the features and symptoms of sleep apnea. Experiments have demonstrated that the delta power through frequency bands using Wavelet Method can actually be related to the body autonomous system of sleep apnea patients and homeostasis regulation. These phenomena happened to sleep apnea patients due to the drop of oxygen. Based on HHT decomposition method, we could observe that there is energy waveform in low frequencies to justify the occurrence of sleep apnea. These findings of having delta power during the decomposition stage can be explained on the body autonomous system. In this study, the Hilbert-based decomposition methods, namely Bivariate, EEMD and EMD methods were deployed to analyse, process, and identify the feature of sleep apnea.

[1]Faculty of Engineering & Information Technology, MAHSA University, Malaysia

3.1 Introduction

Sleep disorder has become the common issue that has affected healthy and daily life. There are many common types of sleep disorders; some sleep issues are serious enough to affect our daily activities, working, social works, mental, and emotional functions. The symptoms include sleep deprivation, heavy snoring, sleep insomnia, and restless legs syndrome. Other sleep disorder symptoms include unaware sleepwalking, night terrors, and bed wetting. The sleep disturbances could be managed via mental consultation, medical procurement, and the substance abuse disorders should focus on the underlying conditions. Based on the analysis and survey, the study shows that more than 7% or 1.9 million Malaysians suffer from sleep apnea [1]. The characteristic of Obstructive Sleep Apnea Syndrome or sleep apnea is mainly because of breathing difficulty and collapse of the upper airway especially during sleeping [2]. The airway calibre of sleep apnea is generally smaller, also the tongue area and soft palate in the mouth are actually bigger [2]. These physical issues actually cause blocking of the airway, resulting in both sleep apneas and hypopneas. These issues would result in depression, daytime sleepiness and neurocognitive defects. The whole symptoms affect every system in the physical body; this will cause stroke, cardiovascular disease, hypertension, pulmonary hypertension, altered immune function, and cardiac arrhythmias. The sleep disorder issue will also cause the risk of having an accident, due to somnolence [3–5].

According to normal practice, the sleep apnea could be diagnosed and observed via overnight polysomnogram study. The specially designed split-night studies are becoming common; these will allow for quicker implementation of therapy and solution at a reduced cost. The general treatment options for sleep apnea include positional therapy, weight loss, oral devices, continuous positive airway pressure, and upper airway surgery. One of the major components of polysomnography (PSG) is the adaptation of EEG analyses. The EEG study is able to investigate different electrical brain activities. The first recording of the electric field of the human brain was made by the German psychiatrist Hans Berger in 1924 in Jena. The recording was named Electroencephalogram (EEG). In particular, EEG used to measure spontaneous activities, evoked potential events, and bio-electric activities produced by single neurons [6].

During the experiment, the general 10- to 20-range international electrode placement system was adopted. The researcher located 21 electrodes on different locations on the scalp (Figure 3.1). These 21 selected electrode positions were chosen from different reference points, consisting of nose (top), eyes level, and inion. All these points were the bony lump at the base of the skull on the midline at the back of the head. From these 21 electrode points, the skull perimeters were measured in the transverse and median planes. All the electrode locations were determined by dividing these perimeters into 10% and 20% intervals. Three other electrodes were located on each side equidistant from the neighbouring points.

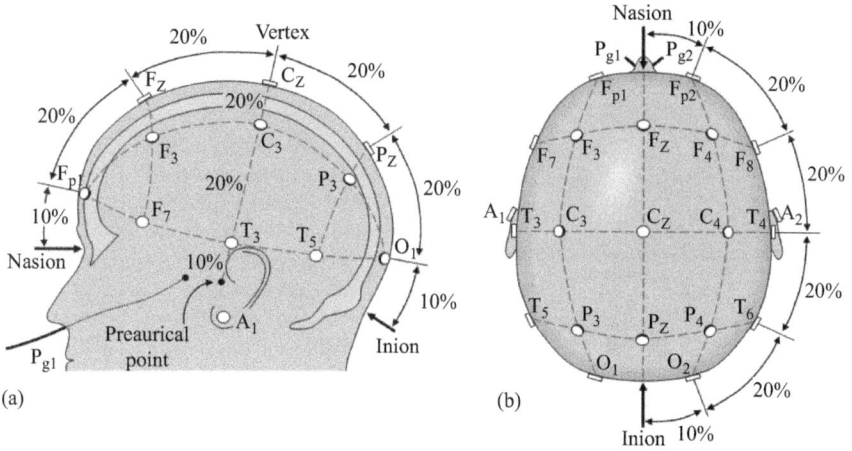

Figure 3.1　The location placement of 10–20 electrodes [6]

3.2　Literature review

There are many research works on sleep order. In particular, the microsleep events refer to short bursts of sleep without noticeable behavioural responsiveness [7]. In general, the EEG data are acquired to detect and investigate the microsleep events. Peiris *et al*. [8] used EEG to investigate the microsleep activities. The relationship between the microsleep events and Fractional Dimension EEG were investigated. During the experiment [7,8], the research data of 15 normal healthy male subjects, aged between 18 and 36 years with a mean of 26.5 years, were recorded. None of them had a history of neurological or sleep disorder symptom. All of them had visual acuities of (20/30) or better in each eyes. The EEG signals were recorded from electrodes at 16 scalp locations and digitised at 256 Hz with a 16-bit A–D converter. The following bipolar derivations were used in the analysis: Fp1–F7, F7–T3, T3–T5, T5-O1, Fp2–F8, F8–T4, T4–T6, T6–O2, Fp1–F3, F3–C3, C3–P3, P3–O1, Fp2–F4, F4–C4, C4–P4, P4–O2.

Peiris *et al*.'s study [8] has shown that all subjects were asked to conduct a special tracking duty. The study involved the sensory-motor tests program SMTests, which displayed a continuous target signal on a computer screen. Subjects controlled a steering wheel to move an arrow-shaped cursor, located at the bottom of the screen. The subject had to follow closest to the pseudo-random target. There was also video recording to capture head and facial features of a subject during the session. These tests were conducted twice on different days, with each session lasting from 12.30 to 5.00 p.m.

In this study, the EEG signals were used to detect abnormalities and microsleep events. These studies [9–15] illustrated a research outcome to integrate EEG features to detect sleep disorder activities. The extracted features include brain electric events, student population, eyelid, eye, and physical movements.

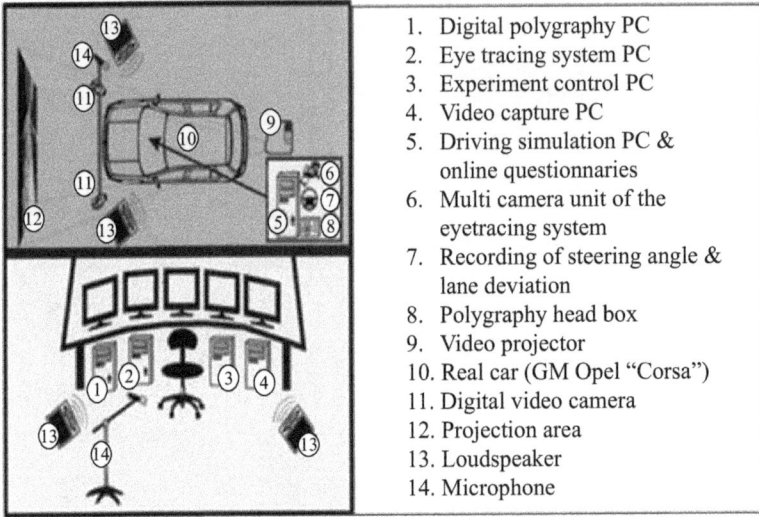

	1. Digital polygraphy PC
	2. Eye tracing system PC
	3. Experiment control PC
	4. Video capture PC
	5. Driving simulation PC & online questionnaries
	6. Multi camera unit of the eyetracing system
	7. Recording of steering angle & lane deviation
	8. Polygraphy head box
	9. Video projector
	10. Real car (GM Opel "Corsa")
	11. Digital video camera
	12. Projection area
	13. Loudspeaker
	14. Microphone

Figure 3.2   The driving simulation setup in Germany [9]

In this study [9], 23 young adults were recruited to join the microsleep research. These subjects were instructed to drive in a Car Driving Monitoring and Simulation Laboratory (see Figure 3.2) starting from 1 a.m. onwards. The basic criteria for the subjects' selection were after a day of usual working activity; all subjects should not have slept for 16 hours. All recruited subjects had to complete the special seven driving sessions continuously for 40 min. All of them have to join 15-min questionnaires and tests with 5-min-long break each. These allocated driving sessions were chosen to support occurrence of microsleep events and drowsiness.

3.3   Research methodology

In this proposed research, the EMD method [16] was adopted to analyse the non-linear and nonstationary EEG signals. The EMD could be used to process the complicated signals and decompose into 'intrinsic mode function' (IMF) followed by Hilbert transforms approach. The decomposition method is adaptive and dynamic where parameters can be modified accordingly. The mentioned decomposition method can process nonlinear and nonstationary data. It was originally used to analyse ocean wave data, later it has discovered more useful application and interest in biomedical signal processing [17].

To start with the proposed EMD method, the original data could be denoted as

$$x(t) = s(t) + n(t) \tag{3.1}$$

where $x(t)$ shows the captured signal, $s(t)$ the actual signal, and $n(t)$ the noise signal.

When a signal $x(t)$ is given, the several steps of the fundamental EMD can be expressed as

(a) Identify all the local extrema of $x(t)$;
(b) Interpolate between minima (resp maxima), ending up with some envelope $e_{min}(t)$ (resp $e_{max}(t)$);
(c) Compute the mean $m(t) = (e_{min}(t) + e_{max}(t))/2$;
(d) Extract the details $d(t) = x(t) - m(t)$;
(e) Iterate on the residual $m(t)$.

The main working principle of EMD is to locally identify the most rapid oscillations in the signal, defined as a waveform interpolating interwoven local maxima and minima. The local maxima points and, respectively, the local minima points are interpolated with a cubic spline, to determine the upper (and, respectively, the lower) envelope. The mean envelope is then subtracted from the initial signal, and the same interpolation scheme is reiterated on the remainder. The sifting process stops when the mean envelope is reasonably zero everywhere, and the resultant signal is designated as the first IMF.

The higher order IMFs are iteratively extracted, applying the same procedure for the initial signal, after removing the previous IMFs [16]. For a set of data, for first iteration, the mean is set to be m_1, and the difference between the data and mean will give us the first component, h_1. The formula to s is as follows:

$$x(t) - m_1 = h_1 \tag{3.2}$$

To continue the sifting process, h_1 is treated as data and iteration continues as shown in (3.3). The sifting process serves to remove riding waves; and to make the wave-profiles more symmetric. The sifting process has to be reiterated more times to achieve this. Equation (3.3) is the second sifting process

$$h_1 - m_{11} = h_{11} \tag{3.3}$$

The sitting procedures can be for k times, until h_{1k} is an IMF, which is as shown in the (3.4)

$$h_{1(k-1)} - m_{1k} = h_{1k} \tag{3.4}$$

To ensure that the IMF components retain enough physical information of both amplitude and frequency modulations, there must be a stopping criterion for the sifting process to stop. This can be done by limiting the size of the standard deviation, SD, computed from the two consecutive sifting results as shown in (3.5):

$$SD = \sum_{t=0}^{T} \left[\frac{|h_{1(k-1)}(t) - (h_{1k}(t))|^2}{h_{1(k-1)}^2(t)} \right] \tag{3.5}$$

The SD is usually set to be between 0.2 and 0.3. This is a very rigorous limitation for the difference between siftings. Huang *et al.* [16] did a comparison and found that Fourier spectra, computed by shifting of only 5 out of 1,024 points from the same data, can have an equivalent SD of 0.2–0.3 calculated point-by-point.

With any stoppage criterion, the c_1 should contain the finest scale or the shortest period component of the signal. This is to allow the first IMF, $c_1 = h_{1k}$, to be removed from the rest of the data by [16].

$$x(t) - c_1 = r_1 \tag{3.6}$$

This gives the residue r_1, which contains all longer period variations in the data; it will become a new data and it is shifted, giving r_2 as shown in (3.7):

$$r_1 - c_2 = r_2 \tag{3.7}$$

The repeated processes will continue and expressed as shown in (3.8) [16]:

$$r_{(n-1)} - c_n = r_n \tag{3.8}$$

Summing up, (3.9) is obtained [16];

$$x(t) = \sum_{j=1}^{n} c_j + r_n \tag{3.9}$$

3.4   Experimental results

3.4.1   *The experimental setup of sleep apnea study*

Figure 3.3 shows the data acquisition and processing stages for the sleep apnea study. During the initial stage, the data acquisition adopts the EEG electrodes onto sleep apnea subjects to collect EEG signals. The subjects were recruited to join the study. The process involved the preparation and briefing of the sleep apnea subjects and placing of electrodes to the right location. The selected experimental laboratory should be appropriate so that the subjects could sleep comfortably and not worried about the surrounding environment. The second stage actually involved data processing with the three proposed decomposition methods, namely the fundamental EMD [16], Ensemble EMD [18], and Bivariate EMD [19]. The pre-processing and post-processing can be conducted to understand the performance effectiveness of the three proposed decomposition methods. The third stage is to analyse the extracted data and identify the special features of sleep apnea. This process is to determine the features of normal sleep and sleep apnea. The performance analysis for three methods could be determined.

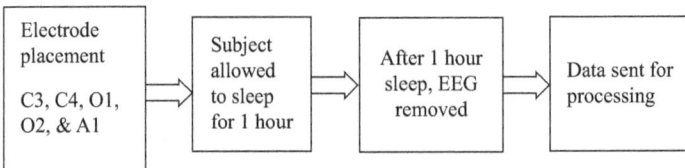

Figure 3.3   The stages of data acquisition and process using EEG placement system

The proposed Actiwave EEG equipment is a simplified and portable biomedical signal waveform recorder. It is designed to identify and record the biomedical EMG, EEG, and ECG signals online. These waveform recordings are done without the need for a large belt or lengthy wires. The device can be attached to the human skin near to the position placement of the electrodes. The equipment is mobile and portable allowing the subjects to capture the signals and would not be restricted to the laboratory experiment. The system allows a maximum 13 h of recording.

First, to start the experiment, the identified areas for electrode placed were marked. The marker can be cleaned by abrasive skin preparation gel called test subject preparation. Then, the adhesive and conductive paste were used to attach the electrode onto scalp. The electrode was secured by adhesive tape. The subjects were advised not to consume any stimulants or depressants, such as nicotine, alcohol, and caffeine, during the 4 h prior to the experimental session. The subjects were asked to relax as usual when they attempted to sleep as done in studies before.

The electrodes used to detect the signals should be placed according to the 10–20 electrode placement system as shown in Figure 3.1. In this study, the electrodes were placed in position C3, C4, O1, O2, and A1, and were recorded by the CamNtech Actiwave EEG. The CamNtech Actiwave 4-channel Recorder (Figure 3.4) was used to collect and record the EEG signal. CamNtech Actiwave Interface Dock is used as interface between the EEG recorder and the computer system. The Embedded system in the EEG device has a feature to filter the undesirable noise and interference from the surrounding environment to provide a more accurate and precise result for clinicians and researchers to carry out the analyses.

The C3 and C4 locations were chosen because these regions consist of electrical activity in somatosensoric and motoric brain areas. The locations O1 and O2 are related to the primary and secondary visual areas to detect Rapid Eye

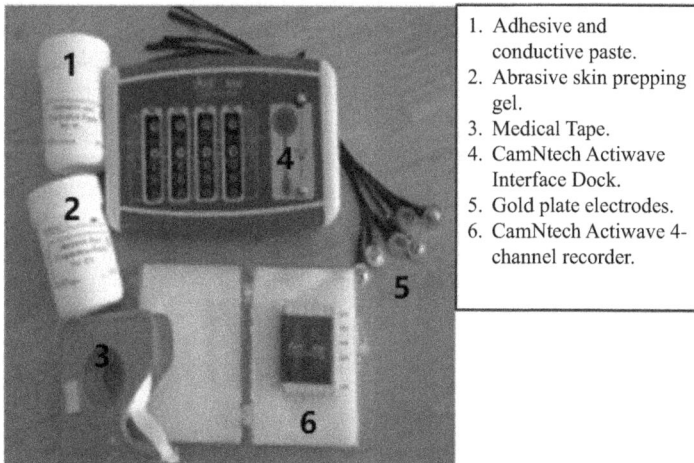

1. Adhesive and conductive paste.
2. Abrasive skin prepping gel.
3. Medical Tape.
4. CamNtech Actiwave Interface Dock.
5. Gold plate electrodes.
6. CamNtech Actiwave 4-channel recorder.

Figure 3.4   List of equipment and materials to conduct the sleep apnea experiment

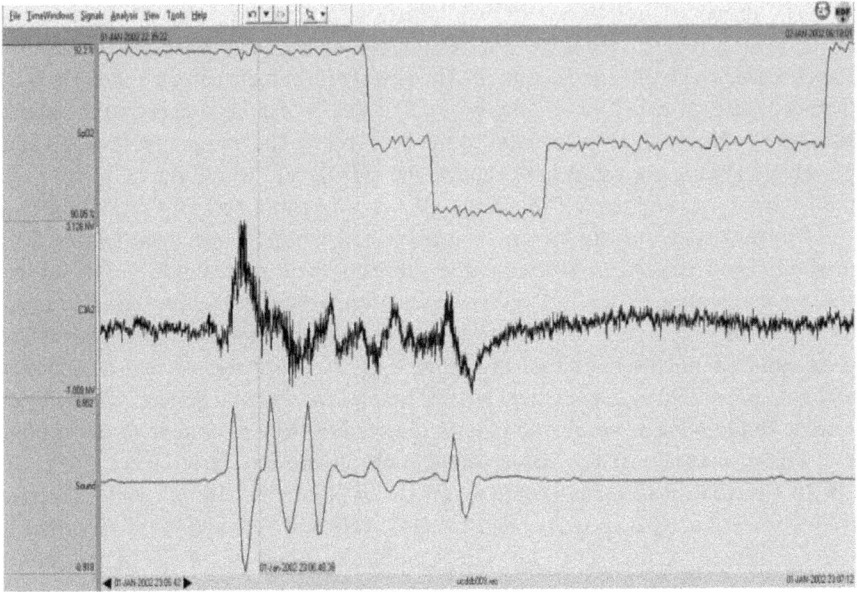

Figure 3.5   Scenario of clear EEG and clear sound

Movement. A1 is served as the reference electrode so that all the other electrodes can be referenced with. The EEG was sampled at 265 Hz.

3.4.2   Effect of forebody

Generally, a sleep research study normally lasts for a few hours. The studies and steps involved consist of processing the whole data of sleep, followed by selecting the data and features, which is quite time consuming. So this study will only look for data areas where there is a drop in oxygen level. A drop in oxygen level would indicate that an apnea might have happened. The second indicator would be to check whether there are rises in sound level. Rises in sound level would indicate snoring or difficulty in breathing, also another characteristic of apnea. After these two indicators are matched, the EEG timing is noted and the portion of EEG is then extracted for analysis.

There are three scenarios where this study tested the ability to identify the feature of sleep apnea in EEG when dealing with sound data. The first would be when it would be very clear when there is only one significant rise in sound and also only one significant rise in EEG as seen in Figure 3.5.

Using different decomposition methods to process the data, the results have been investigated. As the data have been decomposed into different IMFs, it is useful to check the completeness of the decomposed data. The whole idea is to check how much of the feature has remained and been retained. To identify the feature, the index of orthogonality is adopted, to check the degree of orthogonality or perpendicular properties of the data. Based on the result, a lower index

Table 3.1   *Performance measurement for three decomposition methods using index of orthogonality approach*

Decomposition method	Index of orthogonality
EMD	0.2579
EEMD	0.189
Bivariate EMID	0.2026

would show a better result: the data would be more orthogonal or perpendicular like a pure IMF.

3.4.3   Performance analysis using index of orthogonality

In Table 3.1, the extracted data consist of 1,500 samples captured from C3 channel: the data were sampled at 256 Hz. The data were tested via all three proposed algorithms, namely the fundamental EMD, Ensemble EMD, and Bivariate EMD methods, using the Index of Orthogonality approach.

The higher the value of index of orthogonality means that the severity of leakage will also be higher. The value of index of orthogonality obtained should be as low as possible (nearly to 0) to ensure the accuracy and efficiency of the analysed result. In this study, the performance of IMF components that was generated by EMD and EEMD methods, respectively, was compared to determine the reliability of the results. From the index of orthogonality values, it can be seen that EMD performed the most poorly with a value of 0.2579. This shows there was most leakage of data in EMD when the EEG data were decomposed. Bivariate performance was in the middle between EMD and EEMD.

From Figure 3.6, it can be seen from the original data that there are very high peaks as well as low peaks. These raw data present a problem for analysis because there is no mean zero for reference. The local minima can be above zero and local maxima can be below zero. One thing can be said of this character is that the waveform is not uniform. After applying the decomposition methods it can be seen that the waveform became more uniform primarily. Thus, it is now an IMF. Looking into the first iteration or first IMFs in Figures 3.7–3.9 the difference even after the first decomposition is quite considerable compared to the original in Figure 3.6. It can be seen that all local maximas and minimas are above zero and below zero, respectively. Now the waveforms are more uniform and analysis can be done.

Based on the research, there were differences in the first iteration when comparing all three proposed decomposition methods. When comparing first IMF of EMD and Bivariate, the features were highlighted in the labelled red box. There were actually two regions of peaks in the Bivariate method compared to only one in the EMD. The results have shown that more information were retained using the Bivariate method. Another obvious issue when comparing these two methods was that the peaks were higher using the Bivariate method. When comparing the EEMD with the rest it is noticeable that the peaks are not as high as the others. However,

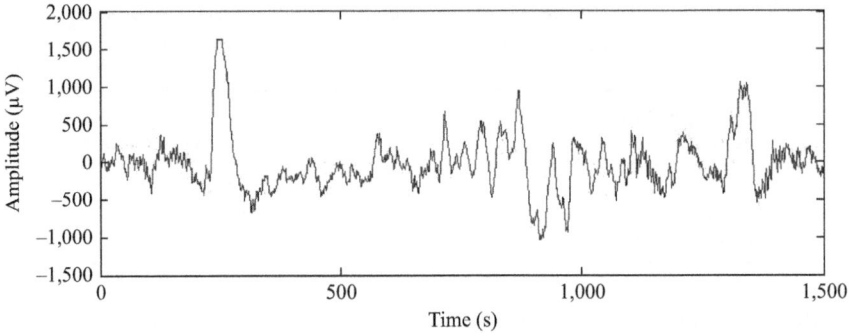

Figure 3.6   The original EEG data were captured from the subject

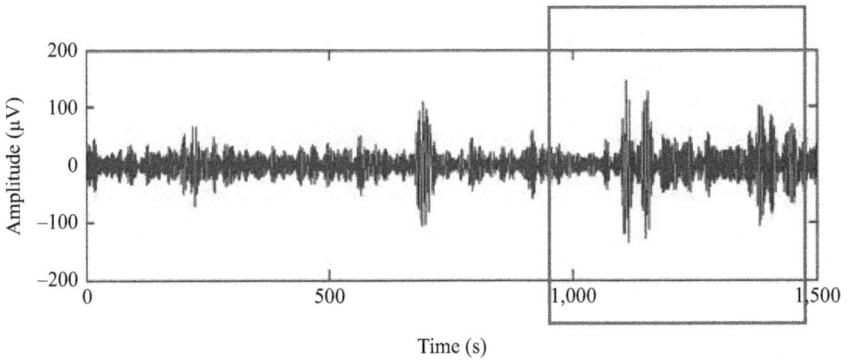

Figure 3.7   First IMF was analysed from the fundemental EMD method

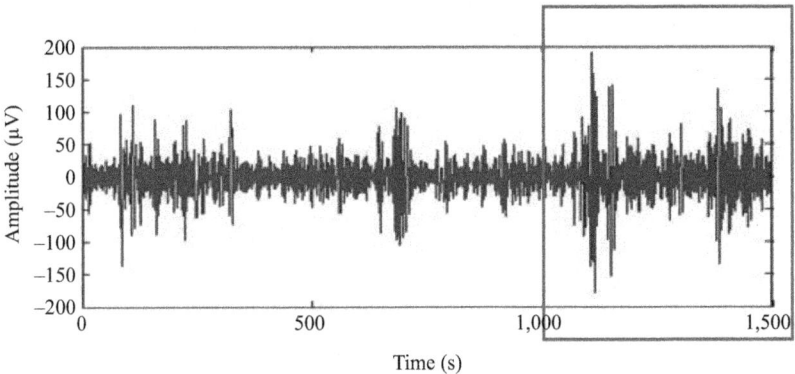

Figure 3.8   First IMF of bivariate EMD method

there are more regions of peaks compared to the other methods. The first iteration alone is unable to identify the differences amongst the three proposed methods. In the third example, the difference has become clearer and supported the initial results of using index of orthogonality.

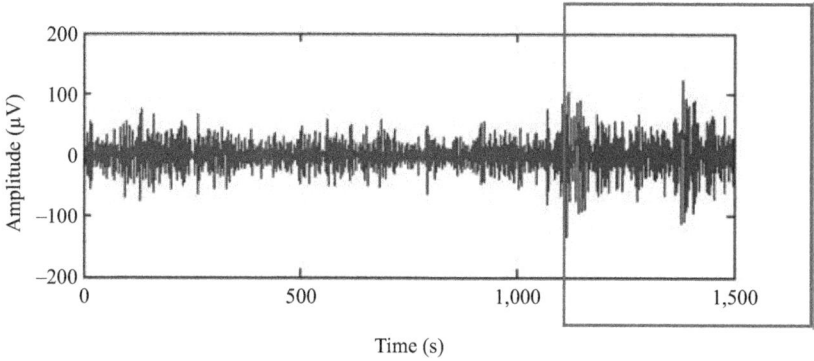

Figure 3.9   First IMF of EEMD method

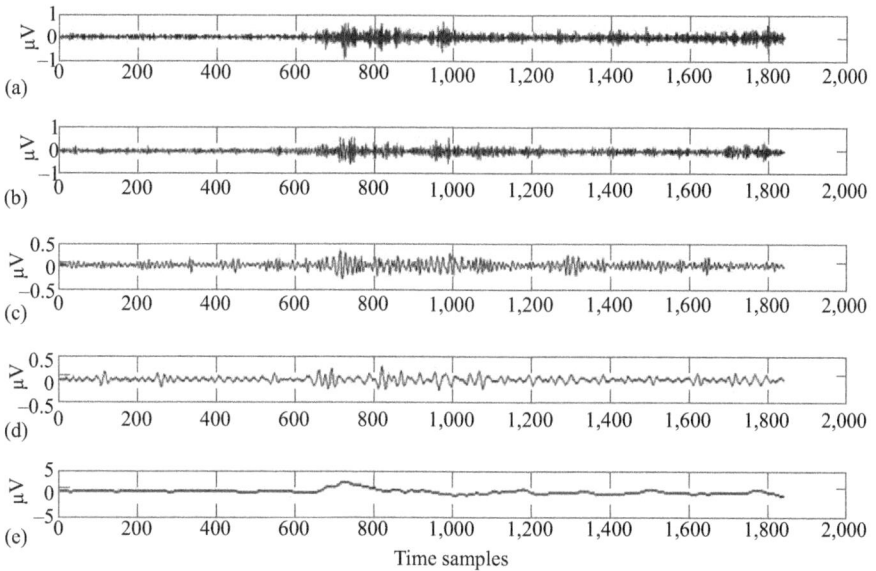

Figure 3.10   Frequency bands of sleep data using Wavelet Transform method: (a) Gamma, (b) Beta, (c) Alpha, (d) Theta, and (e) Delta

3.4.4   Extracting sleep bands using wavelet

Next the common features of sleep study that are able to be extracted are the bands of sleep from the processed signals. Wavelet is the most readily used method to extract the frequency bands of sleep and therefore is used as the reference method to compare the extracted bands of suitable frequency. Sleep bands are a common feature of sleep to see the brain activeness in different stages. Figure 3.10 shows all

Table 3.2   The analysis of 10 IMFs showing the decrease of frequency

IMF	Frequency (Hz) EEMD	Band
1st	43.36186352	Gamma
2nd	21.26384365	Beta/Beta + Alpha
3rd	10.56243214	Alpha + Theta
4th	4.56243214	Theta
5th	2.2931596.9	Delta
6th	0.903365907	Delta
7th	0.41693811	Delta
8th	0.208469055	Delta
9th	0.069489685	Delta
10th	0.069489685	Delta

the five bands that could be extracted from the same original EEG data using Wavelet transformation.

The wavelet transforms the frequency of the original signal into half and each transform further transform into another half. Therefore, as the frequency is 128 Hz using wavelet, the frequency is transformed from 128 to 64 Hz for Gamma band, 64 to 32 Hz for Beta band, 32 to 16 Hz for Alpha band, and 16 to 8 Hz for Theta band. The Delta band is obtained reconstructing from the coefficients of the Theta band, which is the fourth level of decomposition. Therefore, four levels of decomposition are only needed to obtain the five bands (Figure 3.10).

3.4.5   Extracting sleep bands using EMD

Unlike wavelet transform method, EMD, Bivariate, and EEMD approaches of finding the sleep bands are not as straightforward as the wavelet. The basic principle of decomposition method is different from wavelet transform. The frequency after each level of decomposition does not change in a fixed rate of halves as the Wavelet method. The frequency definitely decreases after decomposition. However, the decrease is usually less than half the frequency, therefore it cannot straightaway be utilised for all levels of decomposition for the energy bands as in wavelet method. The first method is to determine the frequency of all IMFs of each method. Another constraint is that as there is no fixed numbers of IMFs per method, therefore the parameters of frequency have to be changed when changing data. Therefore, the frequency of each IMF must be evaluated to see how they can be represented into energy bands (Table 3.2).

Figure 3.11 explains the performance of EMD, EEMD, and Bivariate methods; the results show the trend of frequency decreases over a number of IMFs using the three different methods. Bivariate method uses less number of IMFs for feature detection compared with EMD and EEMD.

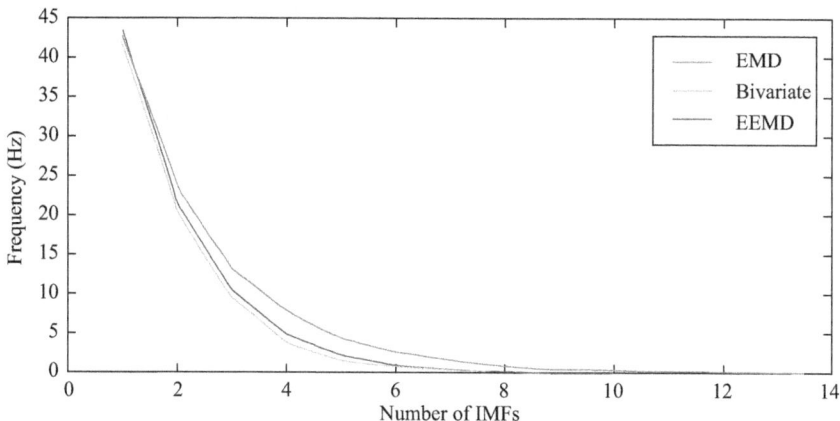

Figure 3.11 Frequency versus IMFs using EMD, EEMD, and Bivariate methods

3.5 Conclusion

These studies show the features and symptoms of sleep apnea using the decomposition-based bivariate EMD, EEMD, and EMD methods. The EEG data were extracted from sleep apnea patients, to understand the features of the data. To understand the performance of the feature extraction capability, the amplitudes, signal energy, index of orthogonality measurement, signal spectrum, instantaneous frequency, and sleep bands classification of the proposed three decomposition methods were compared. The research study shows that the bivariate EMD has better feature extraction capability than EMD, but the performance is lower than EEMD. All three decomposition-based methods are actually managed to illustrate the sleep apnea features and abnormalities. The proposed three methods have shown the occurrence of apnea symptoms, sleep bands, signal correlation with waveform, and delta power of the IMFs. These methods are effective in showing the occurrence of sleep apnea. The Bivariate method is more favourable on data extraction in this study. The EEMD has better performance at specific IMFs and the fundamental EMD method extract better feature at Delta power only.

Some limitations and challenges have been observed in this work. To conduct the research the special approval and ethics clearance are required in order to acquire the EEG for the recruited patients. The approval process needs proper planning and is quite a careful and laborious task. Hence, prior planning efforts and lengthy time need to be considered to complete the clearance process. The process of acquiring the data must also be consistent so that the results consist of similar parameters. The study should not be influenced by the surrounding environments. The next challenge in this study would be identifying and detecting the abnormalities and features of the acquired EEG signals. The EEG data consist of noise and various uncertainties are difficult to be interpreted. Therefore, proper planning and project timeframe need to be considered in this project.

The research study can be further improved by establishing a controlled experiment to analyse and compare the research results generated. The controlled research must be free and independent from any other variables that might directly lead to sleep apnea identification, detection, and prediction. For instance, the female subject tends to have less suffering from sleep apnea. In general observation, subjects suffering from obesity usually have higher probability of having sleep apnea. Therefore, the subject recruitment for the research must be specially considered and pre-selected.

References

[1]   Pack, A. I., 2002. Sleep Apnea: Pathogenesis, Diagnosis and Treatment. 1st ed, CRC Press.

[2]   Tung, R., & Leong, W. Y., 2013, Processing obstructive sleep apnea syndrome (OSAS) data. *Journal of Biomedical Science and Engineering*, 6, 152–164. doi: 10.4236/jbise.2013.62019.

[3]   Caples, S. M., Gami, A. S., & Somers, V. K., 2005. Obstructive sleep apnea. *Annals of Internal Medicine*, 142(3), pp. 187–197.

[4]   *Sleep Well.* TheStar Publications, 2011. Retrieved from: https://www.thestar.com.my/lifestyle/health/2011/10/09/sleep-well/.

[5]   Leong, W. Y., Mandic, D. P., Golz, M., & Sommer, D., 2007. Blind Extraction of Microsleep Events, 2007. *15th International Conference on Digital Signal Processing*, pp. 207–210.

[6]   Harrison, Y., & Horne, J. A., 1996. Occurrence of 'microsleeps' during daytime sleep onset in normal subjects. *Electroencephalogr. Clin. Neurophysiol.*, 98, pp. 411–416.

[7]   Peiris, M. T. R. *et al.*, 2006. Detecting Behavioral Microsleeps from EEG Power Spectra. Engineering in Medicine and Biology Society. *EMBS'06. 28th Annual International Conference of the IEEE*, p. 5723.

[8]   Peiris, M. T. R. *et al.*, 2006b. Fractal Dimension of the EEG for Detection of Behavioural Microsleeps. *Shanghai, IEEE*, pp. 5742–5745.

[9]   Poudel, Govinda R. *et al.*, 2010. The Relationship Between Behavioural Microsleeps, Visuomotor Performance and EEG Theta. *Bueno Aires, IEEE*, pp. 4452–4455.

[10] Leong, W. Y., Mandic, D. P., & Liu, W., 2007. Blind Extraction of Noisy Events Using Nonlinear Predictor, ICASSP 2007. *IEEE*, pp. 657–670.

[11] Poudel, G. R., Innes, C. R., Bones, P. J., & Jones, R. D., 2010. The Relationship Between Behavioural Microsleeps, Visuomotor Performance and EEG Theta. *2010 Annual International Conference of the IEEE Engineering in Medicine and Biology*, pp. 4452–4455.

[12] Leong, W. Y., Mandic, D. P., Golz, M., & Sommer, D., 2007. Blind Extraction of Microsleep Events. *15th International Conference on Digital Signal Processing*, pp. 207–210.

[13] Leong, W. Y., 2006. *Implementing Blind Source Separation in Signal Processing and Telecommunications*, The University of Queensland.

[14] Leong, W. Y., & Mandic, D. P., 2007. Noisy component extraction (noice). *IEEE International Symposium on Circuits and Systems, IEEE*, pp. 3243–3246.

[15] Leong W. Y., & Mandic, D. P., 2006. Towards Adaptive Blind Extraction of Post-Nonlinearly Mixed Signals. *Proceedings of the 16th IEEE Signal Processing Society Workshop on Machine Learning for Signal Processing*, pp. 91–96.

[16] Huang, N. E. *et al.*, 1998a. The empirical mode decomposition and the Hilbert spectrum for nonlinear and nonstationary time series analysis. *Proceedings of the Royal Society of London. Series A: Mathematical, Physical and Engineering Sciences*, 454(1971), pp. 903–995.

[17] Huang, W. *et al.*, 1998b. Engineering analysis of biological variables: an example of blood pressure over 1 day. *Proceedings of the National Academy of Sciences*, 95(9), pp. 4816–4821.

[18] Rilling, G. *et al.*, 2007. Bivariate empirical mode decomposition. *Signal Processing Letters IEEE*, 14(12), p. 9360939.

[19] Wu, Z., & Huang, N. E., 2009. Ensemble empirical mode decomposition: A noise-assisted data analysis method. *Advances in Adaptive Data Analysis*, 1(1), pp. 1–41.

Chapter 4

Person authentication using electroencephalogram (EEG) brainwaves signals

Siaw-Hong Liew[1], Yun-Huoy Choo[1], Yin Fen Low[2], and Zeratul Izzah Mohd Yusoh[1]

This chapter starts with the introduction to various types of authentication modalities, before discussing on the implementation of electroencephalogram (EEG) signals for person authentication task in more details. In general, the EEG signals are unique but highly uncertain, noisy, and difficult to analyze. Event-related potentials, such as visual-evoked potentials, are commonly used in the person authentication literature work. The occipital area of the brain anatomy shows good response to the visual stimulus. Hence, a set of eight selected EEG channels located at the occipital area were used for model training. Besides, feature extraction methods, i.e., the WPD, Hjorth parameter, coherence, cross-correlation, mutual information, and mean of amplitude have been proven to be good in extracting relevant information from the EEG signals. Nevertheless, different features demonstrate varied performance on distinct subjects. Thus, the Correlation-based Feature Selection method was used to select the significant features subset to enhance the authentication performance. Finally, the Fuzzy-Rough Nearest Neighbor classifier was proposed for authentication model building. The experimental results showed that the proposed solution is able to discriminate imposter from target subjects in the person authentication task.

4.1 Introduction

Person authentication or verification is different from person identification. Person authentication or verification result is a one-to-one matching and it gives a yes or no answer (as shown in Figure 4.1). Meanwhile, person identification system is one-to-N matching where an individual identity is determined from a group of persons who are being evaluated [1]. Most of the past literature have focused on

[1]Computational Intelligence and Technologies (CIT) Research Group, Faculty of Information and Communication Technology, Universiti Teknikal Malaysia Melaka (UTeM), Malaysia
[2]Machine Learning and Signal Processing (MLSP) Research Group, Centre for Telecommunication Research and Innovation (CeTRI), Faculty of Electronics and Computer Engineering, Universiti Teknikal Malaysia Melaka (UTeM), Malaysia

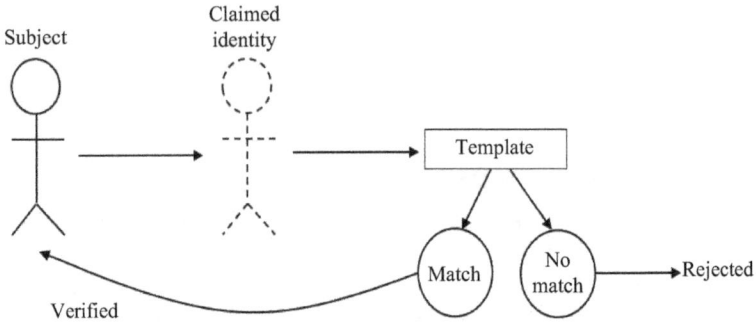

Figure 4.1   The principle of person authentication; one-to-one matching [2]

person identification. However, person authentication is increasingly catching the researcher's attention in line with the emergence of security as one of the important research topics recently. Applications of person authentication such as airport security checking, building gate control, passport confirmation, computer login, internet banking, ATM access, etc., are widely used. An identity authentication system has to deal with two kinds of events: either the person claiming a given identity is the one who he or she claims to be (in which case, he or she is called a client), or he or she is not (in which case, he or she is called an impostor). Moreover, the system may generally take two decisions: either accept the client or reject him or her and decide whether he or she is an impostor.

Several types of methods can be used to authenticate a person from others. Traditional methods of authentication such as knowledge-based and token-based are widely used methods. A password-based system is one of the examples of systems that are established on knowledge-based method while signature is an example of the system established on token-based method. With many new methods of person authentication, most of the people still prefer the use of signature and password as an authentication method because it is easier and does not need any maintenance [3]. Unfortunately, password model and signature are no longer considered reliable enough to satisfy the security requirements because password can be stolen and guessed easily by shoulder surfing and signature can be forged easily. The traditional authentication methods suffer from their inability to differentiate between an authorized person and an impostor who fraudulently acquires the access privilege of the authorized person [4].

Biometric authentication systems were introduced to overcome traditional authentication methods. Biometric is any measurable, physical or physiological feature or behavioral trait that can be used to authenticate the claimed identity of an individual [5]. The major difference between biometric and traditional authentication method is the way how it authenticates a person based on the physical characteristic. It relies on "something that you are" to differentiate between an authorized person and a fraudulent imposter [4]. Physiological biometrics include fingerprint, face, iris, hand geometry, retina, and body odor, while behavioral biometrics include voice, keystroke dynamics, and gait [6]. Nevertheless, these modalities are still facing many challenges. A biometric authentication as long as it satisfies the following requirements [7]:

- **Universality:** Every person should have the characteristics.
- **Uniqueness:** Every person should have different characteristics.
- **Constancy:** The characteristic should remain fairly constant with time.
- **Collectability:** The characteristic can be measured quantitatively.

Fingerprint authentication system considers one of the most popular and oldest biometrics authentication systems. However, due to the advancement of technologies and the evilness of human beings, fingerprint can be imitated, which brings down the uniqueness of it. Apart from that, fingerprint system depends largely on the surface of one's finger. People with physical disabilities or severe injuries such as missing hands or burned fingers are unable to use this system. Other than that, fingerprint nowadays is not secure due to the advancement of technology. There is some research showing that fingerprint can be forged and various algorithms are being developed to detect fingerprint forgery [8]. Fingerprint is public as we place it everywhere when we touch something. Fingerprint authentication system can be forged using artificial fingers and fingerprints made from readily available materials (e.g., silicon, gelatin) or even cadaver fingers (finger of a dead person) [5].

Meanwhile, facial recognition is a computer application that uses face to distinguish an individual from another. It is the most natural means of biometric authentication [9]. Nevertheless, it is less reliable because the human face structure will evolve and change throughout the lifecycle of human due to genetic or environmental factors. Besides, face recognition is not a perfect biometric authentication method because it is dependent on light, facial expression, resolution, and form of hair of an individual [10]. Individual features may not be easily distinguished in poor light condition. Most of the facial recognition systems require the user to stand a specific distance away from the camera and look straight at the camera. This is to ensure that the captured image of the face is within a specific size tolerance and keeps the features in as similar position each time as possible.

Voice can also act as a biometric method in person authentication because every person has a different pitch and it is unique. The sound is produced when air leaves the body of an individual through oral cavity (mouth), nasal cavity (nose), and larynx. Obstructions such as lips, teeth, tongue, size, and position are used to produce sound [10]. However, with the advancement of technology, voice can be easily recorded and forged by an attacker. In addition, voice recognition can be easily affected by environmental factors such as background noise. It might take hours to record the voice, but the system tends to make error.

Hand geometry recognition system was once popular 10 years ago, but it is seldom used nowadays [10]. This recognition system is based on the shape of the hand of an individual, which differs from another person, and the shape of hand does not change after certain age [9]. The main advantages of hand geometry recognition are ease of use, low cost, and simplicity. Environmental factors such as dry skin cannot have influence on the results. Unfortunately, it is less reliable because the measurements of this method are measuring and recording only the length and height of the fingers, shape of the knuckles, distance between joints, and surface area of the hand. Hand geometry recognition system is ideal for adults but not for growing children as their hand characteristics can change in time.

Palmprint refers to an image required of the palm region of the hand. It can be used as a biometric for authentication system. In 1858, palmprint was first introduced by Sir William Herschel in India [11]. Palmprint carries similarities with fingerprint and it consists of some properties such as universality, uniqueness, stability, and collectability for authentication. Every person has a different palmprint; even the palmprints of twins are different. Palmprint area is larger than fingerprint area and hence it provides more information about the person. The features include the principal lines, wrinkles, minutiae, ridges, and delta points of the palms. Palmprinting does not bring any harm to the health of people. Palmprint can be easily captured with low-resolution (at most 400 dpi) devices and thus the devices are not expensive [11]. However, the palmprint authentication system has limitation to mobile users as the size of the palmprint is bigger.

Iris recognition nowadays is with the combination of technologies from several fields such as pattern recognition, optics, and computer vision. Iris is a small internal organ and it is protected by cornea, eyelid, and aqueous humor. It is a unique characteristic of an individual and it does not change during the whole life. As iris is a small internal organ, it is hard to scan from a distance. Furthermore, individuals with eye problems such as cataracts and blindness will have problem using this kind of system due to the inability to scan their iris [10].

Retina scan also acts as biometric authentication, which is based on the blood vessel pattern in the retina of the eye. Retina scan technology is older than iris scan technology, which also uses a part of the eye. It is rarely used nowadays as it is not user friendly and the equipment remains very expensive. The retina scanning system is believed to be very accurate as it has reputedly never falsely verified an unauthorized user so far. However, the main disadvantage of the retina scan is its intrusiveness. The way to obtain retina is personally invasive and the operation of the retina scanner is not easy. A laser light must be directed through the cornea of the eye.

With the shortcomings that have been mentioned above, there is a need to use a biometric that is unique, confidential, and impossible to duplicate in person authentication. Thus, EEG signals is one of the biometric systems that can be used to overcome this problem.

4.2   The human brain

Human brain consists billions of nerve cells that make a large complex neural network. Each of the nerves in the human brain is connected to about 10,000 other nerves. The average human brain weighs around 1,400 g [12]. Human brain can be divided into four portions: brain stem, cerebral cortex, cerebellum, and diencephalon (hypothalamus and thalamus). Cerebral cortex can be divided into two hemispheres and these are connected to each other via corpus callosum. Each

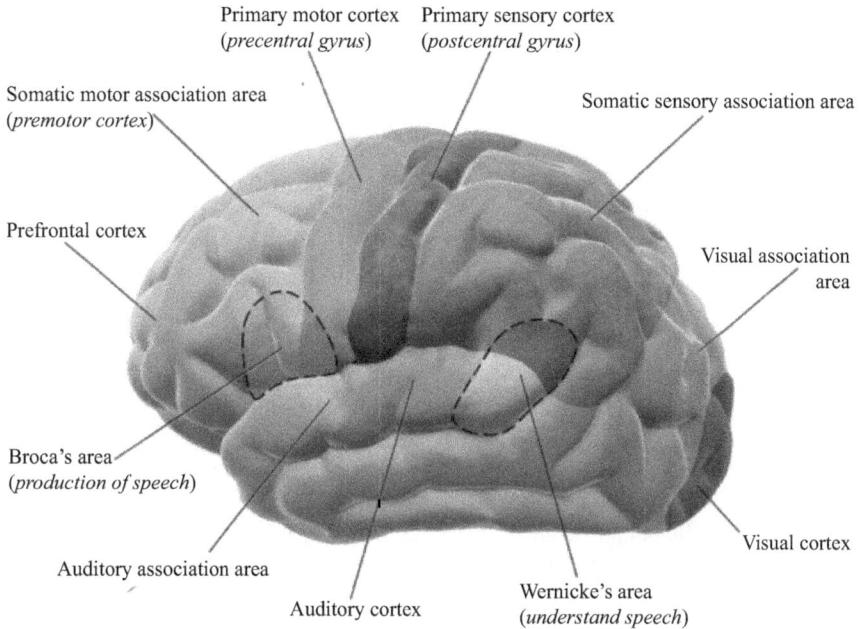

Figure 4.2   The function of the brain [13]

Table 4.1   Cortical area of the brain and their function [13]

Cortical area	Function
Primary Motor Cortex	Initiation of voluntary movement
Somatic Motor Association Cortex	Coordination of complex movement
Prefrontal Cortex	Problem solving, emotion and complex thought
Broca's Area	Speech production and articulation
Auditory Cortex	Detection of sound quality (loudness, tone)
Auditory Association Area	Complex processing of auditory information
Wernicke's Area	Language comprehension
Visual Cortex	Detection of simple visual stimuli
Visual Association Area	Complex processing of visual information
Sensory Association Cortex	Processing of multisensory information
Primary Somatosensory Cortex	Receives tactile information from the body

hemisphere can be divided into four lobes: frontal, parietal, occipital, and temporal. The cerebral cortex can be divided into several areas as shown in Figure 4.2.

The functions of cerebral cortex are problem solving, processing of complex visual information, and language information. The functions of each cortical area are described in Table 4.1.

4.3   Electroencephalogram (EEG)

In 1929, the first signal of electroencephalogram (EEG) was recorded by Berger. EEG signals are brain activities that are recorded from electrodes mounted on the scalp. EEG signals are the product of ionic current flows that happen in the brain's neurons. Some of the connections are excitatory while others are inhibitory. EEG signals have been categorized into six basic rhythms [12] as shown in Table 4.2: Gamma (γ), Beta (β), Mu (μ), Alpha (α), Theta (θ), and Delta (δ). With the advancement in hardware devices, EEG is the most practical method that can be used in biometric. EEG is the most practical capturing method that can be used in biometrics due to the advances in its hardware devices.

The advantages of using brain electrical activity in EEG signals are unique and confidential; the recorded brain response cannot be duplicated, and a person's identity is therefore unlikely to be stolen. A research work done by [7] shows that the EEG signals of a person is unique and differ from person to person, even when they are performing the same task or thought when responding to same visual stimuli. EEG signals can be easily affected, but they cannot be easily reproduced under conditions of stress, fatigue, anxiety, drowsiness, medication, environment, etc. [14]. For example, a person who has been forced or pointing a gun to the head will create different EEG signals from a normal person who is in a relaxed state. In the security aspect, the EEG-based authentication system is not immune to phishing attacks. EEG signals are not 100% identical [15]. With the strength and uniqueness of EEG signals, we believe that the EEG signals are reliable and suitable to be used as a biometric in authentication system.

The EEG recording electrodes and their function are critical for obtaining high-quality data for interpretation [16]. One important problem of EEG signals recording is the artifacts. Examples of the artifacts in EEG signals recording are blinking, head movements, muscle activity, and electrocardiogram. Due to the very low amplitude of EEG signals, artifacts often contaminate the recordings restricting or making difficult in analysis or interpretation. Therefore, the position of subjects

Table 4.2   EEG signal rhythms [12]

Rhythm	Bandwidth	Description
Gamma (γ)	[30,40] Hz	Low in amplitude; can indicate event brain synchronization; and be used to confirm some brain disorders.
Beta (β)	[13,30] Hz	Indicates an alert state, with active thinking and attention.
Mu (μ)	[8,13] Hz	Locates in the motor and sensorimotor cortex; the amplitude varies when the subject performs movements.
Alpha (α)	[8,12] Hz	Indicates a relaxed state, with little or no attention, mainly appear at occipital lobe.
Theta (θ)	[4,8] Hz	Indicates creative inspiration or deep meditation; can also appear in dreaming sleep (REM stage).
Delta (δ)	[0.5,4] Hz	Primarily associated with deep sleep or loss of body awareness, but can be present in the waking state.

during EEG recording should be comfortable enough to avoid unwanted activities; a lying position diminishes the occurrence of some artifacts caused by feeble motion.

Research work done by [1] has obtained highest accuracy of 93.4% for person authentication with a dataset of nine normal subjects performing three tasks during twelve non-feedback sessions over 3 days, which is four sessions per day. A modality for biometric authentication based on EEG signals done by [17] has three tasks of classification accuracy: reading task (97.3%), relax task (94.4%), and multiplication task (97.5%). They analyzed a dataset of 8-channel EEG recordings from 40 volunteer subjects when performing simple tasks such as resting with eyes open and resting with eyes closed. In addition, research work done by [18] used the BCI competition 2003 dataset with the EEG recording from a 64-channel and sampled in 250 Hz. The authentication classification result obtained by [18] ranged from 75% to 85%.

4.3.1 Event-related potentials

Event-related potentials (ERPs) are the potential changes in the EEG signals that occur in response to "event" or stimulus. The changes of the EEG signals are very small and the EEG signals have to be averaged from many trials in order to reveal them. ERPs can be divided into two categories: exogenous (involuntary) and endogenous (voluntary). Exogenous ERPs normally occur up to about 100 ms after the stimulus onset while endogenous ERPs occur from 100 ms onward. It depends on the properties of physical stimulus and behavioral processes related to the event.

The most commonly studied ERP is P300. P300 indicates that positive deflection in EEG occurs approximately 300 ms after the stimulus onset. This effect was present for visual (light flashes) and auditory (clicks) stimuli [19]. P300 is commonly recorded during an "oddball paradigm" where a target stimulus is presented infrequently among more common distracter stimuli. On the other hand, evoked potentials (EPs) is a subset of the ERP, which rise in response to a certain physical stimulus such as visual-evoked potential (VEP), auditory-evoked potential (AEP), and somatosensory-evoked potential (SEP).

Motor imagery is one of the ERP activities. The subjects performed three tasks such as left-hand movements, right-hand movements, and word generation beginning with the same random letter. The classification accuracy achieved about 80% in the research work [20]. One of the ideas that combined EEG signals with authentication system was proposed by [21]. The authentication system was designed by using pass-thoughts, which is reliable and could work as EEG signals are unique and impossible to duplicate.

4.3.2 Visual-evoked potential

EEG signals can be recorded in several types of condition, for example, baseline activity, math activity, letter composing activity, and VEP [22]. The EEG signals recorded when an individual is in a relaxed condition is called baseline activity. The EEG signals recorded in [5] when people were in baseline activity are used to identify the people. Math activity is a simple mathematical equation such as addition, subtraction, multiplication, and division, which a person had to solve without vocalizing and making any movements. A person who was asked to compose a letter to a friend without vocalizing is called letter composing activity. Furthermore, VEP is one of the ERPs that are brain activities that respond to visual stimuli and recorded from the occipital scalp electrode.

VEP is the operational measurement of the visual journey from the retina to the visual cortex of the brain using the optic nerves. The main advantages of VEP signals are short training time, high data transmission rate, and no significant effect on the subjects. VEP may compromise several components such as texture, color, objects, motion, readability (i.e., text vs non-text), and others. Each of these components produced different frequency bands due to the impact in special dispersion of the VEP through the scalp. Therefore, production of VEP should be the focus and stimulate in the same brain area.

Research work in [23] proposed a new method to identify individuals using VEP signals. A dataset of 61-channels placed on the scalp is taken from 20 subjects. The average VEP classification accuracy obtained for identification is 94.18%. Furthermore, the classification accuracy ranged from 95% to 98% for a personal identification experiment based on VEP signals that were recorded from 102 subjects [24]. Malinka [25] designed and implemented VEP as a biometric characteristic. The author proved that VEP is fully suitable for the biometric recognition and the result showed that eight occipital channels are enough to build the biometric authentication system.

The authors in [7] proposed to use brainwave signals that respond to visual stimuli for the purpose of verification. Typically the active electrode is placed over the occipital cortex defined by the International Standard 10–20 EEG System. Research work in [7] considered 8 occipital channels from a total of 64 channels available in dataset for building their authentication system. They presented an EEG authentication system by conducting experiments to investigate the similarities and differences during picture recognition process. A standard set of 260 black-and-white line pictures from [26] will be used in the experiment. The result showed that eight occipital channels are enough to build the biometric authentication system.

EEG signals are unique and particularly strong when a person is exposed to visual stimuli [15]. The main advantage of EEG signal is that it can detect changes over milliseconds. In the research work [15], the authors interviewed a neurologist and EEG expert, Dr Jesper Ronager, who worked at the national hospital of Denmark, Rigshospitalet in Copenhagen. Dr Jesper Ronager mentioned that the visual cortex area of the brain is located at the occipital area and it is the best place to measure EEG signals and the most informative for finding picture recall thought patterns. According to Dr Jesper Ronager, it should not be a problem if the sensors or electrodes are not placed millimeter-precise.

Because EEG signals are highly sensitive to the emotional state, Lee *et al.* [27] studied in EEG-based authentication using three different tasks, i.e., the resting state, the visual stimuli, and the movement or the mental tasks to reduce the high

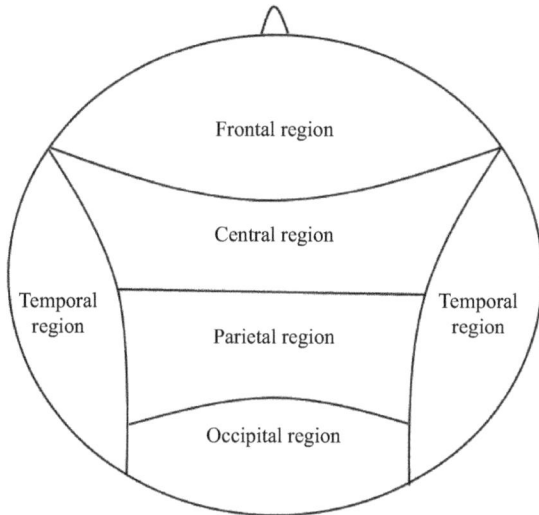

Figure 4.3 Six primary brain regions [28]

sensitivity of the EEG signals on emotional state. The EEG recording measured during resting state by using two channels gained the classification accuracy in the range from 87.5% to 98.1%. Next, the EEG signals recorded from two channels in mental task had the classification accuracy in the range from 91.6% to 97.5% in classification rate. Last but not least, the studies on the VEP gained the best result compared to resting state and mental tasks. The classification result ranged from 92.9% to 98.1%.

4.3.3 Electrode placements

The EEG signals are recorded with electrodes mounted on the scalp. The electrodes are small, conduct electricity, and provide electrical contact between the EEG recording apparatus and the skin by transforming the ionic current on the skin to the electrical current in the wires. Different tasks associated different functional regions in the brain are depicted in Figure 4.3. The frontal region is responsible for problem solving and movement control; the central region manages the initiation of voluntary movement and coordination of complex movement; the parietal region receives sensory information from the body; the temporal region detects sound and performs auditory processing; while the occipital region detects visual stimuli and processes the visual information.

The arrangement of the electrodes is normally based on the International 10–20 system (Figure 4.4). The distance between the electrodes is 10% and 20% and the system consists of 21 electrodes. Each electrode position has a letter and a number to identify the location. The letters C, F, O, P, and T stand for central, frontal, occipital, parietal, and temporal lobes, respectively. Odd numbers indicate the

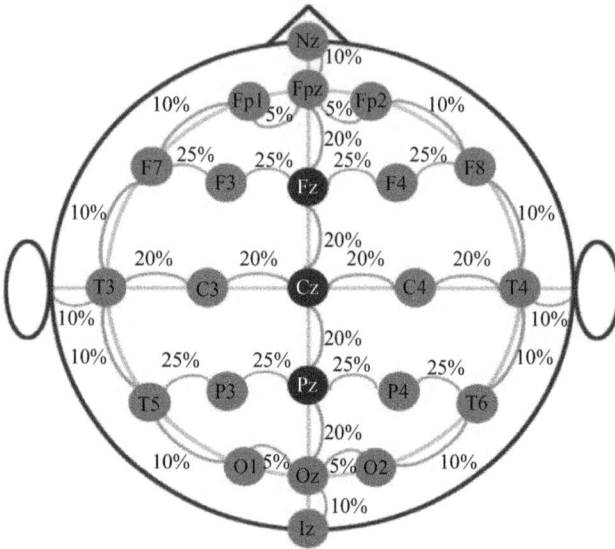

Figure 4.4   International 10–20 electrode placements [29]

electrode position on the left side and even numbers indicate the electrode position on the right side. Z stands for zero and refers to the electrode placements at midline.

Nevertheless, the system allows the use of additional electrodes. The new letter codes for intermediate sites are: AF—intermediate between frontal pole and frontal, FC—between frontal and central, FT—intermediate between frontal and temporal, CP—intermediate between central and parietal, TP—intermediate between temporal and parietal, and PO—intermediate between parietal and occipital. Figure 4.5 shows the 64 EEG electrodes placements.

4.4   Experimentation

A simple flow chart as illustrated in Figure 4.6 describes the person authentication model. It consists of several steps that are EEG signal recording, segmentation, filtering, artifact rejection, feature extraction, feature selection, and classification. Finally, users are classified as client or impostor according to the classification algorithm.

4.4.1   *EEG signal recording and segmentation*

Collected raw EEG data are non-stationary, noisy, complex, and difficult to analyze. Thus, segmentation according to trials must be performed prior to further analysis such as feature extraction, feature selection, and classification. On the other hand, filtering and artifact rejection are also important to avoid misleading information on signal interpretation. The reading with excessive body movements or others types of artifacts will be discarded.

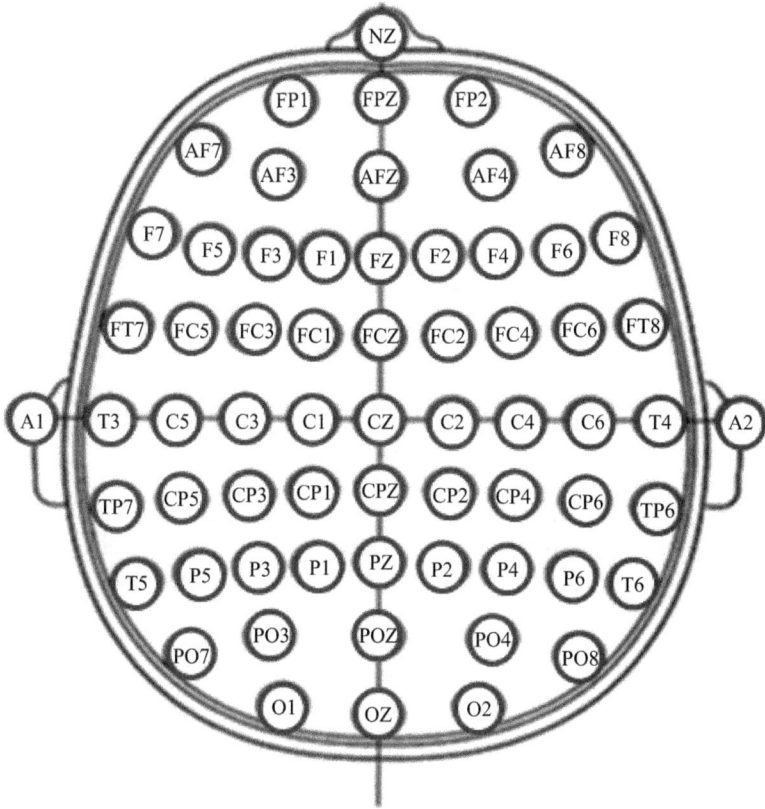

Figure 4.5   The 64 EEG electrode placements [29]

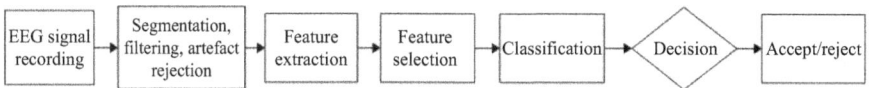

Figure 4.6   EEG-based authentication model

4.4.2   Feature extraction

Feature extraction is to extract the relevant information or characteristics from the EEG signals. Features extracted from EEG signals are unique between subjects and sufficient for person authentication [18]. Different features provide different discriminative power for different subjects. Most of the authentication system will make use of features combination architecture. The results were able to demonstrate significant improvement in the system performance [30]. The feature extraction methods used in this study are as follows:

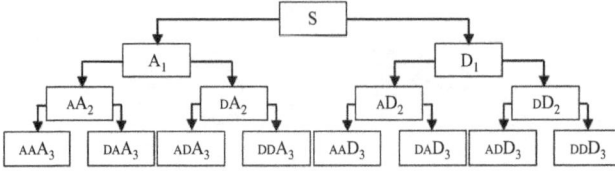

Figure 4.7   Level 3 of wavelet packet decomposition (WPD) tree

4.4.2.1   Wavelet packet decomposition

In [31], the authors have demonstrated wavelet packet decomposition (WPD) is an excellent feature extraction method for non-stationary signals such as EEG signals and it is very appropriate for EEG signals analysis. WPD provides a multilevel time–frequency decomposition of signals and is able to provide more significant features. The wavelet decomposition splits the original signal into detail and approximation coefficients, respectively. After that, the approximation is split into next level approximation and detail. This process will be repeated until n-level. On the other hand, the detail also is split into the next level to yield more than different ways to encode the signal. Figure 4.7 shows a complete decomposition tree of a signal.

Research work by [32] has proven that Daubechies with order 4 (DB4) wavelet and sixth level of WPD is an appropriate parameter in order to analyze the EEG signals with 256-Hz sampling rate. As the frequency of useful EEG signals is lower than 50 Hz, we use 25 sub-bands in each channel. The combination with the time domain and frequency domain can provide more significant features; we characterized the time–frequency distribution of EEG signals by combining the features below:

Average coefficients in sixth sub-band: A total of 8 channels were selected from 64 available channels in the dataset and the sampling rate for each channel is 2^8, the sub-band means (M_j) at jth level is defined as in (4.1):

$$M_j = \frac{1}{2^j} \sum_{k}^{2^8} d_j(k) \tag{4.1}$$

where $d_j(k)$ represents the coefficient of WPD at jth level and kth sample. Twenty-five sub-bands were used for WPD as the frequency of useful EEG signal is lower than 50 Hz. Therefore, the dimensions of feature vector for average coefficients are 200.

Wavelet packet energy in each sub-band: In the perspective of wavelet packet energy, WPD decomposes signal energy on different time-frequency plain; the integration of square amplitude of WPD is proportional to signal power. The sub-band entropy is defined as in (4.2):

$$E(j, n) = \int |S(t)|^2 dt = \sum_{k} \left(d_j^n(k) \right)^2 \tag{4.2}$$

where $n = 0, 1, 2, \ldots, 2^j$. As eight channels were selected in this research, the dimensions of feature vector for wavelet packet energy was 200.

4.4.2.2   Hjorth parameter

Hjorth parameter is essential to analyze EEG signals in both time and frequency domains. It can extract the property of EEG signals efficiently [33]. Hjorth parameters are used to compute the quadratic mean and the dominant frequency of EEG signals on each side of the brain: we used the first two Hjorth descriptors in 1970 and 1973, namely activity and mobility. From the activity and mobility in the EEG signals, it reflects the global trend of a signal, for visual analysis. Hjorth parameters were used in various online EEG analyses, such as in sleep staging in order to compute the amplitude and the main frequency of a signal. These descriptors are chosen because they have a low calculation cost [34].

Let us consider the spectral moment of order 0 and 2:

$$m_0 = \int_{-\pi}^{\pi} S(w)dw = \frac{1}{T}\int_{t-T}^{t} f^2(t)dt \qquad (4.3)$$

$$m_2 = \int_{-\pi}^{\pi} w^2 S(w)dw = \frac{1}{T}\int_{t-T}^{t} \left(\frac{df}{dt}\right)^2 dt \qquad (4.4)$$

where $S(w)$ represents the power density spectrum and $f(t)$ represents the EEG signal within an epoch of duration T. The first two of Hjorth parameters are given by

$$\text{Activity}: h_0 = m_0 \qquad (4.5)$$

$$\text{Mobility}: h_1 = \sqrt{\frac{m_2}{m_0}} \qquad (4.6)$$

where h_0 is the square of the quartic mean and h_1 reflects the frequency of dominant. These quantities are in discrete forms, where $h_0(k)$ and $h_1(k)$ at a sampled time of k are calculated within a sliding window of 1s length using the open source software library BioSig.

Besides that, Hjorth parameter has also used the fourth-order spectral moment m_4 to define a measure of the bandwidth of the signal called complexity.

$$\text{Complexity}: h_2 = \sqrt{\frac{m_4}{m_2} - \frac{m_2}{m_0}} \qquad (4.7)$$

The first parameter is Activity, which represents the signal power; Mobility represents the mean frequency; and Complexity represents the change in frequency.

4.4.2.3   Coherence

Coherence is a feature used to measure the degree of linear correlation between two signals. The correlation between two time series at different frequencies can be uncovered by coherence. Coherence is normally used for analyzing the condition of different cognitive disorders. It has been proved that EEG-based coherence analysis can be used in biometrics [15]. The range value for the magnitude of the squared coherence estimate is between 0 and 1, which quantizes how well x corresponds to y at each frequency. The value of 0 for the coherence function means the independence between two signals. The value of 1 for the coherence function means the complete linear dependence. The formula of coherence is given as follows:

$$C_{xy}(f) = \frac{|P_{xy}(f)|^2}{P_{xx}(f)P_{yy}(f)} \tag{4.8}$$

where $C_{xy}(f)$ is a function of the power spectral density $(P_{xx}$ and $P_{yy})$ of x and y, and the cross-power spectral density P_{xy} of x and y.

4.4.2.4   Cross-correlation

The main idea of the cross-correlation, also known as sliding dot product, is to measure the similarity of two channels. Cross-correlation is used to find occurrences of a known signal in unknown one [35]. Additionally, it is a function of the relative delay between the signals, which can be applied in pattern recognition and cryptanalysis. Two input signals will be used to compute the cross-correlation:

- Channel 1 with itself: ρ_X
- Channel 2 with itself: ρ_Y
- Channel 1 with channel 2: ρ_{XY}

The correlation ρ_{XY} between two random variables x and y with expected values, μ_x and μ_y, and standard deviation, σ_x and σ_y, is given as:

$$\rho_{X,Y} = \frac{\mathrm{cov}(X, Y)}{\sigma_X \sigma_Y} = \frac{E((X - \mu_X)(Y - \mu_Y))}{\sigma_X \sigma_Y} \tag{4.9}$$

where $E(X)$ is the expectation operator and $\mathrm{cov}(X)$ is the covariance operator.

4.4.2.5   Mutual information

In information theory and probability theory, the mutual information is used to measure the relationship between two signals that are sampled simultaneously. In other words, mutual information measures how much the information is communicated in one input signal about another. The common unit of mutual information measurement is the bit when we used logarithms of base 2 in its computation [30].

4.4.2.6   Mean of amplitude

Mean, also known as average, is the sum of all EEG potential value and divided by the number of samples. The expression of the mean is given in (4.10):

$$\bar{x} = \frac{1}{n} \cdot \sum_{i=1}^{n} x_i \tag{4.10}$$

where n is the number of data and x_i is the value of data.

In our earlier work in [36], we have compared the performance of three feature extraction methods (coherence, cross-correlation, and mean of amplitude) and

six feature extraction methods (WPD, Hjorth parameter, mutual information, coherence, cross-correlation, and mean of amplitude). The six feature extraction methods are good to extract important attributes for person authentication.

4.4.3 Feature selection

The WPD method tends to induce large vector set especially when the selected EEG channels increase. Thus, the feature selection process is important to reduce the features set before combining the significant features with the other small feature vectors set. Feature selection plays an important role especially for the large dataset. Three common models for feature selection are the filter model, the wrapper model, and the embedded model. Filter methods investigate the prior knowledge among features to select the best discriminating subset. Therefore, understanding the data features is important to produce a good filter model. On the other hand, wrapper methods employ a predetermined induction algorithm to find a subset of features with the highest evaluation quality by searching through the feature subsets space. The wrapper method is more time consuming than the filter method because it is strongly coupled with an induction algorithm. It calls the induction algorithm repetitively to evaluate the performance of each feature's subset [37] during the performance evaluation process.

The Correlation-based Feature Selection (CFS) often referred as cfsSubsetEval in WEKA is a correlation-based feature selector. CFS is a good feature selection method that is able to reduce dimensionality without affecting accuracy [37]. It is a fast and correlated-based filter algorithm that is applicable in discrete and continuous problems. The CFS algorithm evaluates the feature subset according to the correlation-based heuristic merit. A good feature subset contains high correlation between features and the class [38]. In our earlier work in [36], the experiments were designed in two levels, i.e., select the attributes from WPD feature vectors using CFS algorithm before combining with other feature vectors; and to apply the CFS feature selection across all feature vectors at the same time. The experiment results showed that the feature selection applied on the WPD only gained better classification accuracy and AUC.

4.4.4 Classification

Fuzzy-Rough Nearest Neighbor (FRNN) classifier was proposed in our previous work [36,39] and used to evaluate the performance for person authentication. It is a fuzzy-rough version of WEKA data mining tools. FRNN classifier was first introduced by Jensen and Cornelis [40], which combined the strength of fuzzy sets, rough sets, and nearest neighbors classification approach motivated by human decision making. In FRNN algorithm, the nearest neighbors are used to construct the fuzzy lower and upper approximations to quantify the membership value of a test object to determine its decision class, and test instances are classified based on their membership to these approximations. FRNN algorithm follows the fundamental of fuzzy-nearest neighbors approach in classifying objects into the most probable decision class. However, instead of using the fuzzy membership function, FRNN capture the uncertainty with the fuzzy-rough approximations. FRNN classification approach used in [36] and [39] have gained good results for person authentication using EEG signals.

Fuzzy logic connectives play important role in the development of fuzzy-rough set theory. A triangular norm (t-norm), T is any increasing, commutative, and associative $[0,1]^2 \rightarrow [0,1]$ mapping, satisfy $T(1, x) = x$, for all x in $[0,1]$. On the other hand, an implicator is any $[0,1]^2 \rightarrow [0,1]$ mapping $\mathscr{F}$ satisfying $\mathscr{F}(0,0) = 1$, $\mathscr{F}(1, x) = x$, for all x in $[0,1]$. In [40], they have used Kleene–Dienes implicator for x, y in $[0,1]$.

Various types of performance measurements such as accuracy, recall, precision, and area under receiver operating characteristics curve (AUC) are used to evaluate the efficiency of the results. Accuracy and AUC were selected based on literature review. Although accuracy is commonly used to analyze results, it is not a good performance measurement at all the times because it provides less meaningful information by omitting false positives in its measurement. False positives provide useful information on tolerance up to a certain extent. In addition, AUC is gaining more popularity for judging classifier properties by providing a graphical method. It is a very useful performance measure by calculating AUC learning curves for very large datasets. It cannot be denied that AUC curves are provided very meaningful of both theoretical and empirical justification. AUC is found to have a more discriminating value and statistically consistent compared to the accuracy.

4.5   Results and discussion

A EEG dataset from UCI Machine Learning and EEG dataset from UCI Machine Learning Repository were used in the experiments. Large dataset was used in this research and it consists of 10 subjects with 64 channels electrode placement. Each individual is completed with a total of 60 trials and sampled at 256 Hz. Due to many redundant trials in one of the subjects; it was replaced by another subject from the full dataset. This is necessary to ensure that the prediction ability is not biased due to the redundant data in both training and testing phase. Instead of treating the classification as a ten-class problem, the classifier was trained with only two outputs, i.e., the client and the imposter. The data were split into 80% of training and 20% of testing. In this study, we have considered the electrodes at occipital area. The eight electrodes are PO7, PO3, POZ, PO4, PO8, O1, OZ, and O2 as suggested in [7].

Table 4.3 shows the classification performance of FRNN in person authentication modeling. The classification accuracy and AUC obtained in the experiment were 92.67% and 0.951, respectively. From the results shown in Table 4.3, we can conclude that the FRNN model is suitable for EEG signals classification for person authentication modeling.

Table 4.3   Classification performance of FRNN in person
           authentication modeling

Person	True positive rate (TPR)	False positive rate (FPR)	Accuracy (%)	AUC
Person 1	0.967	0.226	96.67	0.976
Person 2	0.917	0.157	91.67	0.954
Person 3	0.908	0.381	90.83	0.950
Person 4	0.900	0.604	90.00	0.894
Person 5	0.992	0.075	99.17	1.000
Person 6	0.875	0.458	87.50	0.921
Person 7	0.900	0.530	90.00	0.926
Person 8	0.950	0.302	95.00	0.981
Person 9	0.900	0.307	90.00	0.928
Person 10	0.958	0.301	95.83	0.981
Average	0.927	0.334	92.67	0.951

4.6   Conclusion

In this chapter, we discussed the different types of person authentication models. All the mentioned person authentication models have their strengths and shortcomings. Therefore, the EEG signal was proposed to overcome the shortcomings. The EEG signals are unique but highly uncertain, noisy, and difficult to analyze. VEPs can be found in the past literature and showed that the VEPs are suitable for person authentication modeling. Thus, feature extraction such as WPD, Hjorth parameter, coherence, cross-correlation, mutual information, and mean of amplitude are proven good to extract the relevant information or characteristics from the EEG signals. Different features provide different discriminative power for different subjects. On the other hand, feature selection also plays an important role in reducing the dimensionality of feature vectors. FRNN acts as classifier was implemented to measure the performance of uncertainty modeling in EEG signals analysis. The experimental results showed that FRNN is able to be used for person authentication modeling.

References

[1]   S. Marcel and J. D. R. Millán, "Person Authentication using Brainwaves (EEG) and Maximum A Posteriori Model Adaptation.," *IEEE Trans. Pattern Anal. Mach. Intell.*, vol. 29, no. 4, pp. 743–752, 2007.
[2]   K. Fladby, "Brain Wave Based Authentication," Gjovik University College, 2008.
[3]   A. H. Lashkari, S. Farmand, D. O. Bin Zakaria, and D. R. Saleh, "Shoulder Surfing Attack in Graphical Password Authentication," *Int. J. Comput. Sci. Inf. Secur.*, vol. 6, no. 2, pp. 145–154, 2009.

[4]   A. K. Jain, L. Hong, S. Pankanti, and R. Bolle, "An Identity-Authentication System using Fingerprints," *Proc. IEEE*, vol. 85, no. 9, pp. 1365–1388, 1997.

[5]   T. K. Neela and K. S. Kahlon, "A Framework for Authentication using Fingerprint and Electroencephalogram as Biometrics Modalities," *Int. J. Comput. Sci. Manag. Res.*, vol. 1, no. 1, pp. 39–43, 2012.

[6]   M. Ekinci and M. Aykut, "Human Identification Using Gait," *2006 IEEE 14th Signal Process. Commun. Appl.*, vol. 14, no. 2, pp. 267–291, 2006.

[7]   A. Zuquete, B. Quintela, and J. P. Silva Cunha, "Biometric Authentication using Brain Responses to Visual Stimuli," in International Conference on Bio-inspired Systems and Signal Processing, 2010, pp. 103–112.

[8]   Y.-N. Shin, M. G. Chun, and W. Shin, "A Reproducible Performance Evaluation Method for Forged Fingerprint Detection Algorithm," in International Conference on Information Science and Applications (ICISA), 2010, pp. 1–8.

[9]   V. Matyáš Jr and Z. Riha, "Biometric Authentication Systems," Czech Republic, 2000.

[10]   A. Babich, "Biometric Authentication. Types of biometric identifiers," 2012.

[11]   A. Bera, D. Bhattacharjee, and M. Nasipuri, "Hand Biometrics in Digital Forensics," in *Computational Intelligence in Digital Forensics: Forensic Investigation and Applications*, 2014, pp. 145–163.

[12]   J. Lehtonen, "EEG-based Brain Computer Interfaces," Department of Electrical and Communications Engineering, Helsinki University of Technology, Espoo, 2002.

[13]   E. H. Chudler, "Functional Divisions of the Cerebral Cortex." [Online]. Available: https://faculty.washington.edu/chudler/functional.html. [Accessed: 02-Feb-2018].

[14]   I. Svogor and T. Kisasondi, "Two Factor Authentication using EEG Augmented Passwords," in 34th International Conference on Information Technology Interfaces, 2012, pp. 373–378.

[15]   H. Olesen, J. Klonovs, and C. K. Petersen, "Development of a Mobile EEG-Based Feature Extraction and Classification System for Biometric Authentication," Aalborg University: Copenhagen, 2012.

[16]   M. Teplan, "Fundamentals of EEG Measurement," *Meas. Sci. Rev.*, vol. 2, no. 2, pp. 1–11, 2002.

[17]   C. R. Hema, M. P. Paulraj, and H. Kaur, "Brain Signatures: A Modality for Biometric Authentication," in 2008 International Conference on Electronic Design, 2008, pp. 1–4.

[18]   J.-F. Hu, "Multifeature Biometric System Based on EEG Signals," in Proceedings of the 2nd International Conference on Interaction Sciences Information Technology, Culture and Human - ICIS '09, 2009, pp. 1341–1345.

[19]   M. J. M. Alexandra, P. Fonaryova Key, and G. O. Dove. "Linking Brainwaves to the Brain: An ERP Primer," *Dev. Neuropsychol.*, vol. 27, no. 2, pp. 183–215, 2005.

[20]   R. B. Paranjape, J. Mahovsky, L. Benedicenti, and Z. Koles', "The Electroencephalogram as a Biometric," in Canadian Conference on Electrical and Computer Engineering 2001, 2001, vol. 2, pp. 1363–1366.

[21] J. Thorpe and P. C. Van Oorschot, "Pass-Thoughts: Authenticating With Our Minds," in Proceedings of the 2005 Workshop on New Security Paradigms, 2005, pp. 45–56.

[22] R. Palaniappan, "Two-Stage Biometric Authentication Method using Thought Activity Brainwaves," *Int. J. Neural Syst.*, vol. 18, no. 1, pp. 59–66, 2008.

[23] R. Palaniappan and K. V. R. Ravi, "A New Method to Identify Individuals Using Signals from the Brain," in International Conference Proceedings of the 2003 Joint Conference of the Fourth, 2003, pp. 1442–1445.

[24] R. Palaniappan and D. P. Mandic. "Biometrics from Brain Electrical Activity: A Machine Learning Approach," *IEEE Trans. Pattern Anal. Mach. Intell.*, vol. 29, no. 4, pp. 738–742, 2007.

[25] K. Malinka, "Usability of Visual Evoked Potentials as Behavioral Characteristics for Biometric Authentication," in 2009 *Fourth International Conference on Internet Monitoring and Protection*, 2009, pp. 84–89.

[26] J. G. Snodgrass and M. Vanderwart, "A Standardized Set of 260 Pictures: Norms for Name Agreement, Image Agreement, Familiarity, and Visual Complexity," *J. Exp. Psychol. Hum. Learn. Mem.*, vol. 6, no. 2, pp. 174–215, 1980.

[27] H. J. Lee, H. S. Kim, and K. S. Park, "A Study on the Reproducibility of Biometric Authentication Based on Electroencephalogram (EEG)," in *2013 6th International IEEE/EMBS Conference on Neural Engineering (NER)*, pp. 13–16, 2013.

[28] X. L. Zhang, H. Begleiter, B. Porjesz, W. Wang, and A. Litke, "Event Related Potentials during Object Recognition Tasks," *Brain Res. Bull.*, vol. 38, no. 6, pp. 531–538, 1995.

[29] "10/20 System Positioning Manual," Hong Kong, 2012. Trans Cranial Technologies Idt. Hong Kong. Manual.

[30] H. Jian-feng, "Biometric System Based on EEG Signals by Feature Combination," in International Conference on Measuring Technology and Mechatronics Automation, 2010, pp. 752–755.

[31] W. Ting, Y. Guo-zheng, Y. Bang-hua, and S. Hong, "EEG Feature Extraction Based on Wavelet Packet Decomposition for Brain Computer Interface," Measurement, vol. 41, no. 6, pp. 618–625, 2008.

[32] D. Y. Hu, W. Li, and X. Chen, "Feature Extraction of Motor Imagery EEG Signals Based on Wavelet Packet Decomposition," in The 2011 IEEE/ICME International Conference on Complex Medical Engineering, 2011, pp. 694–697.

[33] S.-H. Oh, Y.-R. Lee, and H.-N. Kim, "A Novel EEG Feature Extraction Method Using Hjorth Parameter," *Int. J. Electron. Electr. Eng.*, vol. 2, no. 2, pp. 106–110, 2014.

[34] T. Cecchin, R. Ranta, L. Koessler, O. Caspary, H. Vespignani, and L. Maillard, "Seizure Lateralization in Scalp EEG using Hjorth Parameters.," *Clin. Neurophysiol.*, vol. 121, no. 3, pp. 290–300, 2010.

[35] A. Riera, A. Soria-Frisch, M. Caparrini, C. Grau, and G. Ruffini, "Unobtrusive Biometric System Based on Electroencephalogram Analysis," *EURASIP J. Adv. Signal Process.*, vol. 2008, no. 1, pp. 1–8, 2008.

[36] S. H. Liew, Y. H. Choo, Y. F. Low, Z. I. Mohd Yusoh, T. B. Yap, and A. K. Muda, "Comparing Features Extraction Methods for Person Authentication using EEG Signals," in *Pattern Analysis, Intelligent Security and the Internet of Things*, 2014, pp. 196–205.

[37] K. M. Te Shun Chou, K. K. Yen, J. Luo, and N. Pissinou, "Correlation-Based Feature Selection for Intrusion Detection Design," in Military Communications Conference, 2007. MILCOM 2007. IEEE, 2007, pp. 1–7.

[38] X. Lu, X. Peng, P. Liu, Y. Deng, B. Feng, and B. Liao, "A Novel Feature Selection Method based on CFS in Cancer Recognition," in 2012 IEEE 6th International Conference on Systems Biology (ISB), 2012, pp. 226–231.

[39] S. H. Liew, Y. H. Choo, and Y. F. Low, "Fuzzy-Rough Nearest Neighbour Classifier for Person Authentication using EEG Signals," in Proceedings of 2013 International Conference on Fuzzy Theory and Its Application, 2013, pp. 316–321.

[40] R. Jensen and C. Cornelis, "Fuzzy-Rough Nearest Neighbour Classification and Prediction," *Theor. Comput. Sci.*, vol. 412, no. 42, pp. 5871–5884, 2011.

Chapter 5

Handedness detection system

Chuen Rue Ng[1] and Wai Yie Leong[1]

In this project, an algorithm, together with a testing module, has been developed to classify the handedness of a person. Electroencephalogram (EEG) signals at the homologous occipital region were captured when test subjects were asked to rest or expose to some graphical stimulus. Handedness of the person can be determined from the EEG data captured and further confirmed using a simple game as testing module. EEG signals are obtained from three locations, namely A1, O1 and O2 as shown in Figure 5.1. The signals are processed using Wavelet Transform to classify the signal into four different frequency bands, Alpha, Beta, Delta, and Theta, before it is used to find out the Mean EEG Coherence (MEC).

Generally left-handed person has higher MEC, which means that there are more connections between the left and right hemisphere of cerebrums through the corpus callosum (CC). Based on some research, personal non-right handedness has been associated with both increased CC size and increased functional interaction between cerebral hemispheres. To relate the former to the latter, it is suggested that the increased size of CC, which somehow acts as a bridge that passes information between the two sides of the brain, allows greater interhemispheric communication. Handedness is determined based on this criterion. At the end of the research, several methods were investigated to process the signals, which were in turn were analyzed by several different analysis to conclude that the coherence of a left-hander between the two hemispheres of the brain is higher.

5.1 Introduction

Handedness of a subject is vital as it is often related to brain functions that are important and is reflected in various fields, especially neurology, neuropsychology, and academic research. The recognition of handedness was most often done by observing the hand used for writing. This may not be exactly the true handedness of the person, as left handers may have been forced to write using right hand since childhood and have gained a common practice to write using right hand. Besides,

[1]Faculty of Engineering and Information Technology MAHSA University, Malaysia

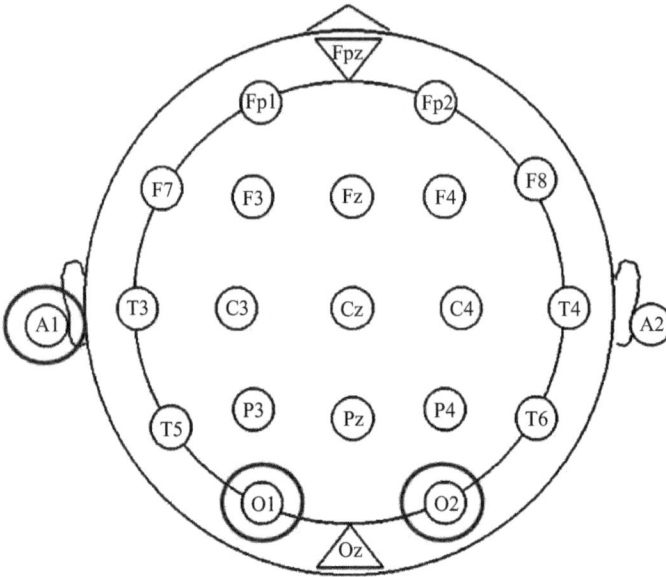

Figure 5.1   The International 10–20 system. The circled electrode placements that are used in this experiment are A1, O1, and O2

environment also plays an important role to alter the natural handedness of a person due to the majority ergonomics of equipment aimed for the right hander, for example, computer mouse, guitar, golf club, and so on. In terms of scientific investigation, and based on [1], the assessment and analysis of handedness are done using the Edinburgh inventory, which includes answering several handedness question on how a person performs daily activities such as writing, throwing, spoon handling, and so on to a total of 10 questions, and from these habits, handedness is then determined.

Although the feasibility of this method is high, it may not be exactly true when a lefty is forced to cope with the right-hander dominant world that they had changed the way they use things naturally or maybe they have been taught to use right hand for various activities since childhood. Another downside of this method is that it needs the subjects to be fully awake and in normal psychological condition so that they can answer those projected questions to its true extent. Therefore, an alternate handedness detection system has been introduced in this research in hope for a better and more accurate handedness determination.

The aim and objective of this research is to establish a system to determine the handedness of a person using data obtained from EEG. Based on the finding from [2], the occipital region gave a higher interhemisphere coherence for a left hander than a right hander. From this discovery, an experiment was set up in this research to determine the MEC of subjects, which is the average connectivity or linkage between the left brain occipital region and the right brain occipital region.

5.2   Methodology

EEG is commonly acquired from a patient or even normal subjects to find out the electrical signal generated by their brain. The basis of this research originated from the findings of [2], which Nielsen found out that the MECs for left handers are higher than those of right-handed subjects in the occipital region. Therefore, an experiment was set up, along with a set of algorithms to determine the handedness of an individual. The EEG signals were obtained from subjects using golden electrodes and then recorded with EEG recorder on the O1, O2, and A1 locations as shown in Figure 5.1.

Before the acquisition of the data, the recorder was configured to capture the EEG signal at a sample rate of 256 Hz with a resolution of 8 bit. The acquisition lasted around 3 min when subjects were asked to watch animation or cartoon to stimulate the image-processing ability of the occipital region. The signals were then gone through a 50-Hz notch filter to get rid of some "hum" from the local mains supply.

5.2.1   Lifting-based discrete Wavelet Transform

After the acquisition of data, signals obtained were processed using the method suggested by [3], which is the lifting-based discrete wavelet transform (LBDWT). The reason for using LBDWT is that we can find the four types of EEG waves, that is, Alpha, Beta, Delta and Theta, after decomposing it to several factors. This is important as we only need these four major brain waves to represent brain signal as a whole and the other excluded waves were deemed to be noises. It is due to the fact that somehow some of the decomposed signals approximate coefficient and/or detailed coefficients, when decomposed using Daubechies four-filter wavelet, will have frequencies almost similar to those of the four types of EEG waves identified at [3]. The similarities are shown in Table 5.1.

Based on the table, the detailed coefficient for the third level of decomposed signal corresponds to the Beta wave, the detailed coefficient for the fourth level of decomposed signal corresponds to the Alpha wave, the detailed coefficient for the fifth level of decomposed signal corresponds to the Theta wave, and finally the approximate coefficient for the third level of decomposed signal corresponds to the Delta wave.

Table 5.1   Similarities between decomposed Daubechies four-filter Wavelet's frequencies and the four types of EEG waves

Decomposed signal	Frequency (Hz)	EEG wave	Frequency (Hz)
D3	12.5–25	Beta	13–30
D4	6.25–12.5	Alpha	8–13
D5	3.125–6.25	Theta	4–8
A5	0–3.125	Delta	1–4

5.2.2   *Reconstructed empirical mode decomposition*

Signal from the subject was being decomposed using Empirical Mode Decomposition (EMD) into several Intrinsic Mode Functions (IMFs). Each of the IMFs contains their distinct frequency bands [4]. The frequency of each IMF is obtained by dividing the number of peaks with time, which in turn is obtained by multiplying the number of time sample with the sampling rate. After each of the IMF's frequency is determined, the IMFs that are within the range of Delta wave brain signal (0.5–4 Hz), Theta wave brain signal (4–8 Hz), Alpha wave brain signal (8–14 Hz), and Beta wave brain signal (14–30 Hz), in other words from 0.5 to 30 Hz, were being reconstructed into a single line of signal, which only contains data in the preferred frequency range.

5.2.3   *Finite impulse response filter*

The Finite Impulse Response (FIR) filter, which was designed in MATLAB®, is an "equiripple" band-pass filter with "fpass" and "fstop" at 0.5–30 Hz, which means it only allows the Delta wave brain signal (0.5–4 Hz), Theta wave brain signal (4–8 Hz), Alpha wave brain signal (8–14 Hz), and Beta wave brain signal (14–30 Hz) to pass.

5.2.4   *Mean EEG coherence*

For Wavelet Transform, after getting the four waves, the coherences between the four waves from O1 and O2 were determined before finally obtaining the mean by adding the four coherences and dividing them by four as suggested by [2]. For Reverse EMD and FIR Filter Method, the coherences between the two signal sources were determined as a whole, without separating them into four waves. According to [5] and [6], coherence is a calculation of the extent of association or coupling of frequency spectra between two different time series. Coherence is related to the measure of phase differences, and the EEG coherence is often used in neurological studies as it epitomizes the interhemispheric communication ability. Coherence is usually defined as follows:

$$\text{Coherence } (f) = \frac{|\text{Cross}-\text{Spectrum}(f)XY|^2}{(\text{Autospectrum}(f)(X))(\text{Autospectrum}(f)(Y))} \tag{5.1}$$

where X and Y = two different channels, which in this research channel are O1 and O2.

The mean of the coherence values from the four types of values is determined and is known as the MEC. This value is used to determine the handedness of the subject according to a set point, which acts as a boundary separating left handers and right handers. The deterministic set point was set by the mean of all MECs. After the set point is set, it was put into test for 16 self-declared left-handed subjects.

5.3   Results and discussion

5.3.1   *Analysis of the MEC*

The MEC was calculated for four left-handed subjects and four right-handed subjects using all three proposed methods. Mean is calculated as an effort to determine the handedness of the subjects.

Table 5.2   Mean EEG coherence for left-handed subjects and right-handed subjects

Subject code	Wavelet	EMD	FIR	Mean
L1	0.7733	0.6915	0.5402	0.6683
L2	0.6985	0.6685	0.6513	0.6728
L3	0.5825	0.3023	0.4500	0.4449
L4	0.4885	0.2206	0.4757	0.3949
R1	0.2768	0.3358	0.2741	0.2956
R2	0.2344	0.1989	0.2233	0.2189
R3	0.2651	0.1695	0.2519	0.2288
R4	0.1537	0.1428	0.2342	0.1769
Mean	0.4341	0.3412	0.3876	0.3876
Range	0.6196	0.5487	0.4280	0.5321
Standard deviation	0.2335	0.2188	0.1631	0.1964

Based on Table 5.2, in which the MEC is obtained from left-handed subjects and right-handed subjects, it can be said that generally left-handed subjects have higher MEC than right-handed subjects. According to [7–13], left handers have larger corpus callosum (CC) than right handers, discovered by either postmortem or using Magnetic Resonance Imaging (MRI). It is due to this that the MEC of the left-handed subject is higher. The CC represents the major commissural tract connecting the two cerebral hemispheres and is supposed to play crucial integrative role in functional hemispheric specialization [8]. Left handers, having bigger corpus callosal areas and better interhemispheric communication, excel in many areas and fields especially those requiring less lateralization.

For Wavelet and FIR methods, the four left-handed and four right-handed subjects were separated correctly and evenly to both sides of the mean, while EMD method had six subjects detected as right handed while two subjects detected as left handed, distributed at the right side of the mean line. One of the reasons for this error was the minor loss of data during the reconstruction of the signals from IMFs. Meanwhile, the mean of all methods correctly determined the handedness of the subjects (Figure 5.2).

5.3.2   Analysis on spectrogram and power spectral density

The analysis on spectrogram was performed on the data obtained. A spectrogram is capable of showing the relationship between time, frequency, and power spectral density (PSD), which is the power of the signal per unit frequency.

Based on Figure 5.3, it can be seen, especially for a left hander, that there are four bands of frequency that fall around 6–8 Hz, 11–15 Hz, 18–21 Hz, and 24–27 Hz from bottom to top. The first band at 6–8 Hz resembles Theta wave brain signal (4–8 Hz). The second band at 11–15 Hz resembles Alpha wave brain signal (8–14 Hz). The third and fourth bands at 18–21 Hz and 24–27 Hz resemble Beta wave brain signal (14–30 Hz). The spectrograms of O1 and O2 for the left-handed subject almost show no difference, signifying high coherence, whereas vast difference is easily spotted for the right hander's O1 and O2 spectrograms.

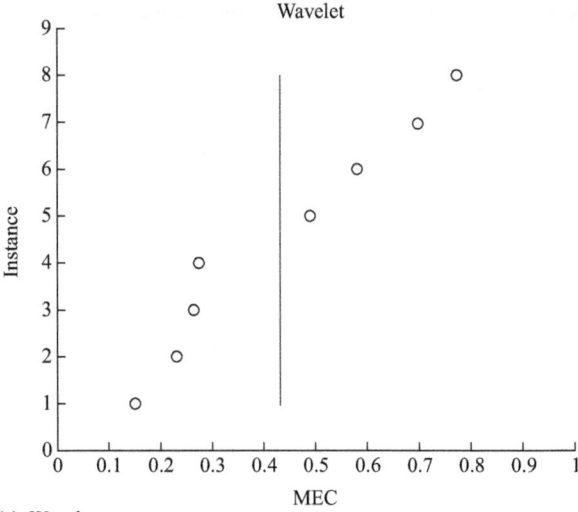

(a) Wavelet

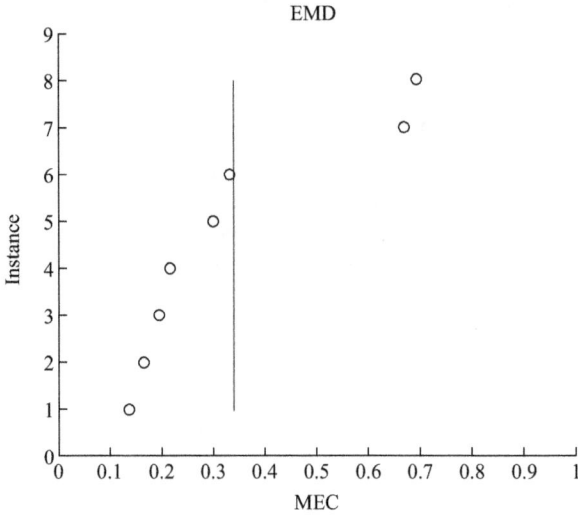

(b) EMD

Figure 5.2   Distribution graph of MEC for all three methods and the mean of all methods for four left handers and four right handers: (a) Wavelet; (b) EMD; (c) FIR; and (d) Mean

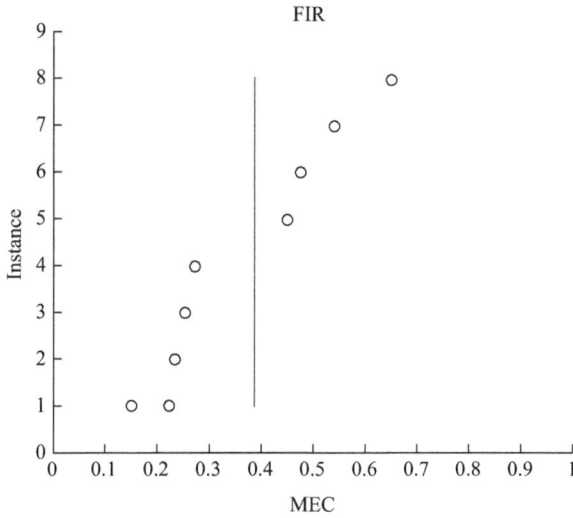

(c) FIR

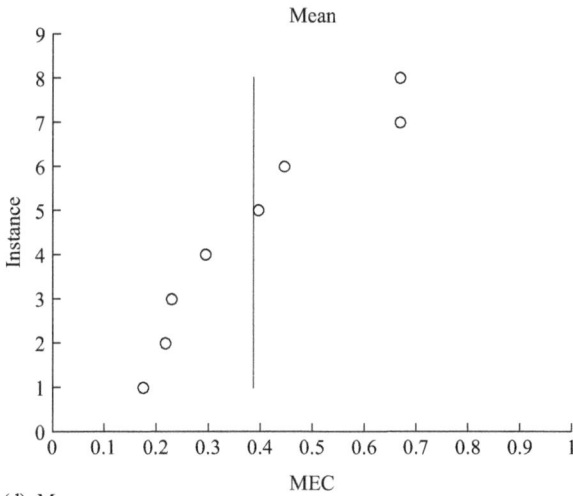

(d) Mean

Figure 5.2 (*Continued*)

As shown in Figure 5.4, semicircle loops have certain frequencies that are high in power, particularly those in the four main brain wave range. Just like the spectrogram, the PSD of O1 and O2 for the left-handed subject almost show no difference, signifying high coherence, whereas vast different is easily spotted for the right hander's O1 and O2 PSD.

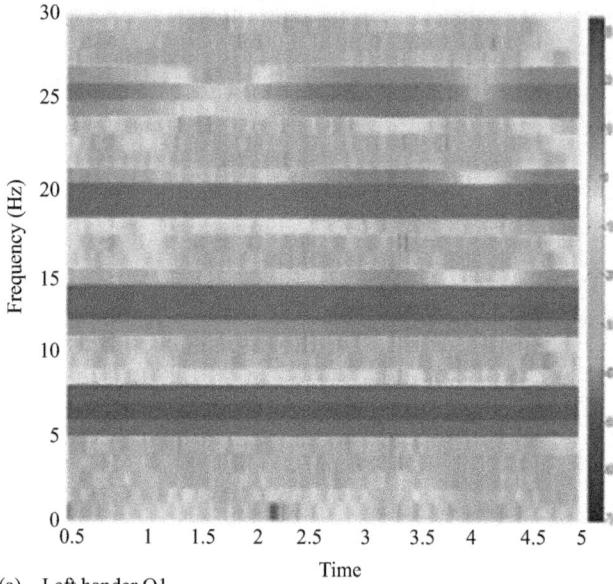

(a)   Left hander O1

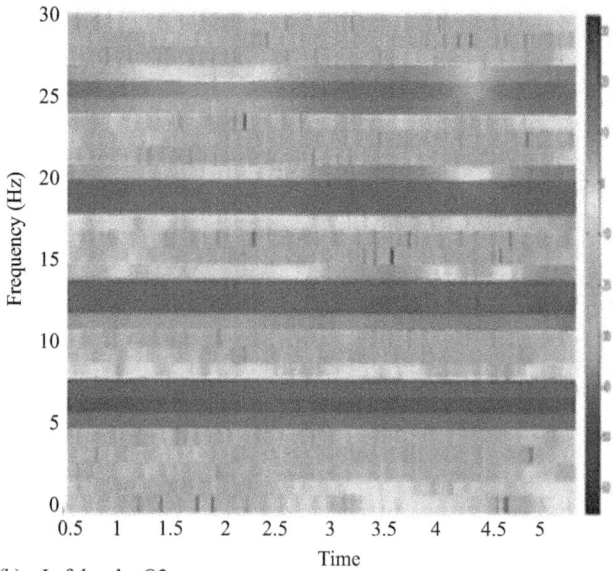

(b)   Left hander O2

Figure 5.3   Spectrograms, frequency versus time graph, (a–d) of O1 and O2 of a left hander and a right hander, respectively

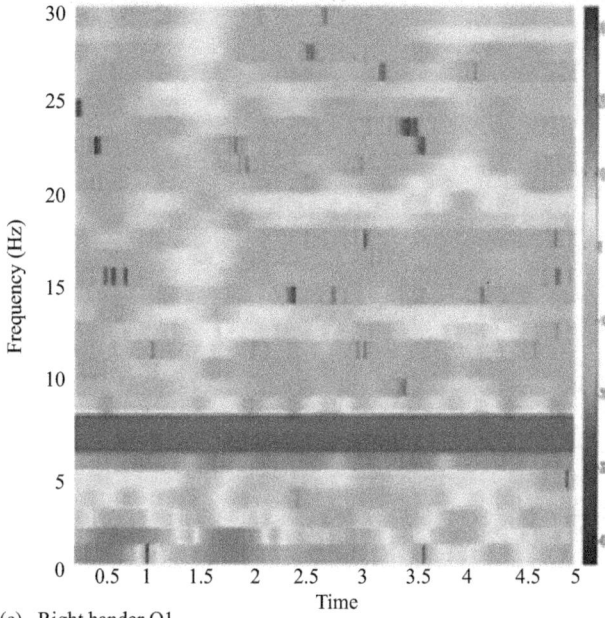

(c) Right hander O1

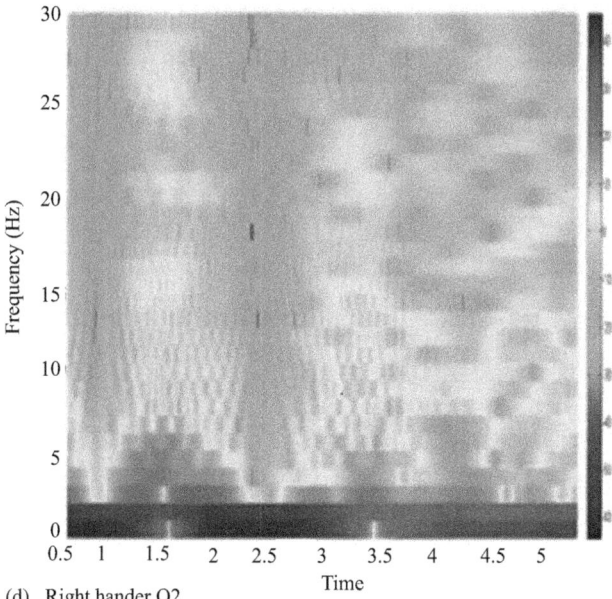

(d) Right hander O2

Figure 5.3 (*Continued*)

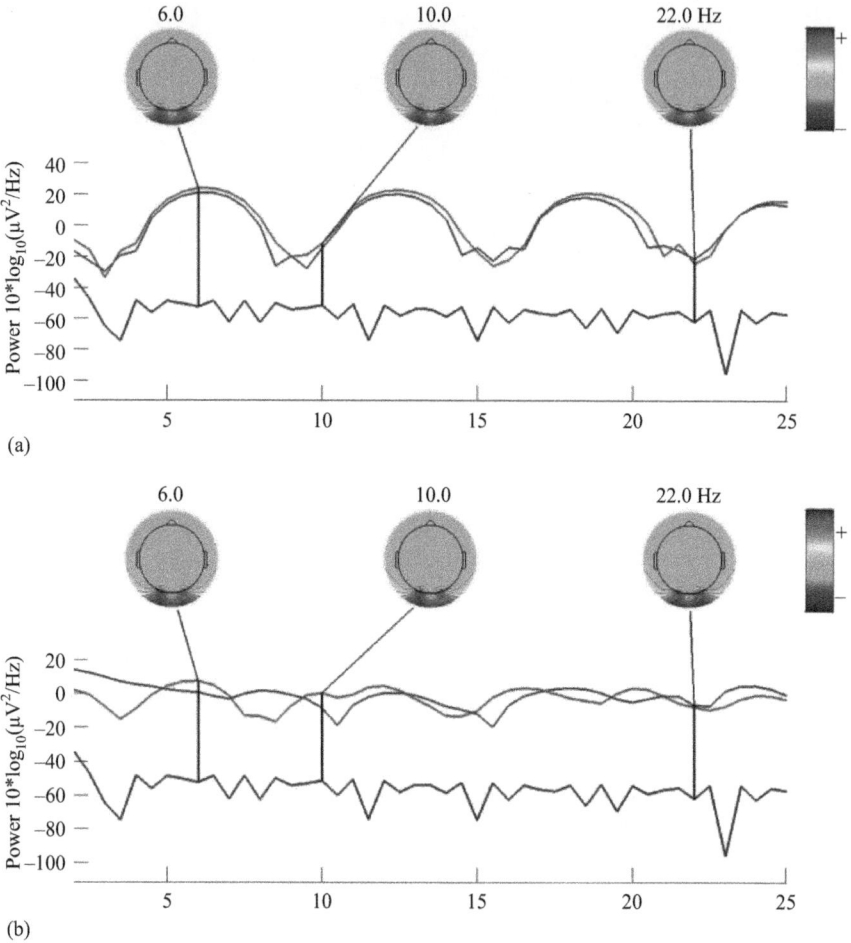

Figure 5.4   *PSD, power versus frequency graph, of O1 and O2 of a left hander and a right hander: (a) Top two curved lines: Left hander O1 and O2. Bottom line: Reference; (b) Top two curved lines: Right hander O1 and O2. Bottom line: Reference*

5.3.3   Analysis on instantaneous frequency

Instantaneous frequency is the frequency calculated at the very instant moment of a time series. It shows the dominant frequency at a particular time.

According to Figure 5.5, the instantaneous frequency graphs of O1 and O2 of the left hander's signal are concentrated on the Beta wave range and show high similarities. On the other hand, the instantaneous frequency graph of O1 and O2 of the right hander's signal are concentrated on the Beta and Delta wave range, respectively, and show low similarities.

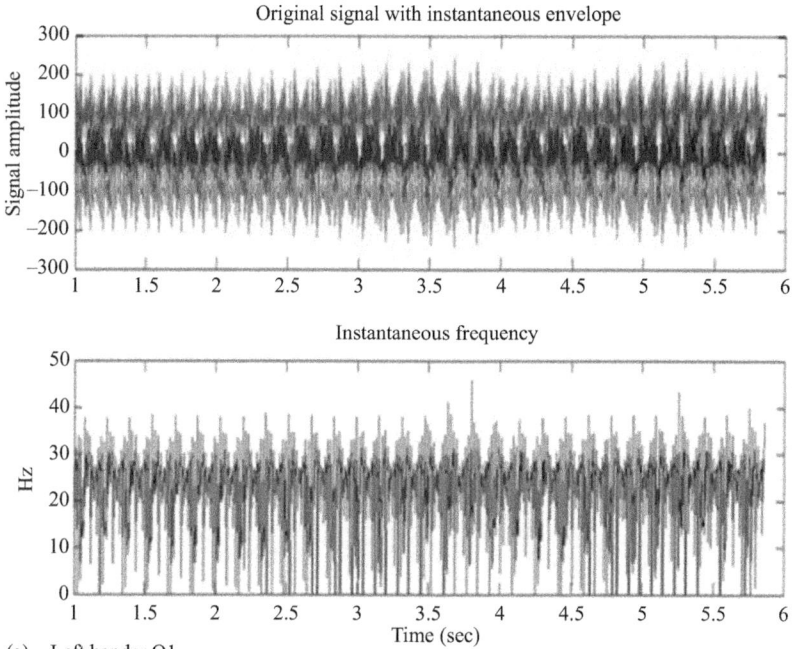

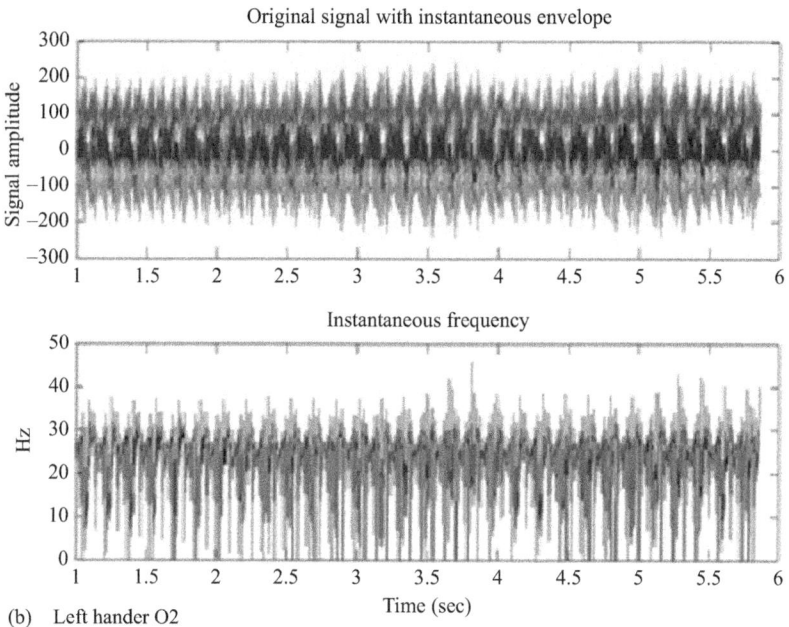

*Figure 5.5   Instantaneous frequency graph of O1 and O2 of a left hander and a
right hander. Original signal with instantaneous envelop graph and
instantaneous frequency graph of (a) left hander O1; (b) left hander
O2; (c) right hander O1; and (d) right hander O2*

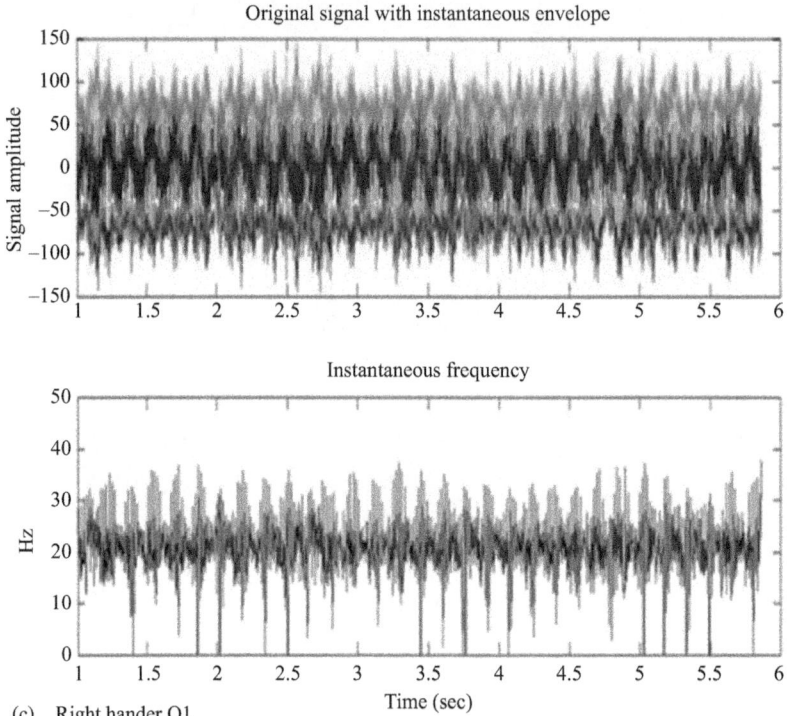

(c)   Right hander O1

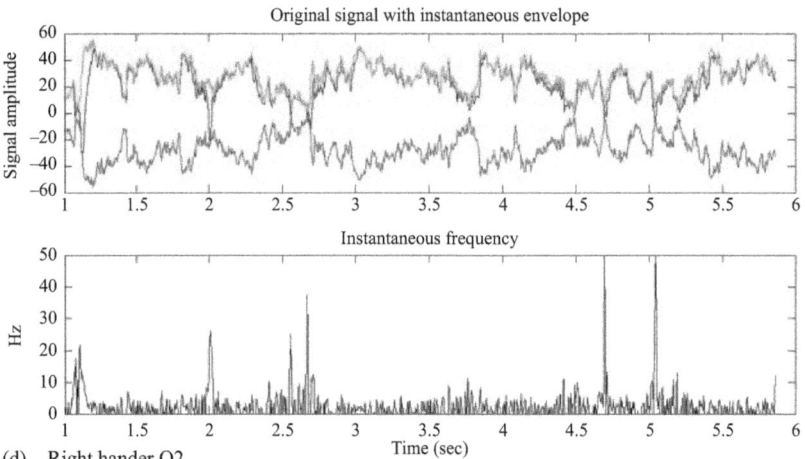

(d)   Right hander O2

Figure 5.5   (Continued)

5.3.4   *Analysis on dynamic time warp*

The function of dynamic time warp (DTW) is to try to merge two temporal signals that may vary in amplitude or time and hence measuring the similarity between them.

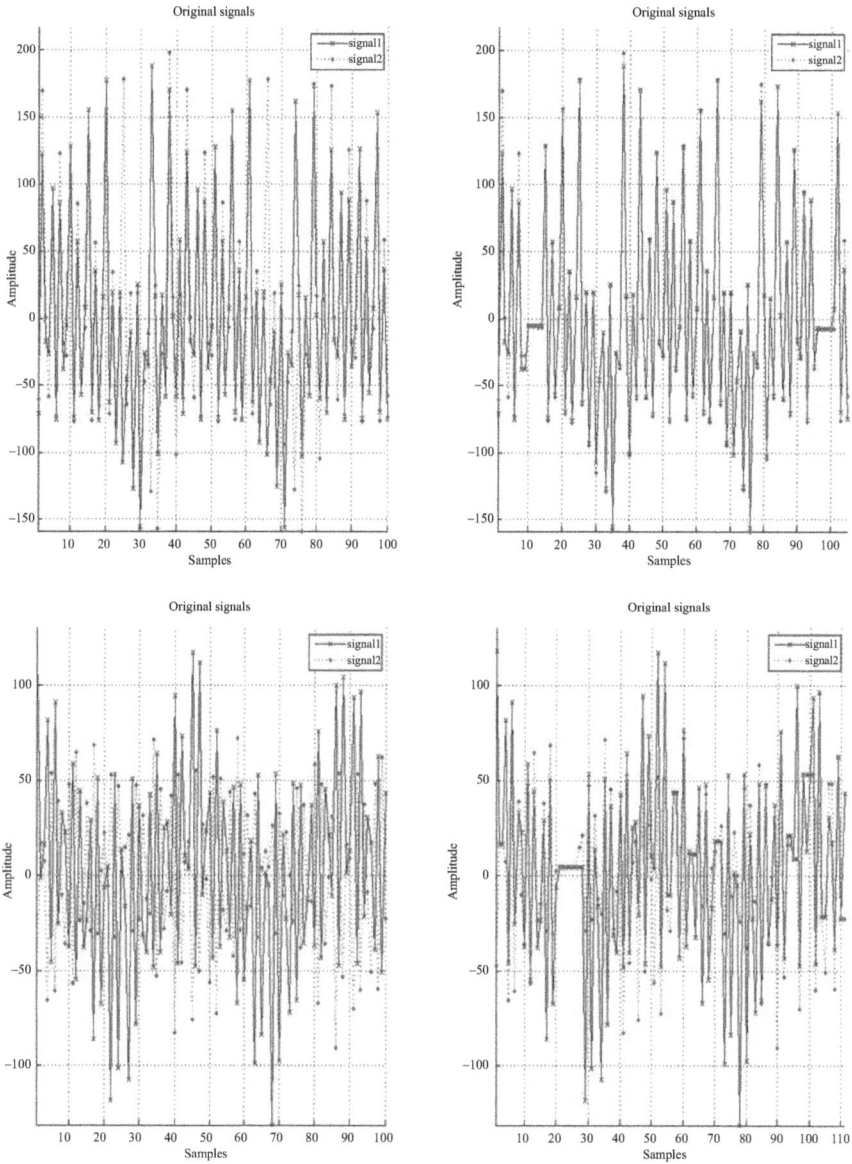

Figure 5.6   DTW graph of O1 and O2 of (a) left hander and (b) right hander: Left: Original signals; Right: Warped signals

The signals from O1 and O2 from a left-handed subject can easily be merged into one, while it is difficult to do so for the signals from a right-handed subject as shown in Figure 5.6.

The similarities can be distinguished by determining the DTW distance between O1 and O2 for all the four left-handed and four right-handed subjects. It is

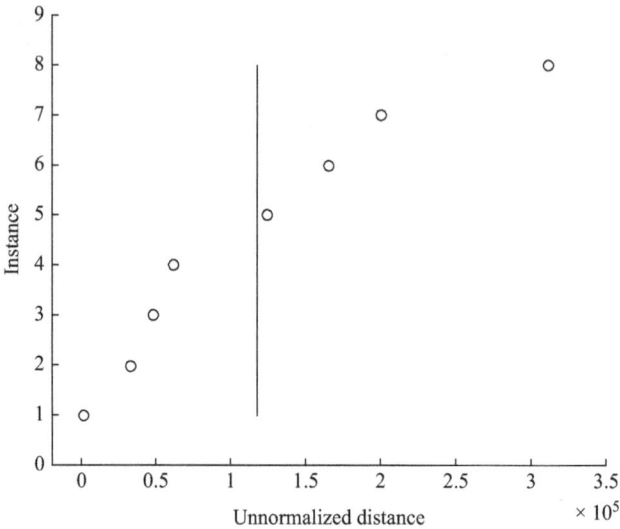

Figure 5.7   Distribution graph of DTW distance between O1 and O2 for four left handers and four right handers

understandable that generally left-handed subjects have less DTW distance for their O1 and O2 signals, showing high similarities and hence coherence in brain functions (Figure 5.7).

5.4   Conclusion

As a conclusion, left hander generally has a bigger CC, which aids in interhemispheric communication that causes the MEC to have a larger number. This ability to use both sides of the brain at once is believed to improve multitasking and let them process information in parallel rather than in linear format, which makes left handers more creative and holistic. Besides, it is also found out that the EEG data obtained from the right side of the brain for left-handed subjects are more rhythmic than those of right-handed subjects, which is chaotic and without a rhythmic pattern. The system created in this experiment is free from habitual constraint, which is the downside of the current inventories. Due to its natural approach, it is recommended to be used on patients who are unconscious or unable to answer a questionnaire. Some does to little kids as to determine their handedness before their development of many habitual handedness distinctive tasks. However, as EEG signals are required for the detection, rather than just a softcopy of attachment that can be sent throughout the Internet, this system is deemed more suitable for clinical use rather than domestic procurement. Following this up, as subjects need to be actually sampled by the EEG equipment individually, it is actually time-consuming and of extreme difficulty to collect a large number of EEG data at the same time, which in contrast can be easily done by inventories or questionnaires. In this system also, due to a single midpoint to distinguish between a left hander and a right hander, it is therefore unable to class subjects to ambidextrous group who can use both hands to perform various tasks including writing. The system developed is in a testing stage and needs more subject data to adjust the MEC midpoint. Due to this fact, the system is more suitable to be a supplement or alternative to the originally available inventories and questionnaires. In the future, the EEG signals are suggested to be loaded into artificial neural network, using the method of back-propagation, to perform the feature extraction of EEG signal and hence distinguish immediately the handedness of a person. It is suggested that experiments should be done in a controlled environment with minimal noises and disturbances.

References

[1] Oldfield, R. C. (1971). The assessment and analysis of handedness: The Edinburgh inventory. *Neuropsychologia*, *9*, 97–113.

[2] Nielsen, T., Abel, A., Lorrain, D., & Montplaisir, J. (1990). Interhemispheric EEG coherence during sleep and wakefulness in left- and right-handed subjects. *Brain and Cognition*, *14*, 113–25.

[3] Subasi, A., & Erçelebi, E. (2005). Classification of EEG signals using neural network and logistic regression. *Computer Methods and Programs in Biomedicine*, *78*(2), 87–99. doi:10.1016/j.cmpb.2004.10.009

[4] Huang, N. E., Shen, Z., Long, S. R., *et al.* (1998). The empirical mode decomposition and the Hilbert spectrum for nonlinear and non-stationary time series analysis. *Proceedings of the Royal Society A: Mathematical, Physical and Engineering Sciences*, *454*(1971), 903–995. doi:10.1098/rspa.1998.0193

[5] Thatcher, R. W., Biver, C. J., & North, D. (2004). EEG coherence and phase delays: Comparisons between single reference. *Average Reference and Current Source*, *33744*(727), 1–15.

[6] Thatcher, R. W., Biver, C. J., & North, D. M. (2007). Hand Calculator Calculations of EEG Coherence, Phase Delays and Brain Connectivity.

[7] Coulson, S., & Lovett, C. (2004). Handedness, hemispheric asymmetries, and joke comprehension. *Brain Research. Cognitive Brain Research*, *19*(3), 275–88. doi:10.1016/j.cogbrainres.2003.11.015

[8] Westerhausen, R., Kreuder, F., Dos Santos Sequeira, S., *et al.* (2004). Effects of handedness and gender on macro- and microstructure of the corpus callosum and its subregions: a combined high-resolution and diffusion-tensor MRI study. *Brain Research. Cognitive Brain Research*, *21*(3), 418–26. doi:10.1016/j.cogbrainres.2004.07.002

[9] Luders, E., Cherbuin, N., Thompson, P. M., *et al.* (2010). When more is less: associations between corpus callosum size and handedness lateralization. *NeuroImage*, *52*(1), 43–9. doi:10.1016/j.neuroimage.2010.04.016

[10] Leong, W. Y. (2006). Implementing blind source separation in signal processing and telecommunications, The University of Queensland, Ph.D. Thesis.

[11] Leong, W. Y., & Homer, J. (2005). Blind multiuser receiver in Rayleigh fading channel, *Australian Communications Theory Workshop (AusCTW'05)*, pp. 145–150, Brisbane, Qld, UQ 2–4 Feb 2005.

[12] Leong, W. Y., Homer, J., & Mandic, D. P. An implementation of nonlinear multiuser detection in Rayleigh fading channel, *EURASIP Journal on Wireless Communications and Networking (EURASIP JWCN)*, 2006, pp. 1–9, Article ID 45647.

[13] Leong, W. Y., & Andrew Ng, C. R. (2014). Left-handedness detection, *International Journal on Smart Sensing and Intelligent Systems*, 7(2), 442–457.

Chapter 6

Parkinson's disease feature extraction

Pooi Chi Quah[1] and Wai Yie Leong[1]

Parkinson's disease (PD) is a growing disease in Malaysia. This disease affects mostly elderly people aged around 60 years and above. Men are one and half times more likely to have PD than women. Many do not realise until they are diagnosed with PD. An estimated 7–10 million people worldwide are living with PD. The loss of dopamine in substantia nigra (SN) in the brain is the main cause of PD. Insomnia and Bradykinesia are the most common symptoms for every PD patient. These symptoms affect their quality of life. A total of 45 participants took part in an experiment where 21 of them were healthy participants and 24 of them were PD patients. Out of these 24 PD patients, 15 suffered from Bradykinesia and 9 experienced insomnia. Electroencephalogram (EEG) was used extensively to collect data. The data were then processed and evaluated using wavelet to segregate PD patients from healthy adults. The expected outcome for this project is mainly to have a better recognition of the signals collected from PD patients and to identify the similar features in the signals.

6.1 Introduction

Parkinson's disease (PD) is a common disorder of the nervous system that affects people later in their lives with tremors, movement instability and rigidity in their limbs. The true reasons for causing PD is still unknown, but many experts and researchers believe that PD could be caused by factors such as genetic, environment, drugs or repeated head injuries [1]. However, PD was characterised primarily by the damage in the SN, which lead to high chances of contracting PD [2,3]. Symptoms of PD can be classified into two different categories: motor and non-motor. The loss of dopamine in SN causes motor symptoms, which affects the mobility of the patients such as tremor, slowness and stiffness. Bradykinesia is one of the common symptoms in motor symptoms category. Bradykinesia means slow movement that affects the patient's mobility and causes difficulty in the person's walking stride. Patients suffering from Bradykinesia mostly walk in a very slow pace because it reduces the synchronous movement between the legs and the body

---

[1]Faculty of Engineering and Information Technology, MAHSA University, Malaysia

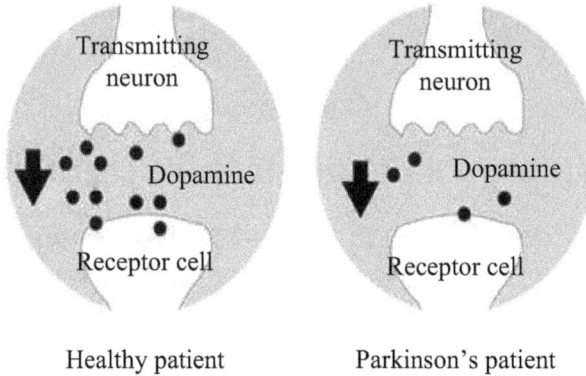

Healthy patient   Parkinson's patient

Figure 6.1   Comparison of the amount of Dopamine between healthy patient and Parkinson's Disease patient [6]

and the chances of falling are higher than healthy adults [4,5]. Figure 6.1 shows the comparison of the amount of Dopamine between healthy patient and PD patient. Healthy patient has considerably more Dopamine compared to PD patient.

Besides motor symptoms, non-motor symptoms such as constipation, insomnia, mood disorders and orthostatic hypotension may happen in the early stages of PD [7]. These symptoms are more serious than the motor symptoms because non-motor symptoms cannot be observed easily. Insomnia happens in the early stages of PD even before motor symptoms appear, and according to Jerry Siegel [8], his study discovered that patients with PD and narcolepsy are likely linked together as both show the symptoms of lack of hypocretin (Hcrt) cells in the brain.

It is estimated that most PD patients are aged between 50 and 90 [9,10], and according to a Dutch study [11], there are 1.4% of chances of getting PD for those aged between 55 and 60 years and 4.3% for those who aged between 85 and 94 years. Currently, there is no laboratory test available to diagnose PD but only positron emission tomography (PET) scan is available to do the imaging test to identify the low level of dopamine in the brain, which is the key of developing PD. Currently not many clinics or hospitals employ PET scan as the cost is still prohibitive [12]. A more common and cheaper diagnosis method available now for PD is neurological interview; any neurologists normally can do this by observing the patients' movement, coordination and balance. The diagnosis might also include some mental and emotional tests [13,14]. However, these diagnoses are judgmental in nature and the results might not be very accurate.

Thus, in order to obtain more accurate results that involve less subjectivity in the diagnosis, for this project, EEG was used on PD patients to analyse their brain waves and compare with healthy adults. According to Harrison and Home [15], the first EEG of human brain was created in Jena, Germany, by a German psychiatrist, Hans Berger, in 1924. EEG is able to record and measure three kinds of activities, which are bioelectrical events produced by a single neuron, spontaneous activity and evoked potentials. Figure 6.2 shows the 10–20 international electrodes placement systems that are used to capture EEG from PD patients [15]. As for this study,

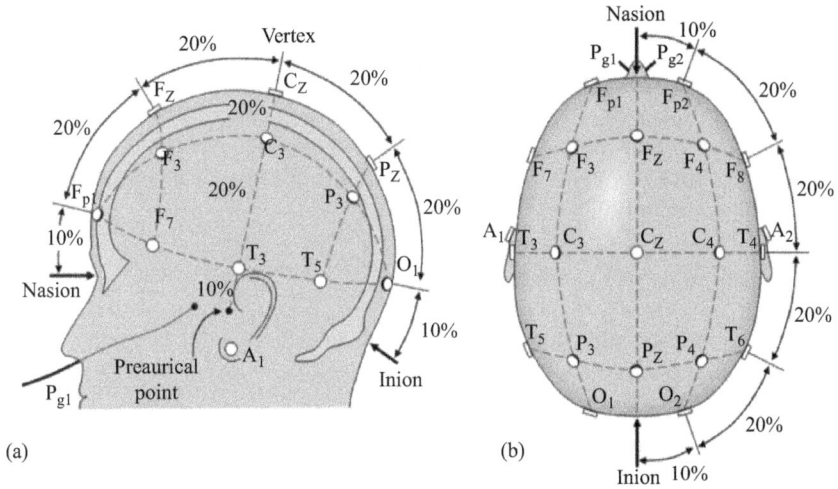

Figure 6.2   10–20 International Electrodes placement [15]. (a) Side view and (b) top view

Table 6.1   Parkinson's disease progression [19]

Stages	Description
Stage 0	No signs of disease
Stage 1	Unilateral disease
Stage 1.5	Unilateral disease plus axial involvement
Stage 2	Bilateral disease, without impaired balance
Stage 2.5	Bilateral disease, with impaired balance
Stage 3	Mild to moderate bilateral disease, some postural instability; physically dependent
Stage 4	Severe disability; still able to walk or stand unassisted
Stage 5	Wheelchair-bound or bedridden

three EEG channels were used, which are F3 or F4, C3 or C4 and O1 or O2, referred to A1 or A2.

6.2   Literature review

Neurological interview is the most commonly used method to diagnose PD patients. Unified Parkinson's Disease Rating Scale (UPDRS) is the most popular tool in neurological interview [16,17]. UPDRS is a complete set of tool to determine the stages of the PD that consists of motor test, non-motor test and Activity Daily Living test. Table 6.1 shows the PD progression stages [18,19]. However, the test results are very subjective because they rely fully on the experience of the neurologist [20].

In a recent study by Costa *et al.* [21], Sample Entropy (SampEn) was introduced to replace Approximate Entropy (ApEn) in the field of biomedical signal analysis due to the inadequacies found in ApEn such as prejudice and the full dependence on sample length. SampEn characterises the consistency of the stride signal and each of the coarse-grained time series was calculated to ease the understanding process for the dynamic properties of time-varying stride [22]. Based on Aboy *et al.* [23], SamEn is much more suitable for biomedical signal analysis because it can avoid counting self-matches to eliminate the ApEn bias, independent on the time series length and is more consistent. Equation (6.1) shows the mathematic form of SampEn

$$\text{SampEn}(m, r, N) = -\log\frac{A^m}{B^m} \tag{6.1}$$

where *m* is the embedding dimension, *r* is the tolerance, *N* is the data point, *A* and *B* are the number of template vector pairs that have

$$d[X_m(i), X_m(j)] < r \text{ of length } m \tag{6.2}$$

$$d[X_{m+1}(i), X_{m+1}(j)] < r \text{ of length } m + 1 \tag{6.3}$$

Furthermore, based on Ylikoski *et al.* [24], PD patients share a lot of similar symptoms with narcolepsy patients. Narcolepsy disease patients are unable to control their sleep and wakefulness. They have symptoms of rapid eye movement (REM), sleep dysregulation and sleep paralysis [25,26]. These symptoms are sleep-related phenomena, which are very similar to non-motor symptoms of PD. These are caused by the loss of Hcrt cells in the brain and based on Thannickal *et al.* and Fronczek with Suzuki [27,28], 28% of the Hcrt cells is lost in stage 1 and the loss keeps increasing until 68% in stage 4. The stages are measured on the Hoehn and Yahr rating scale [19].

6.3   Methodology

Wavelet transform (WT) was used as the main signal processing technique for this project. Based on Lütfü [29], WT is the most frequently used technique in engineering and biomedical field because it can be used to detect, classify and analyse nonlinear and non-stationary data. There are several wavelet functions available. However, Discrete Wavelet Transform (DWT) was selected for this project together with the most popular wavelet properties, Haar and Daubechies wavelet.

6.3.1   Discrete Wavelet Transform

Equations (6.4) and (6.5) show the mathematical equations for Continuous Wavelet Transform (CWT) and DWT. The DWT only uses discrete value in the time-domain of the signal. The reason behind choosing DWT is because it is simpler to implement compared to CWT, and DWT delivers informative data on both analysis and synthesis of the original signals within a short span of time [30].

$$\psi_{s,\tau} = \frac{1}{\sqrt{|s|}} \int x(t)\psi\left(\frac{t-\tau}{s}\right)dt \tag{6.4}$$

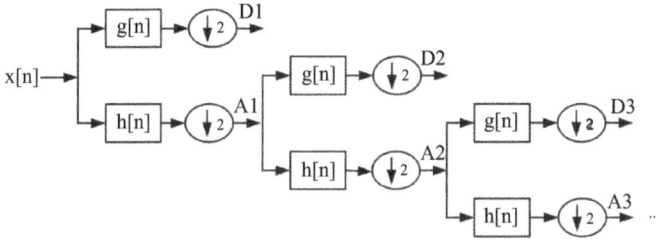

Figure 6.3   Level 3 sub-band decomposition of DWT [30]

$$\psi_{m,n} = \frac{1}{\sqrt{a_o^m}} \left(\frac{t - n b_o a_o^m}{a_o^m} \right) dt \qquad (6.5)$$

In (6.4), ψ is the mother wavelet, s is the scale factor, τ is the translation factor and the factor $s^{-1/2}$ is for energy normalisation across the different scales, t is the time sampling and let $x(t)$ be the signal that will be analysed [30]. In (6.5), ψ is the mother wavelet; m and n control the wavelet dilation and translation, respectively; $a_o > 1$ for specified fixed dilation step parameter and $b_o > 0$ is the location parameter [30]. Figure 6.3 shows the level 3 Sub-band Coding Algorithm.

6.3.2   Haar Wavelet

In 1909, the first DWT Haar Wavelet was invented by Alfred Haar [30]. It uses scaling function together with wavelet to break up or reconstruct signal. Equations (6.6)–(6.8) show the wavelet analysis that are based on Haar Wavelet scaling function.

$$\psi(x) = \begin{cases} 1, \text{if } 0 \leq x < 1 \\ 0, \text{elsewhere} \end{cases} \qquad (6.6)$$

$$\psi(x) = \begin{cases} 1, 0 \leq x < \dfrac{1}{2} \\ -1, \dfrac{1}{2} \leq x < 1 \\ 0, \text{otherwise} \end{cases} \qquad (6.7)$$

$$\psi(x) = \phi(2x) - \phi(2x - 1) \qquad (6.8)$$

6.3.3   Daubechies Wavelet

In 1987, Daubechies Wavelet was invented by Ingrid Daubechies [30] and it is compactly supporting orthonormal wavelets and smoothness when processing the original signal so it makes discrete wavelet analysis practicable. For example, (6.9) shows the equation of Daubechies level 4 where ϕ is the scaling function [31].

$$\phi(x) = \frac{1 + \sqrt{3}}{4} \phi(2x) + \frac{3 + \sqrt{3}}{4} \phi(2x - 1) + \frac{3 + \sqrt{3}}{4} \phi(2x - 1) + \frac{1 - \sqrt{3}}{4} \phi(2x - 1)$$

$$(6.9)$$

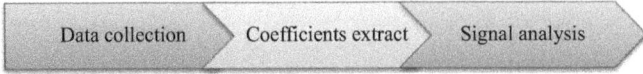

Figure 6.4   Flow chart for overall project

6.4   Experiment setup

Figure 6.4 shows the different stages required to be carried out in this project. The first stage is Data Collection for stride signal data and the sleep EEG signals. Data shared by Harvard Medical Faculty Care Group contained the stride time signal that they captured from a group of PD patients suffering from Bradykinesia. These 15 patients consist of 10 men and 5 women aged from 44 to 79 years with a mean age of 66.8. For comparison purpose, 16 healthy adults were asked to join in this experiment, which included 2 men and 14 women aged from 20 to 74 years with a mean age of 39.9. The stride signals were obtained by placing eight force-sensitivity sensors under their feet.

Sleep EEG data for this project were obtained from a database provided by PhysioBank [32]. The database included EEG data from 9 patients, 4 males and 5 females aged from 47 to 82 years with a mean age of 60.8, suffering from insomnia. For comparison purpose, a total of 9 healthy adults consisting 2 males and 7 females aged from 23 to 42 years with a mean age of 33.3 were used as a control group. Sleep EEG data were obtained by using the Actiwave EEG that are able to record various biomedical waveforms such as electromyography, electrocardiogram and EEG. The placement of the electrodes used to capture the signals follow the 10–20 electrodes international placement system as shown in Figure 6.2.

The second stage is adopting signal processing using different properties of Wavelet, Haar and Daubechies wavelet to extract the coefficients and features from the acquired signals. In this stage, Wavelet Toolbox in MATLAB® came into play. Wavelet Toolbox is packed with many wavelet-based algorithms for signal processing and signal extraction.

Numerical analysis for Haar and Daubechies Wavelet was conducted in the signal analysis stage. To check the efficiency and accuracy of a signal, the index of orthogonality was used. Index of orthogonality checks for the signal leakage after the signals were processed. The higher the index of orthogonality, the higher the amount of data loss in a signal. In addition, distortion measurement was calculated to measure the performance for Haar and Daubechies Wavelet. Besides that, sleep bands were extracted using Daubechies Wavelet.

6.5   Results and discussion

6.5.1   Index of orthogonality

Data collected, which is 15,360 times of samples from C4 channel with 100 Hz samples, were used to run on Haar and Daubechies Wavelet. Table 6.2 shows the index of orthogonality of the algorithms.

Table 6.2   Index of orthogonality for Haar and
Daubechies Wavelet

Decomposition method	Index of orthogonality
Haar	0.9987
Daubechies	0.2097

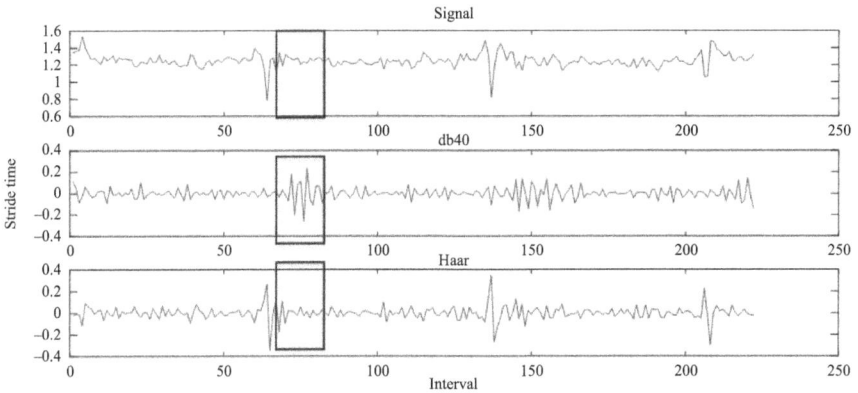

Figure 6.5   PD patient stride time signal

For a better accuracy and efficiency of the results, the value of the index of orthogonality must be as close to zero as possible because the higher the value of index of orthogonality, the higher the data leakage. Table 6.2 shows that Haar has the most data leakage compared to Daubechies when decomposing those signals.

6.5.2   Stride time signal

Figure 6.5 shows the stride time signal processed by the Haar and Daubechies Wavelet. It is clear that the original signals have very high and low amplitude and it is very difficult to analyse because the waveforms were not uniform. However, after applying the Haar and Daubechies Wavelet, it can be seen that the waveform has a minimum difference between the maximum and minimum peak. This means that the waveform is uniform compared to the original. There is an obvious difference in the waveform by comparing the Haar and Daubechies wavelet. Haar Wavelet highlight the extra features from Daubechies Wavelet that have three peak regions compare to no peak in the Haar Wavelet. Thus, this can be concluded that Daubechies Wavelet retained more information compared to Haar Wavelet and this supports my initial result of index of orthogonality.

6.5.3   Sleep EEG

Figure 6.6 shows the EEG data from a PD patient suffering from Insomnia. The box highlights a part that has the most noticeable change in all the three signals.

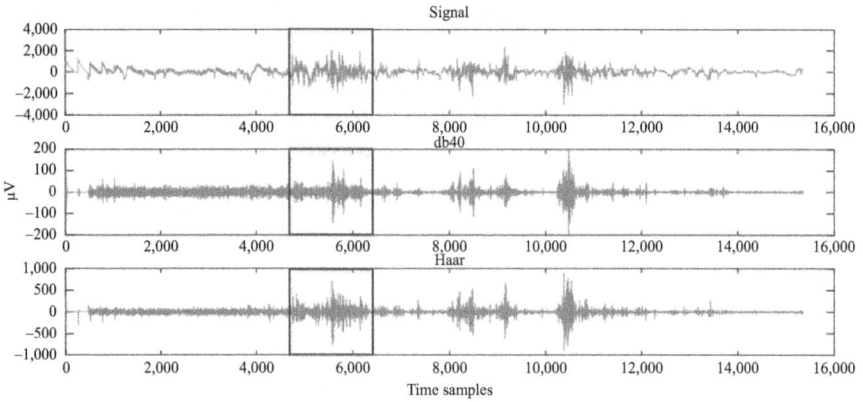

Figure 6.6   Insomnia EEG signals

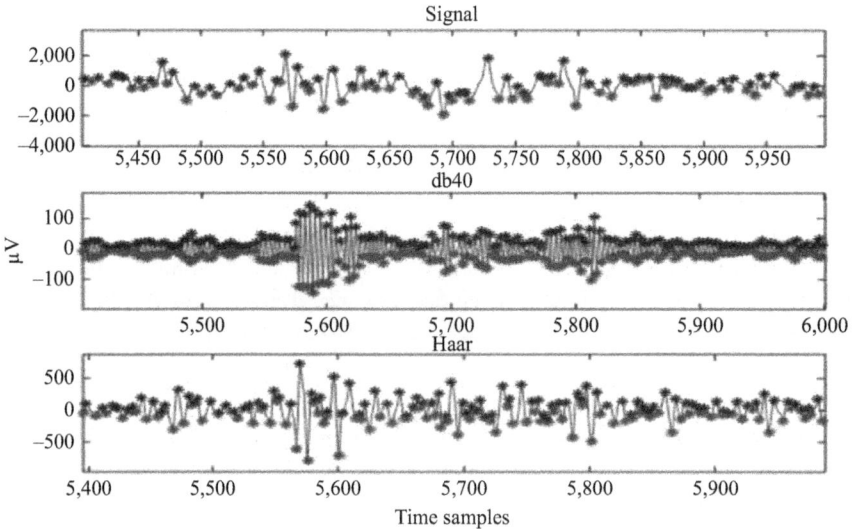

Figure 6.7   Zoomed insomnia EEG signals with maxima and minima indication

The original EEG contains local minima that are above zero and local maxima that are below zero. It means that the EEG waveform is very inconsistence and it is difficult to analyse the data. Figure 6.7 shows the zoomed insomnia EEG signals after applying the Haar and Daubechies Wavelet. Improvement for all local maxima are above zero as indicated in red colour and local minima are below zero as indicated in colour. These improvements decreased the amplitude and uniformed the waveform. From this result, Daubechies Wavelet has lower amplitude compared to Haar Wavelet, which means Daubechies Wavelet waveform is much more uniform compared to Haar Wavelet. However, Haar Wavelet has higher peak

Table 6.3   Distortion measurement

Transformer	Energy retainer	SNR (db)	SD	Cross-correlation	Execution time (s)
Haar	62.8779	13.3075	74.4938	0.153138	0.862
db10	70.2663	25.6716	17.9438	0.004212	0.256
db20	73.7798	26.5144	16.2844	0.010606	0.562
db30	75.6821	26.8055	15.7478	0.00108	0.637
db40	76.8615	26.9736	15.4458	0.003023	0.642

region compared to Daubechies Wavelet. Hence, Daubechies has a uniform waveform but does not manage to retain the data.

Nevertheless, one example will not be sufficient to make the conclusion. Thus Table 6.3 shows a set of more complete results for distortion measurement that include Energy Retainer, signal-to-noise ratio (SNR), standard deviation (SD), Cross-Correlation and the execution time. SNR is the ratio between the signal strength and the noise caused by external interruption. SNR must be as high as possible. The higher the SNR, the higher is the signal efficiency. SD is used to measure how much the signal fluctuates from the mean. Thus, lower SD means less signal fluctuation and more uniform signal. Cross-Correlation is to estimate the degree of two series signals. When the value is close to 1, there are similarity to each other. When the value is 0, it indicates no correlation between the two signals.

6.5.4   Sleep band extraction

Extracting sleep stages is a very common feature for sleep study. Wavelet will be used to extract the frequency bands of sleep from the original sleep EEG data as shown in Figure 6.8. The reason to extract these data is to monitor the brain activities in different stages. Figure 6.8 shows the five stages of the sleep frequency bands.

Daubechies Wavelet filtered out the original EEG signal into half. As the frequency is 100 Hz, therefore, the frequency will be filtered from 100 Hz to 50 Hz for Gamma band (A), 50 Hz to 25 Hz for Beta band (B). For Alpha band (C) is 25 Hz to 12.5 Hz and for Theta band (D) is 12.5 Hz to 6.5 Hz. Special case for the Delta band (E) will be obtained from the reconstructed coefficient of the Theta band. Table 6.4 concludes the sleep stages of the PD patients after extracted the sleep EEG signal [33].

6.6   Conclusion

This chapter shows the signal processing using the Haar and Daubechies Wavelet. Both algorithms are used to analyse on the stride time signal that obtain from a PD patients suffer from Bradykinesia and sleep EEG signals from the PD patients suffer from Insomnia. The outcome could be measured via associating the index of orthogonality, energy retainer, SNR (db), SD, Cross-Correlation and the execution time and sleep band. Both methods successfully show certain features regarding the

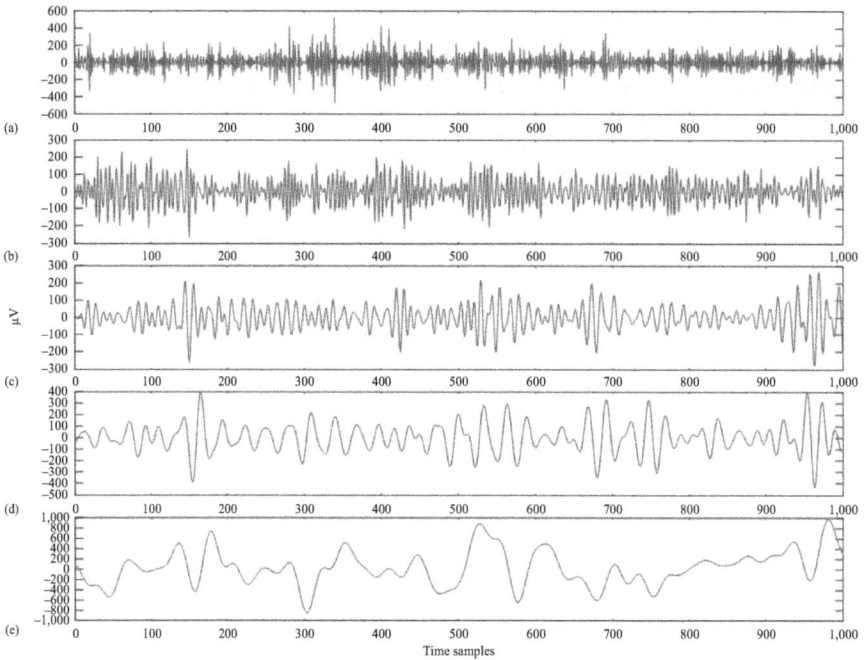

Figure 6.8   Frequency bands for sleep EEG

Table 6.4   Sleep stages [33]

Sleep stages	Frequencies	Description
Awake	31–100 Hz (Gamma band) 16–30 Hz (Beta band)	At this stage, the patient is in a highly awake and consciousness state.
Stage 1 and 2	8–15 Hz (Alpha band)	At Alpha stage, the patient starts to enter sleep stage number 1. In this stage, the patient experiences drowsiness or pre-sleep. Slow rolling of eye movements will be exhibited in this stage.
Stage 3	4–7 Hz (Theta band)	At Theta stage, the patient will be in a deep relaxation state. At this stage, the EEG signal will obviously show an appearance of the sleep spindles or some called it the K complexes. Therefore, spindle is the characteristic feature in stage 3.
Stage 4 and REM stage	0.1–3 Hz (Delta band)	At Delta stage, the patient will be in a deep sleep and unconscious state and REM will occur. When REM occurred, the patient's body will be well paralyzed and the patient will likely to have dreams. Desynchronised EEG is the characteristic featured in this stage.

stride time signal and sleep EEG signal that were important. In conclusion, this report shows the view that Daubechies Wavelet is more accurate and consistent than Haar Wavelet when compared to the index of orthogonality.

Challenges that are faced when conducting this project is that there are no many programs available to read raw EEG data, thus using MATLAB® and sourcing for program is needed. Second is to identify the key features of the data because usually the data are not uniform and normally interrupted. Thus, more time is required to analyse the EEG data.

There are still rooms for improvements in this project. First, it is better to conduct the actual experiment on a PD patient in order to get a pure raw EEG data. This can be done by recruiting PD patients to join in the experiment. Second, gather as much data as possible. More data will translate to more accurate results.

References

[1]   H. Shafique, A. Blagrove, A. Chung, and R. Logendrarajah, 'Causes of Parkinson's disease: Literature review', *Journal of Parkinsonism and Restless Legs Syndrome*, vol. 1, no. 1, pp. 5–7, 2011.

[2]   M. C. Staff, 'Parkinson's disease definition', *Mayoclinic*, 2015.

[3]   J. Meara, 'The Drug Treatment of Parkinson's Disease in the Elderly', *Drugs and the Older Population*, pp. 399–419, 2000.

[4]   'Bradykinesia and rigidity: Parkinson's Victoria – We're in this together', 01-Jan-2003. [Online]. Available: http://www.parkinsonsvic.org.au/parkinsons-and-you/bradykinesia-and-rigidity/. [Accessed: 10-Oct-2015].

[5]   A. E. Gabbey, 'Healthline.' [Online]. Available: http://www.healthline.com/symptom/gait-abnormality. [Accessed: 10-Oct-2015].

[6]   'Early Onset Parkinson's Disease: Symptoms and Treatments', 10-Oct-2015. [Online]. Available: http://www.newhealthadvisor.com/Early-Onset-Parkinson's-Disease.html. [Accessed: 10-Oct-2015].

[7]   W. Poewe and K. N. Chaudhuri, The Non-motor Symptoms Complex of Parkinson's Disease. New York, USA: Oxford University Press, 2009.

[8]   'Parkinson's Disease and Sleep.' [Online]. Available: https://sleepfoundation.org/sleep-topics/parkinsons-disease-and-sleep. [Accessed: 10-Oct-2015].

[9]   J. G. Nutt and G. F. Wooten, 'Diagnosis and Initial Management of Parkinson's Disease', *New England Journal of Medicine*, vol. 353, no. 10, pp. 1021–1027, 2005.

[10] A. Elbaz, J. H. Bower, D. M. Maraganore, *et al.*, 'Risk tables for parkinsonism and Parkinson's disease', *Journal of Clinical Epidemiology*, vol. 55, no. 1, pp. 25–31, 2002.

[11] M. C. de Rijk, M. M. B. Breteler, G. A. Graveland, *et al.*, 'Prevalence of Parkinson's disease in the elderly: The Rotterdam Study', *Neurology*, vol. 45, no. 12, pp. 2143–2146, 1995.

[12] F. Molinet-Dronda, B. Gago, A. Quiroga-Varela, *et al.*, 'Monoaminergic PET imaging and histopathological correlation in unilateral and bilateral

6-hydroxydopamine lesioned rat models of Parkinson's disease: A longitudinal in-vivo study', *Neurobiology of Disease*, vol. 77, pp. 165–172, 2015.

[13] L. Zhao, L. Verhagen-Metman, J. H. Kim, C. C. Liu, and F. A. Lenz, 'EMG activity and neuronal activity in the internal globus pallidus (GPi) and their interaction are different between hemiballismus and apomorphine induced dyskinesias of Parkinson's disease (AID)', *Brain Research*, vol. 1603, pp. 50–64, 2015.

[14] G. S. Watson, B. A. Cholerton, R. G. Gross, *et al.*, 'Neuropsychologic assessment in collaborative Parkinson's disease research: A proposal from the National Institute of Neurological Disorders and Stroke Morris K. Udall Centers of Excellence for Parkinson's Disease Research at the University of Pennsylvania', *Alzheimer's & Dementia*, vol. 9, no. 5, pp. 609–614, 2013.

[15] Y. Harrison and J. A. Horne, 'Occurrence of "microsleeps" during daytime sleep onset in normal subjects', *Electroencephalography and Clinical Neurophysiology*, vol. 98, no. 5, pp. 411–416, 1996.

[16] C. G. Goetz, 'Unified Parkinson's Disease rating scale (UPDRS) and the movement-disorder society sponsored-unified Parkinson's Disease Rating Scale (MDS-UPDRS)', *Encyclopedia of Movement Disorders*, pp. 307–309, 2010.

[17] Á. Jobbágy, P. Harcos, R. Karoly, and G. Fazekas, 'Analysis of finger-tapping movement', *Journal of Neuroscience Methods*, vol. 141, no. 1, pp. 29–39, 2005.

[18] K. L. Chou, J. Zamudio, P. Schmidt, *et al.*, 'National Parkinson Foundation Hospitalization Survey', *PsycTESTS Dataset*, 2014.

[19] C. Owen, 'Parkinson's Disease Staging - Neurosurgical Service - Massachusetts General Hospital.' [Online]. Available: http://neurosurgery.mgh.harvard.edu/ functional/pdstages.htm#UPDRS. [Accessed: 10-Oct-2015].

[20] B. Post, M. P. Merkus, R. M. A. de Bie, R. J. de Haan, and J. D. Speelman, 'Unified Parkinson's disease rating scale motor examination: Are ratings of nurses, residents in neurology, and movement disorders specialists interchangeable?', *Movement Disorders*, vol. 20, no. 12, pp. 1577–1584, 2005.

[21] M. Costa, C.-K. Peng, A. L. Goldberger, and J. M. Hausdorff, 'Multiscale entropy analysis of human gait dynamics', *Physica A: Statistical Mechanics and its Applications*, vol. 330, no. 1–2, pp. 53–60, 2003.

[22] J. S. Richman and J. R. Moorman, 'Physiological time-series analysis using approximate entropy and sample entropy', *Am J Physiol Heart Circ Physiol*, vol. 278, no. 6, pp. H2039–H2049, 2000.

[23] M. Aboy, D. Cuesta-Frau, D. Austin, and P. Mico-Tormos, 'Characterization of Sample Entropy in the Context of Biomedical Signal Analysis'. *29th Annual International Conference of the IEEE Engineering in Medicine and Biology Society*, Aug. 2007.

[24] A. Ylikoski, K. Martikainen, T. Sarkanen, and M. Partinen, 'Parkinson's disease and narcolepsy-like symptoms', *Sleep Medicine*, vol. 16, no. 4, pp. 540–544, 2015.

[25] 'American Academy of Dental Sleep Medicine Continuing Education Offerings', *Sleep and Breathing*, vol. 12, no. 3, pp. 287–288, 2008.

[26] M. Partinen, B. R. Kornum, G. Plazzi, P. Jennum, I. Julkunen, and O. Vaarala, 'Narcolepsy as an autoimmune disease: the role of H1N1 infection and vaccination', *The Lancet Neurology*, vol. 13, no. 6, pp. 600–613, 2014.

[27] T. C. Thannickal, Y.-Y. Lai, and J. M. Siegel, 'Hypocretin (orexin) cell loss in Parkinson's disease', *Brain*, vol. 130, no. 6, pp. 1586–1595, 2007.

[28] K. Suzuki, M. Miyamoto, T. Miyamoto, and K. Hirata, 'Parkinson's disease and sleep/wake disturbances', *Current Neurology and Neuroscience Reports*, vol. 15, no. 3, 2015.

[29] 'Fundamentals of Wavelet Transform', *Chemical Analysis*, pp. 99–146, 2004.

[30] P. S. Addison, 'The Illustrated Wavelet Transform Handbook', *Infinity*, 2002.

[31] S. Malik and V. Verma, 'Comparative analysis of DCT, Haar and Daube-chies Wavelet for Image Compression', *International Journal of Applied Engineering Research*, vol. 7, no. 11, 2012.

[32] M. G. Terzano, L. Parrino, A. Sherieri, *et al.*, 'Atlas, rules, and recording techniques for the scoring of cyclic alternating pattern (CAP) in human sleep', *Sleep Medicine*, vol. 2, no. 6, pp. 537–553, 2001.

[33] M. Hirshkowitz, K. Whiton, S. M. Albert, *et al.*, 'National Sleep Foundation's sleep time duration recommendations: methodology results summary', *Sleep Health*, vol. 1, no. 1, pp. 40–43, 2015.

Chapter 7

Source analysis in motor imagery EEG BCI applications

Aleksandr Zaitcev[1], Wei Liu[1], Greg Cook[1], Martyn Paley[2], and Elizabeth Milne[3]

7.1 Introduction to source localization

Electroencephalography (EEG) represents a continuous voltage measurement from the head skin surface and, hence, measures secondary effects of the electrical brain activity. There is evidence that brain neuronal cells designated to the common task are grouped together into functionally and often anatomically segregated cortical regions [1,2]. During the motor imagery commands the brain-computer interface (BCI) user produces the power variation patterns that are spatially distinctive, due to such anatomical segregation. Cortical locations of event related desynchronization and event related synchronization (ERD/ERS) effects occurring in μ and β bands of EEG can directly indicate the muscles involved in the imaginary task being performed [3,4]. Hence, by finding the motor cortex areas that generate the signal of interest it is possible to infer the imagined type of movement and execute the BCI command associated with it.

As the location of the signal of interest is highly indicative of the brain state, it is relevant to accentuate such spatial properties in the feature extraction process. However, direct analysis of EEG spatial properties is problematic, as the EEG signal acquisition itself suffers from the volume conduction effects. As the neuronal electrical fields propagate from the gray matter to the skin surface, they are distorted and spread. This results in ERD/ERS patterns having high spatial correlation, which impairs the interpretation of the motor imagery task being performed. One of the challenges in motor imagery BCI design is to overcome the low spatial resolution of the EEG.

The cross-electrode correlation due to volume conduction effects can be significantly alleviated by means of EEG source localization (EEG source reconstruction, EEG imaging). The essential idea of source reconstruction is the estimation of primary cortical current densities during the given EEG recording from the head surface. Given the forward head model, which couples the surface voltages to the

[1]Department of Electronic and Electrical Engineering, The University of Sheffield, United Kingdom.
[2]Department of Infection, Immunity & Cardiovascular Disease, The University of Sheffield, United Kingdom.
[3]Department of Psychology, The University of Sheffield, United Kingdom.

Table 7.1   Names, equations, and references of inverse solutions

Name	Equation	References
Minimum norm estimates (MNE)	$\hat{\mathbf{D}}_{\mathrm{MNE}} = \underset{\mathbf{D}}{\mathrm{argmin}}\, \|\mathbf{M} - \mathbf{LD}\|_2 + \lambda\|\mathbf{D}\|_2$	[11,12]
Weighted minimum norm estimates (WMNE)	$\hat{\mathbf{D}}_{\mathrm{WMNE}} = \underset{\mathbf{D}}{\mathrm{argmin}}\, \|\mathbf{M} - \mathbf{LD}\|_2 + \lambda\|\mathbf{WD}\|_2$	[13,14]
Low resolution electrical tomography (LORETA)	$\hat{\mathbf{D}}_{\mathrm{LORETA}} = \underset{\mathbf{D}}{\mathrm{argmin}}\, \|\mathbf{M} - \mathbf{LD}\|_2 + \lambda\|\mathbf{BWD}\|_2$	[15]
Local autoregressive average (LAURA)	$\hat{\mathbf{D}}_{\mathrm{LAURA}} = \underset{\mathbf{D}}{\mathrm{argmin}}\, \|\mathbf{M} - \mathbf{W}_{sens}\mathbf{LD}\|_2 + \lambda\|\mathbf{W}_{source}\mathbf{D}\|_2$	[16]
Least absolute shrinkage and selection operator (LASSO)	$\hat{\mathbf{D}}_{\mathrm{LASSO}} = \underset{\mathbf{D}}{\mathrm{argmin}}\, \|\mathbf{M} - \mathbf{LD}\|_2 + \lambda\|\mathbf{D}\|_1$	[17]
Elastic net (E-NET)	$\hat{\mathbf{D}}_{\mathrm{E\text{-}NET}} = \underset{\mathbf{D}}{\mathrm{argmin}}\, \|\mathbf{M} - \mathbf{LD}\|_2 + \lambda_{sparse}\|\mathbf{D}\|_1 + \lambda_{smooth}\|\mathbf{D}\|_2$	[18]

$\mathbf{W}$, source depth compensation matrix
$\mathbf{B}$, Laplacian operator
Bold capital letters are used to denote matrices; Bold lowercase – vectors; normal letters – scalars

Table 7.1 lists a number of inverse solutions based on a flexible framework of penalized least squares problem. In these methods the solution is obtained by minimizing the cost function, which typically incorporates a residual error term $\|\mathbf{M} - \mathbf{LD}\|_2$ and a regularization term taking the form of $\lambda\|\mathbf{\Gamma D}\|_p$. Here Γ generally represents the linear matrix operator, which implements a certain assumption about the desirable inverse solution and λ is the regularization parameter defining the relative importance of such an assumption. All of the methods listed in Table 7.1 except for LASSO and E-NET can be implemented as a linear operator, which makes them applicable to real-time source analysis. On the other hand, LASSO and E-NET are capable of more accurate and focal reconstruction of sources, which makes them advantageous in source analysis scenarios with no real-time constraints.

7.1.2   Point-spread function

A combination of forward model and an inverse solver comprises an EEG imaging system. One way to characterize such system is to assess its point-spread function, which can be defined as an image produced in response to a single unit active source: in other words, as a spatial impulse response of a system. In this section we use a simulation scenario in order to demonstrate the capabilities of various inverse solvers. In the following examples we utilized the head geometry provided by ICBM 152 head atlas, which was obtained by nonlinear averaging of 152 adult anatomical MRI scans [19–21]. In order to conform to the BEM requirements, the head geometry was defined as a set of boundary surfaces including skin surface, outer skull, inner skull, and a detailed cortical surface comprising 4,504 vertices and 9,000 faces. The source grid was defined at the vertices of the cortical surface with three dipoles oriented along the Cartesian axes set at each point in order to allow for unrestricted source orientations. The EEG electrode locations corresponding to

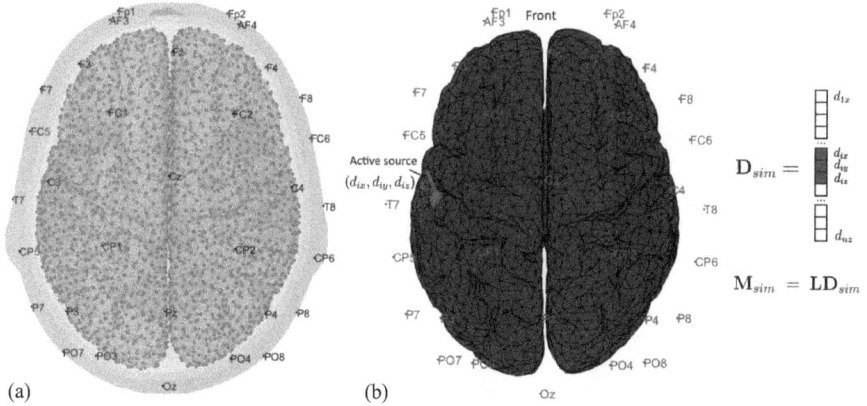

$$\mathbf{D}_{sim} = \begin{bmatrix} d_{1x} \\ \vdots \\ d_{ix} \\ d_{iy} \\ d_{iz} \\ \vdots \\ d_{nz} \end{bmatrix}$$

$$\mathbf{M}_{sim} = \mathbf{L}\mathbf{D}_{sim}$$

(a)   (b)

Figure 7.2   (a) Visualization of the forward head model used in simulations. EEG
sensor locations are marked by channel labels and source locations on
the cortical surface are represented by black dots. (b) Illustration
of the simulation protocol for instantaneous source localization
including triangulated ICBM 152 cortical surface, a single simulated
source with shown orientation and EEG sensor locations (in grey font)
for reference

g.tec's g.Nautilus EEG headset was selected from the standard extended 10–5 electrode configuration provided in Brainstorm suite for MATLAB® [22].

After the necessary prerequisites were defined the symmetric BEM [23] implementation from OpenMEEG software [24,25] was used to obtain the volume conduction model and the resulting lead field matrix. Figure 7.2 provides a visualization of the described forward model including four boundary surfaces, source locations marked by black dots and labeled EEG electrode montage.

In order to estimate the point-spread function it is first necessary to define the simulated sensor measurements. For this purpose we defined a simulated source vector $\mathbf{D}_{sim} \in \mathbb{R}^{3n \times 1}$ with zero values at all locations except for a single active point i. The Cartesian components (d_{ix}, d_{iy}, d_{iz}) of the simulated source were scaled with respect to the orientation of vertex normal at this point. Then, according to (7.1), a vector of simulated sensor measurements $\mathbf{M}_{sim} = \mathbf{L}\mathbf{D}_{sim}$ was calculated. The visualization of this simulation scenario is shown in Figure 7.2.

The power distribution topographies obtained by several different inverse solvers for the described simulation scenario are shown in Figure 7.3. As discussed before, each source location is modeled by a set of three dipoles oriented along the Cartesian axes. The power estimate at location k was calculated as Euclidean norm of (d_{kx}, d_{ky}, d_{kz}). Four methods (MNE, WMNE, LORETA, and LAURA) were implemented as linear inverse operators according to the general framework of Tikhonov regularization. For these solvers parameters λ from the range of $\left[10^{-20}, 10^{10}\right]$ were selected according to the L-curve alternatively generalized cross-validation (GCV) procedures [11,26,27] yielding the most focal solutions possible for these methods.

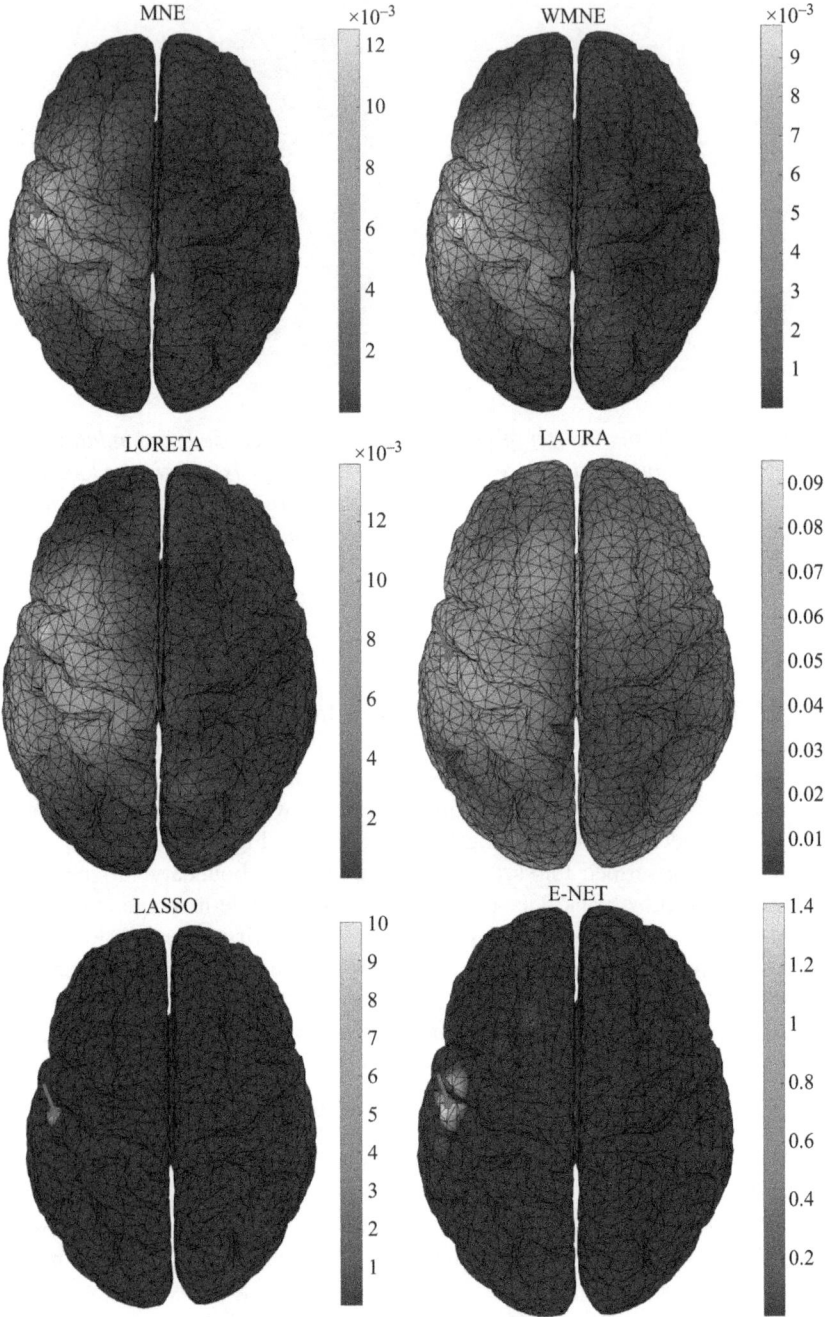

*Figure 7.3   Power distribution topographies of instantaneous source localization
simulation results obtained with different inverse solvers*

Sparse solutions LASSO and E-NET were obtained using the CVX package for MATLAB [28,29]. For these methods the L-curve and GCV selection procedures are not applicable, and therefore, regularization parameters were selected heuristically from the range of $\left[10^{-20}, \; 10^{10}\right]$ with the aim of minimizing the spatial spread of electrically active area, which was calculated as a number of vertices at which the power is more than half of the maximal power within the whole solution. In other words, λ was selected to minimize the full width half maximum area.

As seen from the results, each source localization method has its own limitations and characteristic artifacts. In general, inverse solutions based on $l-2$ norm minimization produce more distributed, "blurry", topographies with Gaussian spatial distribution of source components and negligible calculation time (less than 0.001 s in our settings), which makes them suitable for real-time applications. On the contrary, sparse source localization methods, which employ $l-1$ norm minimization, yield very focal results with exponential spatial priors and capabilities for exact reconstruction of sources in the absence of noise. However, the estimation of such sparse solutions is computationally complex, in our settings taking no less than 5 s per time sample, which in this form makes it inapplicable to real-time applications.

7.1.3 Spatial component decorrelation

One of the common disadvantages of EEG is high degree of cross-electrode coupling. Due to the volume conduction effects, strong electrical activity at any cortical region is observable at all available EEG sensors. In this context source reconstruction is beneficial, as it can effectively reduce the coupling effects and represent the EEG recording segment as a superposition of *spatially independent* components. In this section we present a simulation scenario that demonstrates such useful properties of source localization.

In order to demonstrate the separation capabilities of source reconstruction it is first necessary to define the simulated sensor measurements within the same forward model as described in Section 7.1.3. For this purpose we defined a continuous simulated source matrix $\mathbf{D}_{sim} \in \mathbb{R}^{3n \times q}$ varying over q time samples with zero values at all locations except for three active points i, j and k. At each active vertex a sinusoidal component $\sin(2\pi f t + \phi)$ was set with $t \in [1 \ldots q]$, individual frequencies f_i, f_j, f_k, and phases ϕ_i, ϕ_j, ϕ_k. Then, using the definition in (7.1) a matrix of simulated sensor measurements $\mathbf{M}_{sim} = \mathbf{L}\mathbf{D}_{sim}$ was calculated. With $q = 1500$ $\mathbf{M}_{sim}$ represents 3 s of EEG, recorded with sampling frequency of 500 Hz. Visualization of this simulation scenario with sources i, j, and k and their parameters is shown in Figure 7.4. Figure 7.5(a) illustrates the mixture of simulated frequency components at sensors closest to the active sources.

Next, the WMNE linear inverse operator with regularization parameter $\lambda = 0.01$ was obtained for the given forward model and applied to the simulated sensor data, yielding the matrix of reconstructed source components $\hat{\mathbf{D}}$ [14]:

$$\hat{\mathbf{D}} = (\mathbf{W}^T \mathbf{W})^{-1} \mathbf{L}^T (\mathbf{L}(\mathbf{W}^T \mathbf{W})^{-1} \mathbf{L}^T + \lambda \mathbf{I}_m)^{-1} \mathbf{M} = \mathbf{G}_{WMNE} \mathbf{M}_{sim}. \tag{7.3}$$

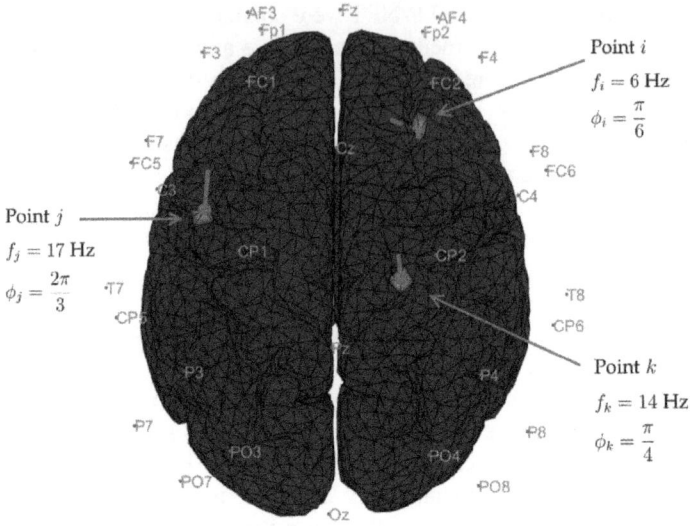

Figure 7.4   Visualization of the simulation protocol for continuous source localization including triangulated ICBM 152 cortical surface, EEG sensor locations, and simulated sources i, j, k with shown orientations and simulated signal parameters

The simulation results, illustrated in Figure 7.5(b), demonstrate two important benefits of source reconstruction. First, this type of processing is capable of isolating the signal components on the basis of their spatial origins. As shown in Figure 7.5(b), each channel of the original simulated data $\mathbf{M}_{sim}$ contained a mixture of all active frequency components, especially at channel FC2. In this scenario the WMNE source localization has achieved evident, although imperfect, reconstruction of the simulated frequency components.

Second, source reconstruction greatly expands the dimensionality of data—the original simulated EEG signal $\mathbf{M}_{sim} \in \mathbb{R}^{32 \times 1500}$ is defined over 32 variables, while the inverse solution $\hat{\mathbf{D}} \in \mathbb{R}^{13,512 \times 1,500}$ represents each time sample by 13,512 variables defined over 4,504 locations. Considering that each of these variables has individually allocated spatial properties, such dimensionality expansion provides for more accurate signal component selection and spatial filter design, which in this case also corresponds to region-of-interest (ROI) selection. With the capability for spatial component segregation, source reconstruction and subsequent ROI extraction achieves the partial cancellation of noise and artifact energy, i.e., improves the SNR of the signal of interest and alleviates the negative effects of muscular artifacts.

7.2   Application of source localization to BCI feature extraction

In the past few decades, there was a large number of proposed BCI design approaches focusing on feature extraction, classification or other aspects with more than 300 designs described only in [30,31]. Considering a wide variety of design choices,

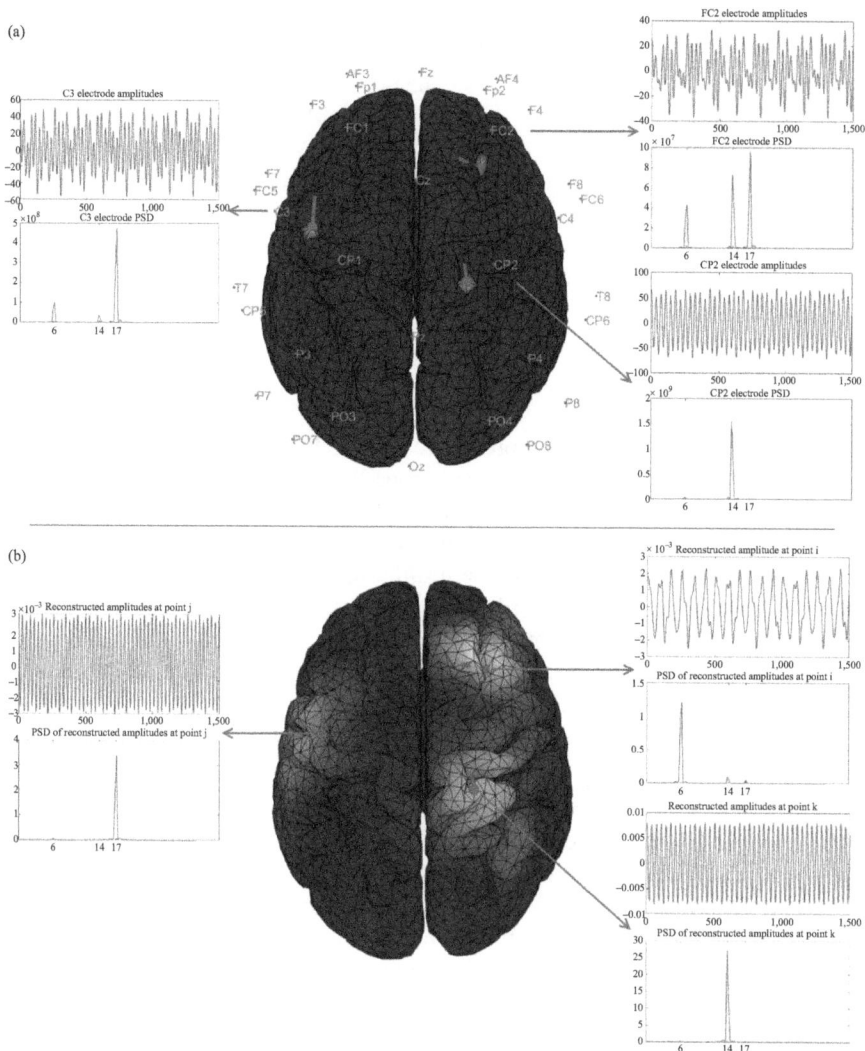

Figure 7.5   *(a) Visualization of continuous simulated EEG data at channels closest to the simulated active points. There is an evident mixture of simulated frequency components at all presented channels, especially at channel FC2. (b) Results of source reconstruction on the simulated data. The topography of variance distribution is shown by bright areas over the cortical surface. Graphs of reconstructed amplitudes at the original active locations and corresponding power spectral densities demonstrate the capabilities for spatial source separation*

including the signal acquisition systems, sensor montages, feature extraction, selection, and classification methods, it becomes almost impossible to reproduce and, thus, validate the reported results. This issue is partially what was behind the idea of BCI competitions organized by the Universities of Berlin, Graz, Freiburg, and Washington over several years from 2001 to 2008. Within these events the competing research groups were given a single common dataset, designed with focus on a specific BCI design challenge, and a common evaluation protocol. Consequently, classification accuracy or ITRs reported in publications using such datasets can be directly compared. The following sections are dedicated to the description of our proposed feature extraction method employing source reconstruction and demonstration of its performance on dataset from BCI competition IV [32].

7.2.1   EEG dataset

The proposed feature extraction procedure was evaluated using the BCI Competition IV EEG dataset 2a [32]. The dataset consists of EEG recordings of four types of mental tasks, namely left-hand, right-hand, feet, and tongue imaginary movement, to which we will further refer to as data of classes 1, 2, 3, and 4, respectively. The motor imagery signals from nine healthy adult subjects with little or no previous BCI experience were recorded over two sessions, one for classifier training purposes and one for evaluation. Each session consisted of $N_{trl} = 288$ trials, each structured in a way to include 2 s of preparation and 4 s of mental task execution. The signal was recorded from $N_{ch} = 22$ gel EEG sensors with 250 Hz sampling frequency and a single common reference at left mastoid.

7.2.2   Overview of the signal processing sequence

At the described BCI competition the design that achieved the highest classification reliability was based on the filter bank common spatial patterns (FBCSP) feature extraction approach [33]. As shown in [3], characteristic frequency of ERD/ERS varies greatly between different motor imagery tasks and the subjects performing them. This observation is taken into account in FBCSP feature extraction, which combines the capabilities of common spatial patterns (CSP) for extraction of ERD/ERS effects of motor imagery with the subject-specific estimation of indicative frequency bands. This method utilizes a set of bandpass filters to decompose the original data into a set of narrow band components. Within each individual band a feature vector is extracted using the conventional CSP method. Feature vectors from separate bands are then concatenated and fed to feature selection and classifier training stages, where a small number of indicative features are selected from the whole set and used to fit a multiclass linear discriminant analysis (LDA) classifier.

Considering the reported high efficiency of such feature extraction method, it was taken as a basis for our proposed signal processing scheme incorporating source reconstruction. From the design architecture perspective, the source localization step may be employed here in two different ways—prior to subband decomposition, or individually within each individual band after filtering. The latter approach provided better results; however, it is extremely computationally

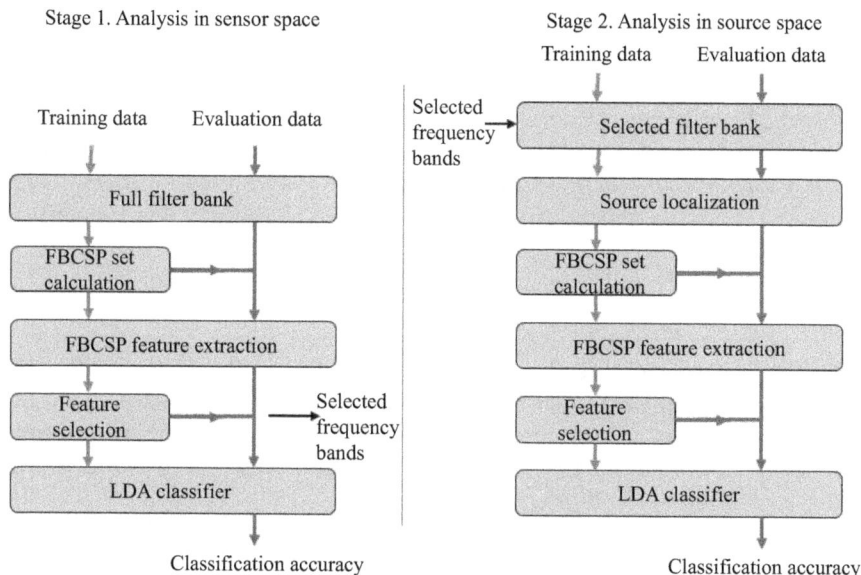

Figure 7.6   Two-stage signal processing scheme for motor imagery classification. At the first stage the indicative frequency bands are selected based on the sensor feature ranking and classifier evaluation procedure. At the second stage, only a small number of bands are used for source reconstruction and subsequent feature extraction

expensive if applied to the whole set of subbands. Considering that this analysis aims to demonstrate the advantages of source reconstruction compared to the conventional analysis in the sensor space, the EEG processing was performed in two separate stages (Figure 7.6). The aim of the first stage was to estimate the subject-specific bands of signal that are indicative of mental state by utilizing the metrics of CSP features from a large number of narrow bands. Based on these results a small number (2–3) of subbands was selected for each subject and at the second stage source reconstruction and ROI extraction were applied as a pre-processing step only within these bands. Alternatively, subband selection can be performed heuristically, based on, e.g., simple visual assessment of trial-averaged time-frequency representations (TFRs) of different mental tasks. However, taking into account the large number of subjects in a dataset, the proposed two-stage scheme is significantly faster and besides more autonomous, facilitating the data-driven estimation of design parameters. The following sections provide a detailed description of the proposed signal processing scheme.

7.2.3   Stage 1. Analysis in sensor space

7.2.3.1   Signal preprocessing

Generally, during EEG recording the trial timing structure is embedded into the data by means of an auxiliary channel containing event triggers, marking the time of trial onset and the type of visual cue shown to the subject. Such markers embedded in dataset 2a were used to segment the continuous session recordings into a set of trials comprising 1-s pre-stimulus interval (before the cue was shown to the subject) and 3 s of mental task execution. The original EEG data were recorded with 250 Hz sampling frequency. Considering that the effects indicative of motor imagery type arise mainly in μ (7–13 Hz) and β (16–31 Hz) bands of EEG and high computational requirements of source analysis, the signal was downsampled to 100 Hz sampling rate.

7.2.3.2   Filter bank

As was explained earlier, FBCSP aims to find subject-specific frequency bands indicative of mental state and process them separately, which employs the separation of the original signal into a set of narrow-band components. Such sub-band decomposition of each trial was achieved by applying the filter bank comprising $N_f = 12$ bandpass FIR filters implemented using Kaiser window method and spanning the 7–33 Hz frequency range. Each filter was designed with 3 Hz passband, 2 Hz transition band, and a stopband attenuation of 60 dB. The magnitude response of the employed filter bank with individual filters is shown in Figure 7.7.

7.2.3.3   CSP estimation and feature extraction

Next the subband data from each trial was used for feature extraction. The CSP algorithm is a method for data-driven spatial filter generation, which contrasts the data of different classes (mental tasks) in terms of variance distribution across channels [34]. The CSP feature extraction is a key method for motor imagery representation as it is capable of extraction of ERD/ERS effects associated with this type of mental tasks, and provides for remarkable classification reliability [35–37]. While the conventional CSP is defined for two-class discrimination problems, the

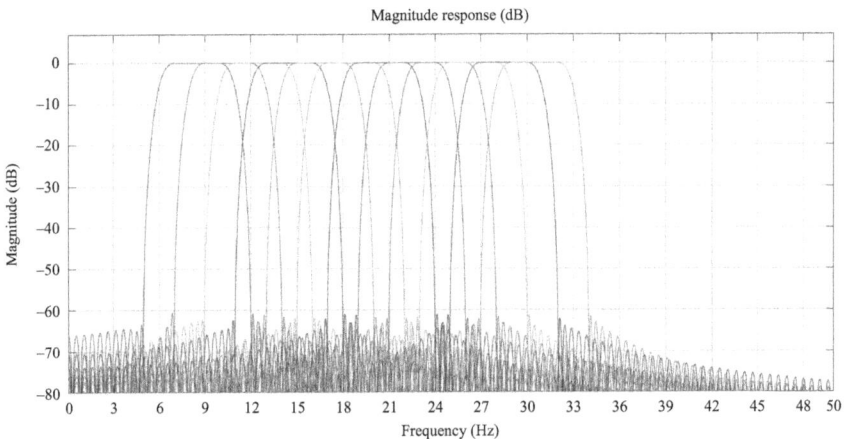

Figure 7.7   Magnitude response of the employed filter bank

dataset contains data from four different classes; therefore, for each subject and within each subband the CSP problem was solved four times, contrasting every class of data separately in the one-vs-rest (OVR) manner. Within the i-th subband the most desirable spatial filter for a certain class, which maximizes the variance contrast with the remaining classes, can be found as a vector that maximizes the following ratio:

$$\hat{\mathbf{w}}_{csp} = \underset{\mathbf{w}_{csp}}{\operatorname{argmax}} \frac{\mathbf{w}_{csp}\mathbf{C}^i_+\mathbf{w}^T_{csp}}{\mathbf{w}_{csp}\mathbf{C}^i_-\mathbf{w}^T_{csp}}, \tag{7.4}$$

where $\mathbf{C}^i_+$ is the average covariance of the data type being contrasted. $\mathbf{C}^i_-$ then denotes the average covariances of the remaining data classes. For example, when estimating the OVR CSP set for right-hand motor imagery (class 2), $\mathbf{C}^i_+ = \mathbf{C}^i_{class\ 2}$, and $\mathbf{C}^i_- = (\mathbf{C}^i_{class\ 2} + \mathbf{C}^i_{class\ 3} + \mathbf{C}^i_{class\ 4})/3$. In practice the spatial filters within each frequency bin are calculated as eigenvectors of the following generalized eigenvalue problem:

$$\mathbf{C}^i_+\mathbf{W} = \Lambda\mathbf{C}^i_-\mathbf{W}, \tag{7.5}$$

with $\mathbf{W}$ denoting the matrix of eigenvectors and Λ representing a diagonal matrix with eigenvalues on the main diagonal. The eigenvector of problem (7.5) corresponding to the largest eigenvalue is the spatial filter that maximizes the ratio in (7.4). Therefore, only two spatial filters corresponding to the largest eigenvalues were selected for each class of data, yielding a total of $N_{csp} = 8$ filters per frequency band. These filters were then combined in the matrix $\hat{\mathbf{W}}^i_{\mathbf{csp}} \in \mathbb{R}^{N_{csp} \times N_{ch}}$, which denotes the multiclass CSP set for the i-th frequency bin. Next, the feature vector $\mathbf{F}_{full}$ that combined the CSP features from all subbands of EEG observation $\mathbf{M}$ was formed in the following way:

$$\mathbf{Z}^i = \hat{\mathbf{W}}_{\mathbf{csp}}{}^i\mathbf{M}^i, \forall i \in [1\ldots N_f]$$

$$\mathbf{f}^i_j = \log\left(\frac{\mathrm{var}(\mathbf{Z}_j{}^i)}{\sum\limits_{p=1}^{N_{csp}}\mathrm{var}(\mathbf{Z}_p)}\right), \forall i \in [1\ldots N_f], \forall j \in [1\ldots N_{csp}] \tag{7.6}$$

$$\mathbf{F}^i = [\mathbf{f}_1, \mathbf{f}_2 \ .. \ \mathbf{f}_{N_{csp}}], \forall i \in [1\ldots N_f]$$

$$\mathbf{F}_{full} = [\mathbf{F}^1, \mathbf{F}^2, \ldots, \mathbf{F}^{N_f}],$$

where $\mathbf{M}^i$ represents the i-th subband of signal observation $\mathbf{M}$ and $\mathbf{Z}^i_j$ denotes the j-th row of $\mathbf{Z}^i$, obtained as a 1-D projection of $\mathbf{M}^i$ onto the j-th row of $\hat{\mathbf{W}}_{\mathbf{csp}}{}^i$. In other words, conventional CSP feature extraction was applied to each subband of trial $\mathbf{M}$ and the full feature vector $\mathbf{F}_{full}$ was obtained by concatenating features from all frequency bands. Considering that $N_f = 12$ and $N_{csp} = 8$ in our settings, this yields a total of 96 predictor variables representing a single observation of motor imagery. For each subject in the dataset this process was repeated over all given EEG trials, resulting in 288 feature vectors per subject.

In order to demonstrate the principle of CSP feature extraction, we show the visualization of CSP filters and corresponding projections for two conditions: left-hand and right-hand motor imagery. Figure 7.8(a) and (b) contains the weight distribution topographies of the most desirable CSP filters $\mathbf{w}_{LH}$ and $\mathbf{w}_{RH}$ for left-hand and right-hand imagery, respectively, displayed over the given electrode montage. These filters were obtained using the data for subject 8 in the dataset and a single subband of 9–12 Hz. The areas of high weight magnitude point to the electrodes with large variance difference between the two conditions. For example, the variance at channel CP4 is significantly lower during the left-hand imagery compared to other mental tasks, and therefore channel CP4 has a large weight

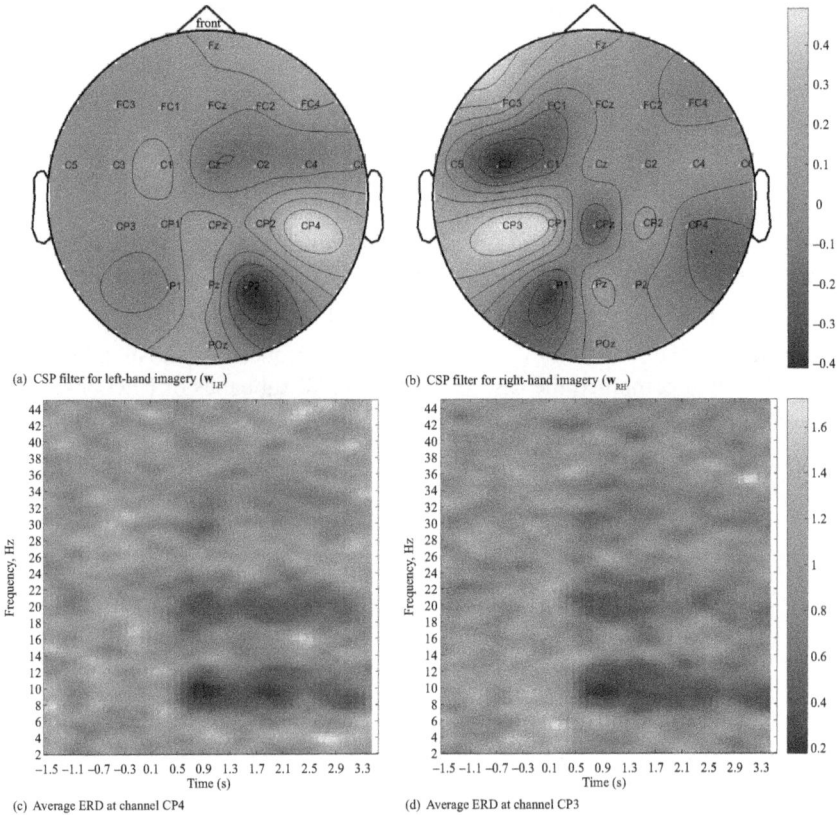

(a) CSP filter for left-hand imagery ($\mathbf{w}_{LH}$)   (b) CSP filter for right-hand imagery ($\mathbf{w}_{RH}$)

(c) Average ERD at channel CP4   (d) Average ERD at channel CP3

Figure 7.8   CSP filters for the left-hand and right-hand motor imagery tasks and characteristic ERD effects. (a) & (b) Spatial filter weight coefficients shown over the given EEG montage. (c) & (d) Average time–frequency maps of the effects that filters $\mathbf{w}_{LH}$ and $\mathbf{w}_{RH}$ aim to extract. On average there was an evident reduction in μ and β band power during the task execution

magnitude associated with it. Figure 7.8(c) and (d) illustrates such variance contrast, which CSP aims to pinpoint. These figures were obtained by averaging the TFRs of raw data from the highlighted sensor and all trials of the corresponding mental task, and normalizing it to the average PSD of the pre-stimulus interval. As a result, Figure 7.8(c) and (d) highlights the relative reduction in μ and β band power during the mental task execution, i.e., the ERD effect, which on average occurred roughly 500 msec after the cue was shown to the user at time point 0. Such visual representations may be used to directly select the bands of interest, in cases when the characteristic effect is as evident as in Figure 7.8(c) and (d).

Next, Figure 7.9 illustrates the projection of EEG data onto the spatial filters $\mathbf{w}_{LH}$ and $\mathbf{w}_{RH}$, described above. For this purpose, we used two arbitrarily selected trials—one of left-hand motor imagery, $\mathbf{M}_{LH}$, and one of right-hand motor imagery, $\mathbf{M}_{RH}$. The four graphs in Figure 7.9 demonstrate how CSP filters may be used to contrast two different conditions on the basis of their projection's variance. Note how the filter produces a low variance projection when the trial matches its desired class, which corresponds to the extraction of ERD effect.

7.2.3.4 Feature selection and classification

Next a set of the most indicative FBCSP features was selected for each subject and used to train and evaluate the classifiers according to the BCI competition IV evaluation protocol. Within both processes of feature selection and classifier training the signal observations were grouped in OVR manner, hence these procedures were repeated multiple times—once for each class of data. In the selection process FBCSP features were first ranked by their class separability. For this purpose we have

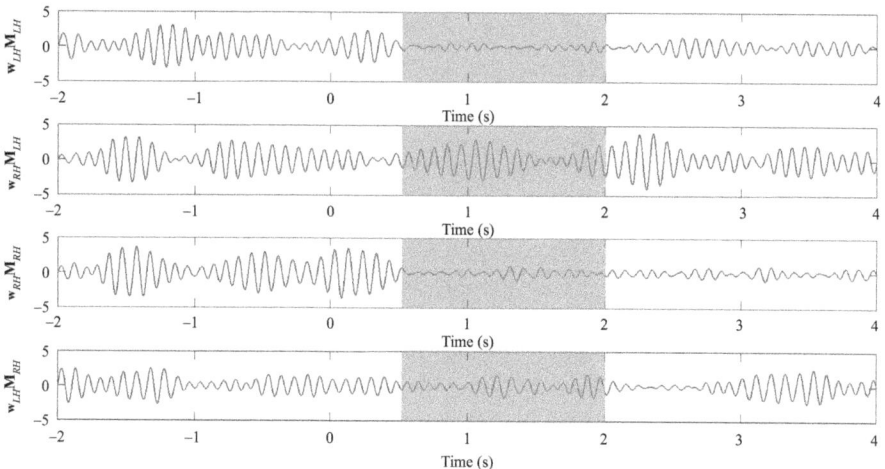

Figure 7.9 Extraction of ERD effects using a set of spatial filters. The figure contains different combinations of left-hand and right-hand imagery signals ($\mathbf{M}_{LH}$ and $\mathbf{M}_{RH}$) projected onto CSP filters $\mathbf{w}_{LH}$ and $\mathbf{w}_{RH}$. The time interval highlighted in gray was used for feature extraction

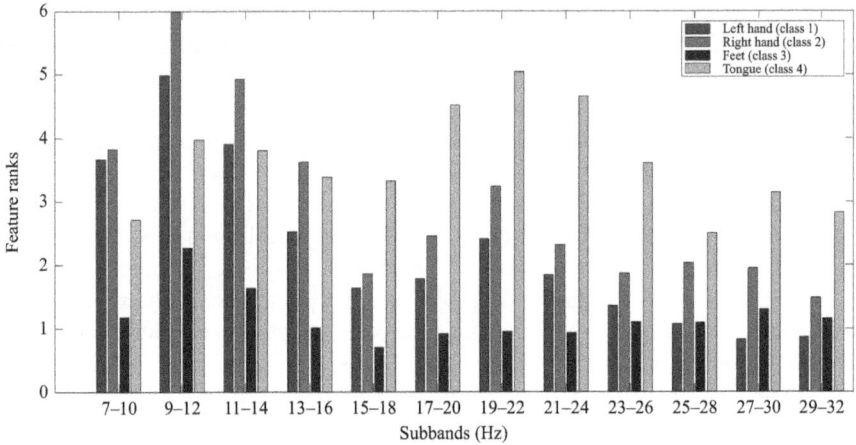

Figure 7.10   The distribution of feature ranks over the subbands estimated for a single subject in the dataset

Table 7.2   Classification accuracy estimates

Subject	CSP sens	FBCSP sens	FBCSP source
1	70.3	74.4	76.9
2	59.7	66.3	65.5
3	80.6	83.5	86.1
4	60.3	68.2	69.3
5	58.9	65.6	66.8
6	57	65.3	68.7
7	77.9	86	87.8
8	78.3	84.3	90.9
9	70.1	76.1	79.2
AVG ± STD	**68.1 ± 9.3**	**74.4 ± 8.5**	**76.8 ± 9.5**

Bold in the bottom row denotes the average accuracy and standard deviation across all subjects

utilized the relative entropy criterion, also known as Kullback–Leibler distance or divergence, which quantifies the distance between two probability distributions [38]. An example of feature ranks over multiple sub-bands estimated for a single subject is given in Figure 7.10.

After the predictor variables were ranked, the sequential forward feature selection was utilized in order to find a subset of features yielding the best classification reliability [39]. Within such selection process, a number of LDA classifiers were trained iteratively using various numbers of the highest ranked features, and their performance was assessed with the evaluation dataset. At the feature selection stage, no more than three subbands were chosen for each subject in the dataset as the further increase in number of bands resulted in reduced classification reliability. The highest achieved classification accuracies for each subject in the dataset are presented in Table 7.2.

7.2.4 Stage 2. Analysis in source space

After the feature selection and classifier training/evaluation stages the selected frequency bands were used to decompose the raw EEG data in preparation for further source reconstruction and analysis in the source space. As mentioned before, band selection may be alternatively conducted by visual assessment of TFRs normalized to the average power during rest, when the ERD/ERS effects are evident. Prior to further source reconstruction, the raw EEG data was segmented and preprocessed as described in Section 7.2.3.1 and filtered into separate subbands selected at the sensor space analysis.

7.2.4.1 Source reconstruction

The source reconstruction was implemented using the forward model comprised by the same ICBM 152 head geometry and source grid as described in Section 7.1.2. However, the employed dataset consists of EEG recordings from a different electrode montage with 22 sensors. The forward model together with the EEG electrode locations is displayed in Figure 7.11. The ROI was defined heuristically as 1,735 locations (38.5% of sources) spanning the expected area of ERD/ERS effects associated with motor imagery.

For source representation, the cortical current estimates were obtained using the WMNE method. The linear inverse operator $\mathbf{G}_{WMNE}$ with regularization parameter $\lambda = 0.01$ was calculated as described in (7.3). Next, this operator was applied to each pre-filtered signal observation and only source magnitudes from the ROI (shown in Figure 7.11) were extracted and used in the following processing.

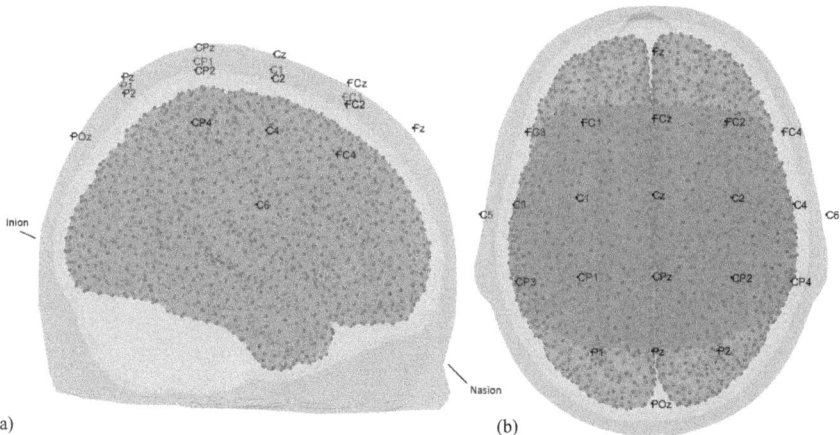

(a) (b)

Figure 7.11 Visualization of forward head model used in simulations. EEG sensor locations are marked by channel labels and source locations on the cortical surface are represented by black dots. (a) Side view from the right. (b) Top-down view with region-of-interest (ROI) highlighted by the darker area

7.2.4.2   CSP estimation and feature extraction

Next the reconstructed source activity from each trial's subband was used to esti-mate a set of CSP filters within the individual bands. This process was identical to the feature extraction described in Section 7.2.3.3 with the difference that only the previously selected subbands were used and the dimension of source representation was much higher compared to the original sensor data. For each subband and subject in the dataset the multiclass set of filters $\hat{\mathbf{W}}_{csp}^{i}$ was calculated by grouping and contrasting the source data in the OVR manner.

Figure 7.12 contains the normalized weight distribution topographies of the most desirable CSP filters for all given classes of mental tasks. These filters were obtained using the data for subject 8 in the dataset and a single subband of 9–12 Hz. For visualization purposes the presented filters were calculated over all sources in the model, without the ROI extraction stage. The reader may notice how closely the filter spatial profiles correspond to the Penfield's sensory homunculus, i.e., the expectations about the relevant muscle-related brain areas (see [40]). The same as with sensor data, only two most desirable CSP filters were selected per class of data and per subband, yielding a set of band-specific unmixing matrices $\hat{\mathbf{W}}_{csp}^{i}$ with a total of 8 filters for each frequency band. Next, the subband filter sets $\hat{\mathbf{W}}_{csp}^{i}$ were used as described in Sec-tion 7.2.3.3 to obtain the feature vectors $\mathbf{F}_{full}$ representing a single motor imagery observation. Taking into account that no more than three frequency bands were used for each subject, the feature vectors $\mathbf{F}_{full}$ contained up to 24 predictor variables.

7.2.4.3   Feature selection and classification

The projection of source trial data onto the CSP projection matrix $\hat{\mathbf{W}}_{csp}^{i}$ greatly reduces the dimension: within our settings $3 \times 1,735$ current dipole moments from the ROI were decomposed into only eight components per subband. Considering that only the indicative frequency bands were used in preprocessing and only the

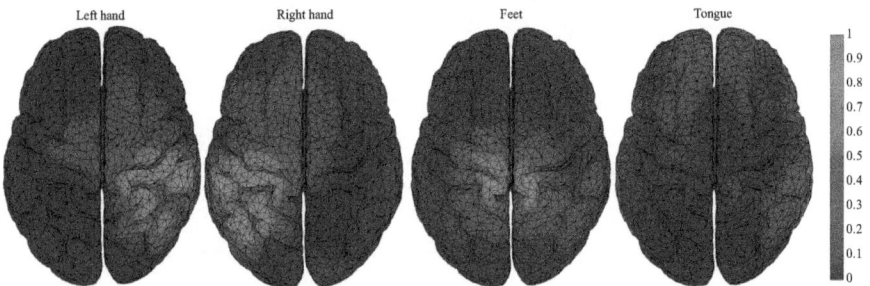

Figure 7.12   The most desirable CSP filters for all four classes of data. Distribution topographies of the normalized filter weights are shown over the standard cortical surface. For display purposes these filters were calculated over all sources in the model without the ROI extraction stage

strongest CSP filters were selected from the full set, the feature selection process was less beneficial in terms of further reduction of feature vector length and classification improvement. However, forward sequential feature selection was still performed for all subjects in the group and a small number of features (1–6 for different subjects) was discarded if it resulted in classification accuracy increase. The same as with sensor data, a separate multiclass LDA classifier was then trained and evaluated according to the same procedure as described for sensor data (see Section 7.2.3.4). The comparison of classification accuracy results for conventional wide band CSP, sensor FBCSP, and source FBCSP methods are given in Table 7.2.

7.2.4.4   Discussion

According to our results, on the whole subjects have shown different capabilities for eliciting strong and consistent BCI control commands, which explains the large variance of the accuracy estimates. Within the 4-class classification paradigm the random classification accuracy is 25%. As can be seen from the table, FBCSP feature extraction applied to reconstructed source components consistently outperforms conventional CSP methods in the sensor space. With source FBCSP features the highest classification accuracy of 90.9% was achieved for subject 8 in the dataset, which was significantly higher than the average rate of $76.8 \pm 9.5\%$ among all 9 subjects.

As described previously, within the SMR BCI paradigm the control signal may be defined as the frequency-specific variation in band power, relative to the resting condition, which is referred to as ERD or ERS effects. Then, the aim of the proposed signal processing scheme is to lock such effects in time, frequency, and space. With the given fixed trial-based dataset the locking in time corresponds to the time window selection, which can be done through visual assessment of averaged data or heuristically, by applying several differently positioned time windows and selecting the one, which maximizes classification performance (or feature metrics). In real-time BCI applications this corresponds to a simple sliding window. Locking of characteristic signal in frequency was done by the application of filter bank and further selection of indicative bands based on feature metrics or classification performance. The CSP filters, estimated from the grouped training data, correspond to locking of the ERD/ERS effects in space. Within such time–frequency–space filtering approach, source reconstruction does not affect the performance of filtering in the time domain. Besides that, the WMNE inverse solutions are linear, and in other words, do not produce new frequency components and, as shown in the simulated example (see Section 7.1.3) are capable of accurate local oscillatory activity reconstruction. Therefore, the employed source imaging affected only the performance of the CSP method by providing it with data of higher dimension and, at the same time, less linear interdependency. Besides, considering the capabilities of EEG imaging for isolation of source components based on their origin, the ROI extraction represents the partial removal of noise energy that appears to be more efficient and flexible compared to the simple channel selection in the sensor space.

The positive effect of source localization can be demonstrated by performing the comparison of features extracted from sensor and source representations of the signal. Figure 7.13(a) and (b) contains the parallel coordinate visualization of all

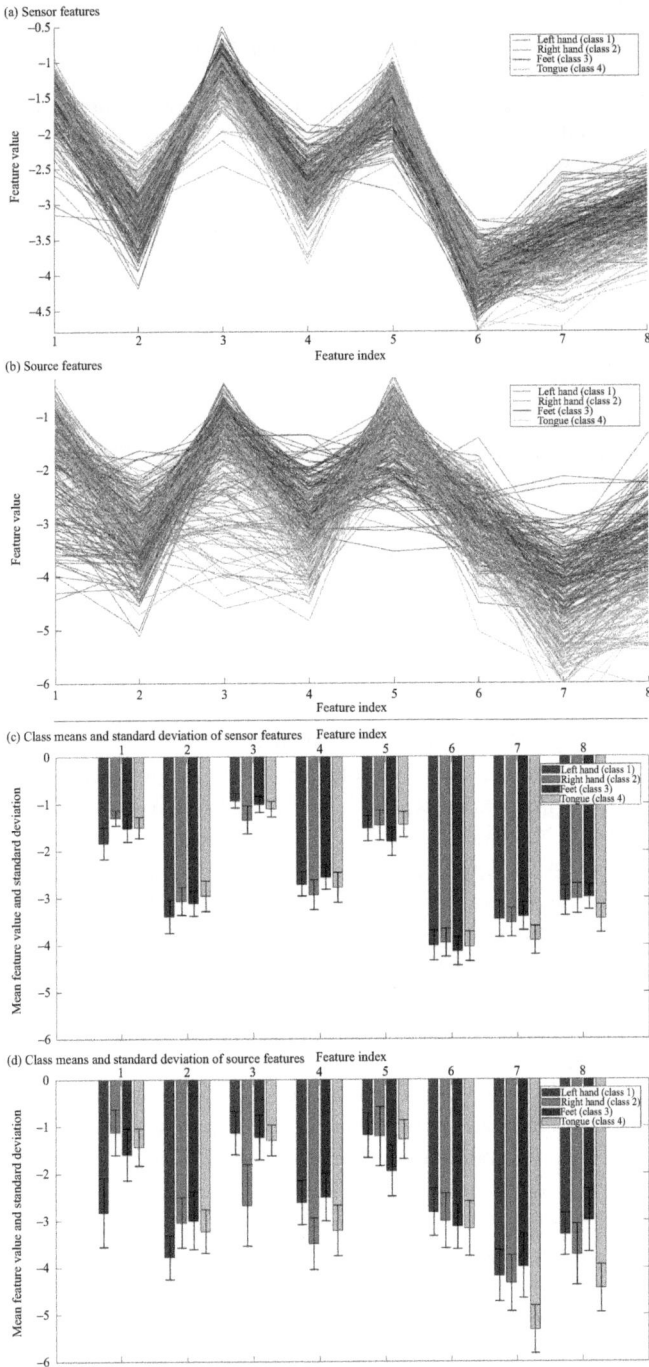

Figure 7.13 (a) & (b) The parallel coordinate visualization of sensor and source
CSP features extracted from a single subject and 9–12 Hz subband.
(c) & (d) Class means and standard deviation of features shown in
figures (a) and (b). The source features have clearly larger distance
between the class means, which explains their better class
separability compared to sensor features

training feature vectors extracted from a single 9–12 Hz band of subject 3 in the dataset. This type of plot is often used to visualize the multidimensional data such as a full set of training feature vectors. Here each line represents the observation (a feature vector) and the line color indicates the class of data, i.e., the type of mental task performed during the observation. The feature values are defined at the labeled points on the x-axis denoting the feature indices. With x denoting data class and y denoting the filter index in the full CSP set the feature values f_{xy} were ordered according to the utilized CSP filters as $(f_{11}, f_{12}, f_{21}, f_{22}, f_{31}, f_{32}, f_{41}, f_{42})$. As was described before, these values represent the logarithm of normalized variance calculated for the signal projections obtained using the selected CSP filters (two filters per class). For example, from the plot it can be seen that the values of features f_{21}, f_{22}, extracted from trials of right-hand imagery (class 2) using the CSP filters designed for this class, generally had lower values than features extracted from different classes with the same filters. This effect, visible in Figure 7.13(a) and (b), corresponds to the extraction of ERD effect during the motor imagery.

Figure 7.13(c) and (d) demonstrates the effect of source reconstruction on feature class separability shown for the same set of feature vectors. This figure shows the class means of the given features and their standard deviation. In our settings the source reconstruction resulted in features with slightly higher variance, although significantly larger distance between the class means, which explains the observed increase in classification reliability.

The presented analysis scenario shows how source reconstruction can be embedded in the EEG classification system and highlights its benefits for BCI performance. Results of the analysis, trained classifiers, and selected feature indices can be directly used in BCI feedback training sessions. Linear inverse operators, such as WMNE, and sparse regions-of-interest are computationally simple enough to be applied in real-time settings. Although the individual head models obtained from anatomical MRIs are known to be advantageous for localization accuracy [41], the utilized ICBM 152 standard head model still provided positive effects of source reconstruction.

References

[1]   Friston KJ. Functional and effective connectivity: a review. Brain Connectivity. 2011;1(1):13–36.

[2]   Sakkalis V. Review of advanced techniques for the estimation of brain connectivity measured with EEG/MEG. Computers in Biology and Medicine. 2011;41(12):1110–1117.

[3]   Pfurtscheller G, Brunner C, Schlögl A, Lopes da Silva FH. Mu rhythm (de) synchronization and EEG single-trial classification of different motor imagery tasks. NeuroImage. 2006;31(1):153–159.

[4]   Kaiser V, Bauernfeind G, Kreilinger A, *et al.* Cortical effects of user training in a motor imagery based brain-computer interface measured by fNIRS and EEG. NeuroImage. 2014;85:432–444.

[5]   Baillet S, Mosher JC, Leahy RM. Electromagnetic brain mapping. IEEE Signal Processing Magazine. 2001;18(6):14–30.

[6]   Hallez H, Vanrumste B, Grech R, *et al.* Review on solving the forward problem in EEG source analysis. Journal of Neuroengineering and Rehabilitation. 2007;4:46.

[7]   Ahn M, Hong JH, Jun SC. Source space based brain computer interface. In: 17th International Conference on Biomagnetism Advances in Biomagnetism–Biomag2010. Springer; 2010. p. 366–369.

[8]   Zaitcev A, Cook G, Liu W, Paley M, Milne E. Application of Compressive Sensing for EEG Source Localization in Brain Computer Interfaces. In: 2014 Loughborough Antennas and Propagation Conference (LAPC). IEEE; 2014. p. 272–276.

[9]   Zaitcev A, Cook G, Liu W, Paley M, Milne E. Feature extraction for BCIs based on electromagnetic source localization and multiclass Filter Bank Common Spatial Patterns. In: 2015 37th Annual International Conference of the IEEE Engineering in Medicine and Biology Society (EMBC). IEEE; 2015. p. 1773–1776.

[10] Edelman BJ, Baxter B, He B. EEG source imaging enhances the decoding of complex right-hand motor imagery tasks. IEEE Transactions on Biomedical Engineering. 2016;63(1):4–14.

[11] Grech R, Cassar T, Muscat J, *et al.* Review on solving the inverse problem in EEG source analysis. Journal of Neuroengineering and Rehabilitation. 2008;5:25.

[12] Pascual-Marqui RD. Review of methods for solving the EEG inverse problem. International Journal of Bioelectromagnetism. 1999;1(1):75–86.

[13] Baillet S. Toward functional brain imaging of cortical electrophysiology Markovian models for magneto and electroencephalogram source estimation and experimental assessments. Orsay, France. 1998.

[14] Hämäläinen MS, Ilmoniemi RJ. Interpreting magnetic fields of the brain: minimum norm estimates. Medical & Biological Engineering & Computing. 1994;32(1):35–42.

[15] Pascual-Marqui RD, Michel CM, Lehmann D. Low resolution electromagnetic tomography: a new method for localizing electrical activity in the brain. International Journal of Psychophysiology. 1994;18(1):49–65.

[16] de Peralta Menendez RG, Murray MM, Michel CM, Martuzzi R, Andino SLG. Electrical neuroimaging based on biophysical constraints. Neuroimage. 2004;21(2):527–539.

[17] Tibshirani R. Regression shrinkage and selection via the lasso. Journal of the Royal Statistical Society Series B (Methodological). 1996;267–288.

[18] Zou H, Hastie T. Regularization and variable selection via the elastic net. Journal of the Royal Statistical Society: Series B (Statistical Methodology). 2005;67(2):301–320.

[19] Collins DL, Zijdenbos AP, Baaré WF, Evans AC. ANIMAL+ INSECT: improved cortical structure segmentation. In: Biennial International

Conference on Information Processing in Medical Imaging. Springer; 1999. p. 210–223.

[20]   Fonov VS, Evans AC, McKinstry RC, Almli C, Collins D. Unbiased non-linear average age-appropriate brain templates from birth to adulthood. NeuroImage. 2009;47:S102.

[21]   Fonov V, Evans AC, Botteron K, *et al.* Unbiased average age-appropriate atlases for pediatric studies. NeuroImage. 2011;54(1):313–327.

[22]   Tadel F, Baillet S, Mosher JC, Pantazis D, Leahy RM. Brainstorm: a user-friendly application for MEG/EEG analysis. Computational Intelligence and Neuroscience. 2011;2011:8.

[23]   Clerc M, Gramfort A, Olivi E, Papadopoulo T. The Symmetric BEM: Bringing in More Variables for Better Accuracy. In: 17th International Conference on Biomagnetism Advances in Biomagnetism–Biomag 2010. Springer; 2010. pp. 109–112.

[24]   Kybic J, Clerc M, Abboud T, Faugeras O, Keriven R, Papadopoulo T. A common formalism for the integral formulations of the forward EEG problem. IEEE Transactions on Medical Imaging. 2005;24(1):12–28.

[25]   Gramfort A, Papadopoulo T, Olivi E, Clerc M. OpenMEEG: opensource software for quasistatic bioelectromagnetics. Biomedical Engineering Online. 2010;9:45.

[26]   Golub GH, Heath M, Wahba G. Generalized cross-validation as a method for choosing a good ridge parameter. Technometrics. 1979;21(2):215–223.

[27]   Hansen PC. The L-curve and its use in the numerical treatment of inverse problems. IMM, Department of Mathematical Modelling, Technical University of Denmark; 1999.

[28]   Grant M, Boyd S, Ye Y. CVX: Matlab software for disciplined convex programming; 2008.

[29]   Grant MC, Boyd SP. Graph implementations for nonsmooth convex programs. In: Recent Advances in Learning and Control. Springer; 2008. pp. 95–110.

[30]   Mason SG, Bashashati A, Fatourechi M, Navarro KF, Birch GE. A comprehensive survey of brain interface technology designs. Annals of Biomedical Engineering. 2007;35(2):137–169.

[31]   Nicolas-Alonso LF, Gomez-Gil J. Brain computer interfaces, a review. Sensors (Basel). 2012;12(2):1211–1279.

[32]   Brunner C, Leeb R, Müller-Putz G, Schlögl A, Pfurtscheller G. BCI Competition 2008–Graz data set A. Institute for Knowledge Discovery (Laboratory of Brain-Computer Interfaces), Graz University of Technology. 2008; p. 136–142.

[33]   Tangermann M, Müller KR, Aertsen A, *et al.* Review of the BCI competition IV. Frontiers in Neuroscience. 2012;6:55.

[34]   Ramoser H, Müller-Gerking J, Pfurtscheller G. Optimal spatial filtering of single trial EEG during imagined hand movement. IEEE Transactions on Rehabilitation Engineering. 2000;8(4):441–446.

[35] Blankertz B, Tomioka R, Lemm S, Kawanabe M, Muller KR. Optimizing spatial filters for robust EEG single-trial analysis. IEEE Signal Processing Magazine. 2008;25(1):41–56.

[36] Grosse-Wentrup M, Buss M. Multiclass common spatial patterns and information theoretic feature extraction. IEEE transactions on Biomedical Engineering. 2008;55(8):1991–2000.

[37] Ang KK, Chin ZY, Wang C, Guan C, Zhang H. Filter bank common spatial pattern algorithm on BCI competition IV datasets 2a and 2b. Frontiers in Neuroscience. 2012.

[38] Bishop CM. Pattern recognition and machine learning. Vol. 4 of Information Science and Statistics. Jordan M, Kleinberg J, Schölkopf B, editors. Springer; 2006.

[39] Theodoridis S, Koutroumbas K. Pattern Recognition, Third Edition. vol. 11; 2006.

[40] Penfield W, Rasmussen T. The cerebral cortex of man; a clinical study of localization of function. American Journal of Physical Medicine. 1950; 33(2):126.

[41] Acar ZA, Makeig S. Effects of forward model errors on EEG source localization. Brain Topography. 2013;26(3):378–396.

Chapter 8

Evaluation for smart air travel support system

CheeFai Tan[1], Wei Chen[2], and Matthias Rauterberg[3]

Long haul air travel passengers will experience different level of physiological and psychological discomfort. It is because the long haul air travel is not a natural activity for human being. The literature review showed that seating comfort and discomfort is subjective and interchangeable. Comfort is an attribute that is highly demanded by most of the aircraft passengers. An aircraft passenger's comfort depends on different features and the environment during air travel. Seat discomfort is a subjective issue because it is the customer who makes the adjustment based on their seating experience. The aircraft passenger seat has an important role to play in fulfilling the passenger comfort expectations. The seat is one of the important features of the aircraft where the aircraft passenger spends most of the time during air travel. A smart support system for long haul air travel has been developed at the Eindhoven University of Technology, the Netherlands. The purpose of the system is to reduce travel discomfort and improve the comfort experience during long haul air travel.

In this chapter, four experiments were reported. The first study is to identify factors of seating comfort. Next, the survey of relationship between seat location and sitting posture is reported. It is followed by the validation of aircraft cabin simulator. Lastly, the validation experiment of Smart Neck Support System is described. The validation experiment is to validate the developed smart systems for neck support in a simulated "real life" setting. The aim of a developed smart system is to support the passenger's head and reduce passenger neck muscle stress during air travel adaptively. An aircraft cabin simulator was utilized to conduct the validation experiment. The calibration experiment was conducted to gain information to be used for the validation experiment. The validation is an important process of Smart Neck Support System (SNes).

[1]Department of Mechanical Precision Engineering, Malaysia–Japan International Institute of Technology, Malaysia
[2]Author Center for Intelligent Medical Electronics, Department of Electronic Engineering, School of Information Science and Technology, Fudan University, China
[3]Department of Industrial Design, Eindhoven University of Technology, The Netherlands

8.1   Introduction

Air travel is becoming increasingly accessible to people both through the availability of cheap flights and because the airlines now are able to cater for individuals of all ages and disabilities. However, long haul air travel is not a natural activity for humans. Many aircraft passengers experience different degrees of physiological and psychological discomfort and even stress during flying. The aircraft passenger's health may endanger by excessive stress that may cause passenger to become aggressive and over-react [1]. A number of health problems can affect aircraft passengers. During the departure process, an aircraft passenger may experience anxiety caused by overcrowded airport and complicated airport departure procedures. After boarding into the aircraft cabin, the aircraft passenger may experience discomfort caused by environmental factors such as humidity, pressure, and noise. Besides, some aircraft passengers also feel discomfort during sitting where the passenger may be affected by the seat location, seat position, and sitting duration. A long haul air travel across different time zones and irregular meal timings may continuously affect the health of an aircraft passenger [2].

Comfort is an attribute that today's passenger demand more and more. An aircraft passenger's comfort depends on different features and the environment during air travel. Seat discomfort is a subjective issue because it is the customer who makes the final determination and customer evaluations are based on their opinions having experienced the seat [3]. The aircraft passenger seat has an important role to play in fulfilling the passenger comfort expectations. The seat is one of the important features of the vehicle and is the place where the passenger spends most of time during air travel. The aviation industry is highly competitive and therefore airlines try to maximize the number of seats [4]. Often this results in a very limited amount of seating space for passengers, especially in economy class [5].

8.2   Seat comfort and discomfort

The Cambridge Advanced Learner's dictionary (2008) defined comfort as "a pleasant feeling of being relaxed and free from pain." Seat comfort is determined subjectively because the user justifies the seat comfort based on his/her subjective experience in using the seat [3]. Helander [6] stressed that a good ergonomic design of the seat is a precondition for seat comfort. De Looze *et al.* [7] described comfort as affected by different factors such as physical, physiological and psychological factors. Helander and Zhang [8] noted that there is a difference between seating comfort and discomfort in office chairs. They described how comfort is related to emotional aspects such as feeling safe and luxury. Their findings described that the physical aspects such as feeling pressure and muscle pain are related to body discomfort.

Table 8.1   Causes of seating discomfort [10]

Human experience mode	Biomechanical		Seat/environment
	Physiology causes	Engineering causes	Source
Pain	Circulation occlusion	Pressure	Cushion stiffness
Pain	Ischemia	Pressure	Cushion stiffness
Pain	Nerve occlusion	Pressure	Seat contour
Discomfort	-	Vibration	Vehicle ride
Perspiration	Heat	Material	Vinyl upholstery
Perception	Visual/auditory/tactile	Breathability Design/vibration	Vehicle cost

The concepts of comfort and discomfort in sitting are under debate. There is no widely accepted definition, although it is beyond dispute that comfort and discomfort are feelings or emotions that are subjective in nature [7]. Seating discomfort has been examined from a number of different perspectives. The problem with evaluating comfort with regard to pressure or any other factor is that comfort is subjective and not easy to quantify. Seating discomfort varies from subject to subject and depends on the task at hand. Comfort, however, is a vague concept and subjective in nature. It is generally defined as lack of discomfort [9]. Discomfort feelings, as described by Helander and Zhang [8], is affected by biomechanical factors and fatigue. The sources of such discomfort are listed in Table 8.1.

8.2.1   Identifying factors of seating comfort

In this subsection, a questionnaire is developed to determine the relationship between the selected factors and comfort in economy class aircraft passenger seat. Zhang *et al.* [11] identified the comfort and discomfort factors of office chair. The research defined 23 comfort factors and 20 discomfort factors in using office chair.

8.2.1.1   Selection of comfort factors

First, all possible comfort factors related to sitting were collected from various journal articles and online journal database. The journal articles were studied to select the possible comfort and discomfort factors. For example, the factors selected from Kolich [12] paper were "breathability" and "styling."

From the literature review, potential factors were selected based on their relationship with seating comfort and discomfort. Next, 28 studies were used to select 41 factors.

8.2.1.2   Methods

There were 55 students ($N = 55$) recruited from Department of Industrial Design, Eindhoven University of Technology, the Netherlands, to volunteer in the main study. The online questionnaire with 41 factors was developed by using QuestionPro systems and send to respondents via electronic mail. The respondents rated the factors in terms of comfort on a 4-point scale (1 = not related to comfort, 2 = slightly related to comfort, 3 = closely related to comfort, 4 = very closely related to comfort). Fifty-five respondents filled in the questionnaire online.

8.2.1.3   Data analysis
In the study, 41 comfort factors were ranked on mean ranks (MR) of their rating score with the Friedman test. The factor that was not rated by the subject was coded as "99" and regarded as a missing value. Next, 41 factors were classified into factors with Principal Components Analysis (PCA) with Varimax Rotation method.

8.2.1.4   Results
The 41 comfort factors were ranked from 1 to 41. The Friedman test, which evaluated differences in medians among the 41 comfort factors, is significant χ^2 (40, $N = 41) = 274$, $p < 0.001$. From the result as shown in Table 8.2, "spacious" (MR = 29.68) exhibited the highest comfort factor level. It was followed by "adjustable" (MR = 28.83), "ergonomic" (MR = 28.62), "head rest" (MR = 28.04), "seat contour" (MR = 26.90), and "neck support" (MR = 26.37). The comfort factors were ranked based on MRs.

A factor analysis was conducted to identify the underlying dimensions of the comfort factors. Scores on the 41 factors were submitted to PCA with Varimax Rotation. The comfort factors were classified into 12 factors with eigenvalues greater than 1. Thus, the six factors solution yielded the best solution (Table 8.3). Factors 1–6 explained 58.69% of the variance in the data. The other six factors explained 19.37%, which showed less variance than the first six factors and will not be further discussed.

The first factor included eight factors that described the "no irritation in sitting," i.e., "no shock," "no strained," "no fatigue," "no pressure," "not tired," "no sore muscles," "not bouncy," and "no heavy leg." The first factor explained 22.92% of the variance in the data. The second factor included eight factors, i.e., "leg support," "side support," "arm rest," "spacious," "neck support," "adjustable," "head rest," and "ergonomic." This factor appeared to reflect the support of economy class aircraft passenger seat and it was labeled as "body support." The third factor included four factors, i.e., "safety," "reliable," "intelligent," and "functionality," and was labeled as "seat function." The fourth factor was labeled as "feeling in sitting" and included five factors, i.e., "no hardness," "no vibration," "firmness of back rest," "warm," and "no stiffness." The fifth factor was labeled as "long hour sitting" and included three factors, i.e., "long duration," "seat cushion firmness," and "fit." The sixth factor included three factors, i.e., "relax," "adaptable," and "restful." Therefore, it was labeled as "relaxing."

Table 8.2   The mean ranks for comfort factors

No.	Factor	Mean rank
1	Spacious	29.68
2	Adjustable	28.83
3	Ergonomic	28.62
4	Head rest	28.04
5	Seat contour	26.9
6	Neck support	26.37
7	Relax	25.59
8	Firmness of backer seat	25.38
9	Seat cushion firmness	25.27
10	Restful	24.67
11	Safety	24
12	Adaptable	23.38
13	Arm rest	22.91
14	Lumbar support	22.9
15	No stiffness	22.6
16	Breathability	22.41
17	No sore muscles	22.4
18	No fatigue	22.37
19	Fit	21.77
20	Side support	21.37
21	Leg support	20.49
22	No hardness	19.78
23	No pressure	19.56
24	Not tired	19.26
25	No shock	19.15
26	No vibration	18.93
27	Reliable	18.79
28	Well being	18.70
29	Warm	18.41
30	No uneven pressure	18.29
31	Functionality	18.24
32	No uneasy	18.01
33	Massage	18.00
34	No heavy leg	17.66
35	No strained	17.41
36	Automatic adjustment	16.28
37	Long duration	16.17
38	Pleasurable	16.07
39	Intelligent	12.72
40	Not bouncy	12.07
41	Short duration	11.55

8.2.1.5   Summary

The comfort factor, namely "spacious," was most related to comfort in experiencing economy class aircraft passenger seat, followed by "adjustable," "ergonomic," "head rest," "seat contour," and "neck support." Next, the Factor Analysis with Varimax Rotation is used to classify the selected comfort factors into

Table 8.3   Factor loading of the comfort factors

No.	Factors	Factor 1 No irritation in sitting	Factor 2 Body support	Factor 3 Seat function	Factor 4 Feeling in sitting	Factor 5 Long hour sitting	Factor 6 Relaxing
1	No shock	0.828					
2	No strained	0.798					
3	No fatigue	0.736				0.470	
4	No pressure	0.689					
5	No tired	0.673					
6	No sore muscles	0.658					
7	No bouncy	0.649					
8	No heavy leg	0.462					
9	Leg support		0.844				
10	Side support		0.786				
11	Armrest		0.774				
12	Spacious		0.682				
13	Neck support		0.647				
14	Adjustable		0.541				
15	Head rest		0.470				
16	Ergonomic		0.463				
17	Safety			0.798			
18	Reliable			0.771			
19	Intelligent			0.638		0.452	
20	Functionality			0.509			
21	No hardness				0.755		
22	No vibration				0.676		
23	Firmness of backrest			0.459	0.596		
24	Warm	0.477			0.575		
25	No stiffness				0.554		
26	Long duration					0.743	
27	Seat cushion firmness					0.635	
28	Fit					0.561	
29	Relax						0.853
30	Adaptable						0.630
31	Restful						0.523
32	Lumbar support						
33	Well being						
34	No uneven pressure						
35	Automatic adjustment						
36	No uneasy	0.551					
37	Seat contour						
38	Short duration						
39	Pleasurable						
40	Massage						
41	Breathability						
	Explained variance	22.92%	12.06%	7.27%	6.38%	5.63%	4.43%
	Cronbach's alpha	0.860	0.840	0.730	0.790	0.660	0.730

Note: Only factor loadings > 0.450 are displayed

factors. The first six factors, which explained 58.69%, were selected. The first six factors were "no irritation in sitting," "body support," "seat function," "feeling in sitting," "long hour sitting," and "adaptability." The main study showed that the factors of the factor "no irritation in sitting" are most related to comfort and the factors of the factor "relaxing" are least related to comfort. From the factor analysis result, it can be assumed that the main perception of respondents about the economy class aircraft passenger seat comfort is "no irritation in sitting." It is followed by "body support," where the respondents felt that the body support of the aircraft passenger seat will improve the seating comfort.

8.2.2 Survey of relationship between seat location and sitting posture

During air travel, passengers can book the preferred seat location or receive an assigned specific seat location during check-in. The seat location in the economy class cabin can be classified to aisle, center, and window seat [4]. The observation method was used in economy class aircraft cabin to investigate (a) the relationship between different economy class aircraft passenger seat location and sitting posture and (b) the relationship between gender and sitting posture. The observation was conducted in the economy class cabin of Malaysia Airlines (Boeing 747-400). The flight was from Kuala Lumpur International Airport, Malaysia, to Schiphol International Airport, the Netherlands. The departure time was 11:55 p.m. on May 27, 2009 and the arrival time was 6:35 a.m. on May 28, 2009. The flight duration was 12 h 40 min. The sitting postures of 12 passengers within observer eye view were observed and recorded.

8.2.2.1 Methods
Observation administration and recording
The observer and observed subjects sat at the location as shown in Figure 8.1. The sitting location of the observer was seat number "35C." The seat numbers of observed subjects were "34B," "34C," "34D," "35A," "35B," "35D," "35E," "35F," "35G," "36D," and "36E." The observed subjects were within the observation range of the observer. The other seats were occupied by passengers as well but they were out of the observation range of the observer. The observer recorded the sitting postures of the subjects in every 15 minutes.

	A	B	C		D	E	F	G
33					SUBJECT 5 (Female)			
34		SUBJECT 1 (Male)	SUBJECT 2 (Male)	Aisle	SUBJECT 6 (Male)			
35	SUBJECT 3 (Female)	SUBJECT 4 (Male)	OBSERVER		SUBJECT 7 (Male)	SUBJECT 8 (Female)	SUBJECT 9 (Female)	SUBJECT 10 (Male)
36					SUBJECT 11 (Male)	SUBJECT 12 (Female)		

Figure 8.1 The sitting location of observer and observed subjects

The sitting posture was pre-defined and coded in seven postures as referred to Table 8.4. The explanation of seven postures are as follows:

1. Sitting posture "A": the passenger's head faces forward.
2. Sitting posture "B": the passenger's head tilts to right.
3. Sitting posture "C": the passenger's head tilts to left.
4. Sitting posture "D": the passenger's head rotates to right.
5. Sitting posture "E": the passenger's head rotates to left.
6. Sitting posture "F": the passenger's head and body rotate to right.
7. Sitting posture "G": the passenger's head and body rotate to left.

If a subject leaves the seat, we code this condition as "others."

8.2.2.2   Results

A Crosstab and Chi-square method was used to analyze the recorded data. The first analysis investigates the relationship between seat location and sitting posture. Next, the relationship between the gender and sitting posture was examined.

For Crosstab analysis on the relationship between seat location and sitting posture, out of 330 postures that are recorded in the aisle seat, 185 postures are position "A" (56%) and 64 postures are position "D" (19%). The results showed that the preferred sitting positions in aisle seat are positions "A" and "D." For the center seat, positions C (10%), D (19%), and E (14%) were preferred by the subjects. For the window seat, out of 110 recorded postures, positions "B" (22%) and "E" (13%) were preferred by the subjects. On average, the seat location of passengers will affect their sitting posture during air travel. A Chi-square test showed that this difference was significant (χ^2 (10) = 43.332, $p < 0.001$). Position A was preferred by 51% of the observed passengers because it is the most comfort position.

For the relationship between gender and seat location, Crosstab and Chi-square methods were used. The observed subjects were seven males and five females. Out of 262 postures that were recorded from female passengers, females preferred positions "B" (12%), "C" (10%), "D" (20%), and "E" (13%). In contrast, males preferred position "A" (58%) as referred to the 374 recorded positions. On average, there was a significant difference between the gender of passengers and their sitting posture during air travel. A Chi-square test showed that this difference was significant (χ^2 (5) = 21.687, $p < 0.05$).

8.2.3   Validation of aircraft cabin simulator

The validation experiment of the aircraft cabin simulator was carried out using the presence questionnaire [13]. The presence questionnaire is used to measure the presence between real and simulated flight experiences in aircraft cabin simulator. The validation experiment was designed by Hao Liu and the author. The validation experiment was conducted as a part of the experiment to validate the developed in-flight entertainment system by Hao Liu *et al.* [14] for SEAT project. The participants were required to sit inside the cabin simulator to simulate a flight from Schiphol International Airport, the Netherlands, to Shanghai Pudong International Airport, China.

Table 8.4   The coding of sitting posture for observation purpose

No.	Sitting posture
A	
B	
C	
D	
E	
F	
G	
Others	Subject leaves the seat

8.2.3.1 Methods
Participants
Twelve participants (six females and six males) were invited to participate in our validation experiments. The age of the participants ranged from 21 to 33 years. The professions in the first experimental group included one reporter, two workers, and three engineers. The professions in the second experimental group included one student, two workers, and three engineers. The participants were recruited through advertisement in regional news (newspaper, radio, and television) and were given €50 upon completion.

Supporting personnel
A former professional flight attendant from Swiss Air was invited to provide cabin service during user experiments. Hao Liu acted as the simulated flight captain. The author provided technical supports. Matthias Rauterberg coordinated and directed the experiments.

Experimental setup
We conducted the validation experiment for the aircraft cabin simulator inside the simulation laboratory in the Main Building of Eindhoven University of Technology. Twelve participants were allocated to two experiments. Each experiment consisted of six participants. The participants were tested at the economy class section in the aircraft cabin simulator. The in-flight entertainment system was installed and used by the participants as well. Both experiments simulated the KLM KL0895 flight from Schiphol International Airport to Shanghai Pudong International Airport. Both experiments were conducted with the same environment and procedure following the real flight schedule.

Questionnaire
Presence is defined as the subjective experience of being in one place or environment, even when one is physically situated in another [15]. In this chapter's context, presence means the "passenger's" subjective experience of being in a long haul flight, even when the "passenger" is physically sitting in the aircraft cabin simulator. The presence questionnaire by Usoh *et al.* [13] is used to measure the perceived presence of participants. It is customized resulting in the following five questions:

1. Please rate your sense of being in the long haul flight on the following scale from 1 to 7.
   I had a sense of "being there" in the long haul flight:

   Not at all ○ ○ ○ ○ ○ ○ ○ **Very much**

        1   2   3   4   5   6   7

2. To what extent were there times during the experience when the laboratory became the "real long haul flight" for you, and you almost forgot about the "real world" of the laboratory in which the whole experience was really taking place?

There were times during the experience when the virtual "long haul flight" became more real for me compared to the "real flight"...

At no time ○ ○ ○ ○ ○ ○ ○ Almost all
          1   2   3   4   5   6   7   the time

3. When you think back about your experience, do you think of the laboratory more as the laboratory that you saw, or more as somewhere that you visited? Please answer on the following 1–7 scale:
    The laboratory seems to me to be more like...

Laboratory that ○ ○ ○ ○ ○ ○ ○ Somewhere
   I saw   that I visited
           1   2   3   4   5   6   7

4. During the time of the experience, which was the strongest on the whole, your sense of being in the long haul flight or of being in the real world of the laboratory?
    I had a stronger sense of being in...

The real ○ ○ ○ ○ ○ ○ ○ The virtual
world of the   reality of the
laboratory 1   2   3   4   5   6   7 Longhaul flight

5. The questionnaire was distributed to participants at the end of the simulated flight.

Apparatus and data recording

The following hardware were used for both experiments:

* Observation camera
* Computer
* Aircraft cabin simulator

A CCTV observation camera was used to record the situations inside the simulator throughout the experiment. Two CCTVs were installed in the economy class section of the simulator. The activity of the participants was observed and monitored. The recorded data were saved in the computer. Two snapshots of the video recordings in the aircraft cabin simulator are shown in Figure 8.2.

Experimental procedure

In order to simulate a real flight experience, the participants were requested to bring along their hand luggage and the mockup air tickets, which were issued beforehand. Before the experiment started, 15 min of briefing was conducted. Next, the participants were positioned to the seat according to the mockup air ticket. The participants were given a drink and snack before the departure. The general simulated procedure in the KLM economy class as well as flight procedure was used. The flight simulation procedure is shown in Figure 8.3. The departure time of the flight is Amsterdam local time 6:18 p.m. The arrival time of the flight is Amsterdam local time 4:55 a.m. + 1 day (Shanghai local time 10:55 a.m.). The flight duration is

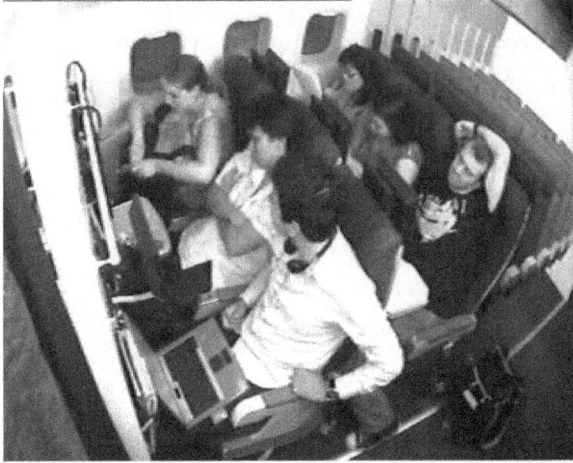

(a)

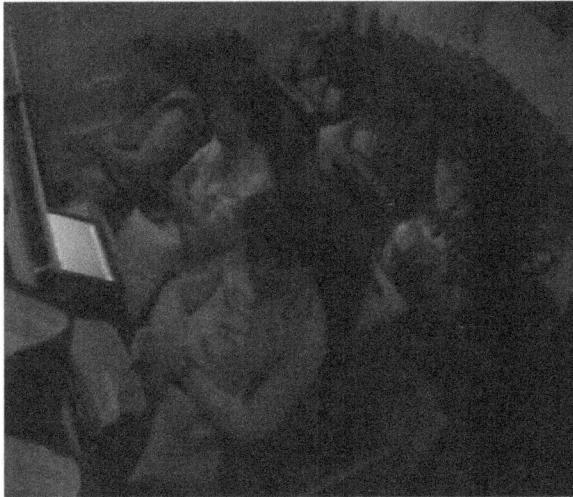

(b)

Figure 8.2   The video recording inside the aircraft cabin simulator: (a) Time: 22:16:49; (b) Time: 03:15:31 (+1 day)

10 h 35 min. The first experiment was conducted on July 31, 2009 (Friday); the second experiment was conducted on August 7, 2009 (Friday).

Safety precaution

The safety precaution provides information intended to prevent personal injury to the participants, the experiment operators and property damage. During the experiment, the participants seated inside the aircraft cabin simulator for more than 10 h. The aircraft cabin simulator setup is equipped with electrical and electronic equipment such as a computer and a beamer. Subsequently, smoke detectors were

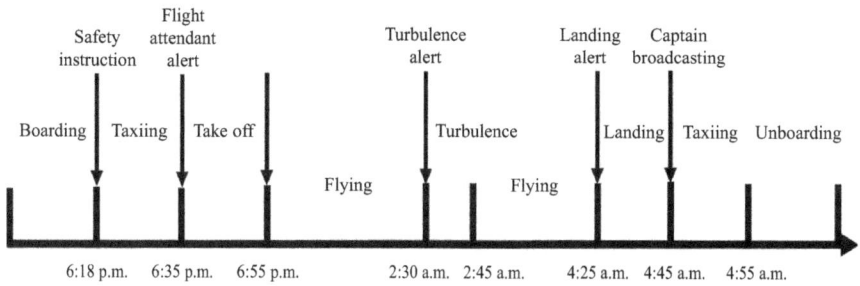

Figure 8.3   Procedure of the flight simulation

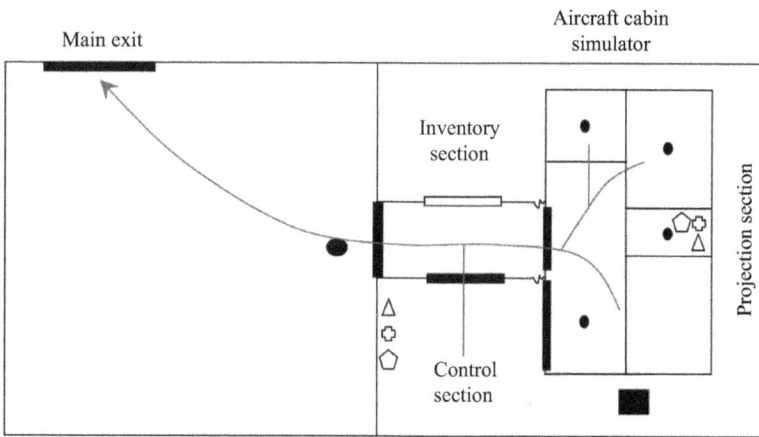

Legend:
⟡ First aid kit   ● Smoke detector
△ Fire extinguisher   ⬠ Telephone

Figure 8.4   The floor plan for emergency evacuation and the location of safety equipment

installed inside the simulator as well as the ceiling of the Simulation Lab. Fire extinguishers and fire blankets were equipped at the control section and inside the simulator. An evacuation plan was also designed for an emergency evacuation. Figure 8.4 shows the evacuation route during emergency as well as the location of the smoke detectors. The university security was informed about the experiment and permission to stay overnight was granted before the experiment started.

Statistical analysis

Applied statistics was used to analyze the questionnaire data. The statistical analysis was carried out with SPSS® version 17.0 for Windows®.

8.2.3.2   Results

The results of the presence questionnaire for 12 participants are described in this section. The raw data analysis of the questionnaire is described in Liu *et al.* [14]. The means and standard deviations of the questionnaire scores are shown in Table 8.5.

Table 8.5   Means (M) and standard deviations (SD) of presence questionnaire

No.	Question	M	SD	N
1	*I had a sense of "being there" in the long haul flight*	4.00	0.74	12
2	*There were times during the experience when the virtual "long haul flight" became more real for me compared to the "real flight"...*	3.75	1.22	12
3	*The laboratory seems to me to be more like...*	3.58	0.79	12
4	*I had a stronger sense of being in...*	3.92	0.79	12
5	*During the experience I often thought that I was really sitting in the laboratory....*	3.50	1.09	12

As referring to Table 8.5, the first question about "*I had a sense of "being there" in the long haul flight*" showed the neutral result (M = 4.000, SD = 0.739). Question 2 is about "*There were times during the experience when the virtual "long haul flight" became more real for me compared to the "real flight"*. The statistical result (M = 3.750, SD = 1.215) showed that the participants tend to experience the real world of the laboratory. Next, the result at Question 3 (M = 3.583, SD = 0.793) showed that the participants think that they felt the simulator is more like the laboratory that they saw than somewhere that they visited. The result of Question 4 (M = 3.917, SD = 0.793) showed that the participants have a stronger sense of being in the real world of the laboratory than in the virtual reality of the long haul flight. Lastly, the result of Question 5 (M = 3.500, SD = 1.087) showed that the participants realized that they were in the laboratory most of the time rather than "never because the long haul flight overwhelmed me".

8.2.3.3   Summary

Based on the results of our presence questionnaire by 12 participants inside the aircraft cabin simulator, they felt that they were experiencing the laboratory environment more than real long haul flight situation. Subsequently, the overall mean ratings (M = 3.750, SD = 0.925) are 0.25 lower than mean rating of neutral (4). The overall result showed that the developed aircraft cabin simulator is able to simulate the average aircraft cabin for research purpose.

8.2.4   Validation experiment for smart neck support system (SNes)

8.2.4.1   Research questions

There are two research questions related to the validation experiment. The first question is to examine subjectively about the comfort experience of the participants with or without the smart neck support system based on the questionnaire. The second question is to examine objectively whether the SNes is able to reduce the SCM muscle stress when supported by our SNes. Both questions are applicable to our treatment group in the validation experiment.

The first question is to examine subjectively about the comfort experiences of the participant with or without the smart neck support system by answering the questionnaire after each experiment (control experiment and treatment experiment).

The second question is to examine whether the SCM EMG values of the participant supported by SNes are lower than without support condition. The result from this hypothesis is important information used to validate the developed smart neck support system subjectively and objectively.

8.2.4.2 Methods

The architecture of the can be roughly sketched as consisting of a bottom sensor layer, a middle network layer and a top application layer. As one of the primary information-acquiring means at the bottom layer of the tags have found increasingly widespread applications in various business areas, with the expectation that the use of RFID tags will eventually replace the existing bar codes in all business areas.

Participant

Three participants ($N = 3$) with no neck pain over the last 3 months were recruited in this experiment. The group consisted of one female and two males aged between 27 and 32 years (mean 29.67 years). They were informed regarding the experiment, which involved questionnaires, sat inside the aircraft cabin simulator for 1 h with SCM electromyography measurement and video recording. The participants were invited for the experiment and were given €20 after completion. The demographic details of the participant are shown in Table 8.6.

Experimental setup

We conducted two experiments inside the aircraft cabin simulator. The location of the experiment is in the simulation laboratory in the main building of the Eindhoven University of Technology. The first experiment was done with the control group where there is no installation of the SNes and the participants had attached EMG electrodes. The first experiment was conducted from 7:00 p.m. to 8:00 p.m. on Friday (first day). The second experiment was done with the treatment group where there is installation of the SNes to the economy class aircraft passenger seat and the participants had attached EMG electrodes. The second experiment was conducted from 7:00 p.m. to 8:00 p.m. after 1 week (second day). Both experiments recruited the same participants and tested under the same experimental conditions. The duration of both experiments is about 1 h. The experimental setup for the treatment group in the aircraft cabin simulator is shown in Figure 8.5.

For observational purposes, CCTVs were installed inside the aircraft cabin simulator. There were two CCTVs used to monitor each participant's activities separately. One CCTV is located in front of the participant and another CCTV is

Table 8.6   Table demographic details of participants

Variable	M	SD	N
Age (years)	29.67	2.52	3
Weight (kg)	64.67	4.51	3
Height (m)	1.72	0.07	3
BMI (kg/m^2)	21.77	0.55	3

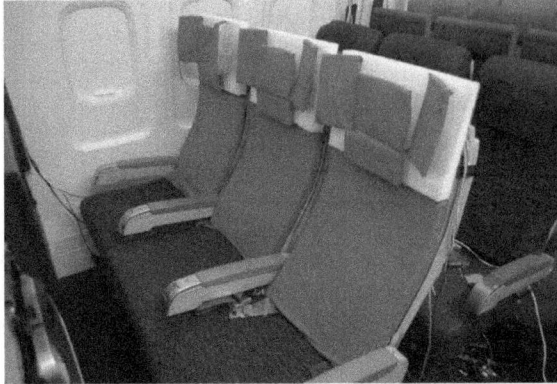

Figure 8.5   The installation of three SNes prototypes in the aircraft cabin simulator for validation experiment with the treatment group

located directly above the head of the participant. There is a CCTV that monitored the overall activities in the cabin.

Questionnaire

A questionnaire was distributed after the experiment with the control group and the experiment with the treatment group. The questionnaire consisted of two sections: (1) questions regarding the comfort factors of the neck support (without SNes in control group, with SNes in treatment group) during the experiment and (2) questions about demographic background. The primary goal of our investigation is to understand the smart neck support effects to the participant after the experiment. The questionnaire had two main parts:

1. The first part examined the comfort factor of the neck support of the economy class aircraft passenger seat during the experiment. It contained 10 questions that evaluated the comfort feeling of the participants during the experiment. Participants could indicate their degree of comfort based on a 9-point Likert scale (1 = "not at all"; 5 = "moderately"; 9 = "extremely").
2. The second part assessed demographic variables of the participants, such as gender, age, height and weight.

Apparatus and data recording

For the first experiment with the control group, the following hardware were used:

- MP150 Biopac system with EMG module (MP150WSW with EMG100C)
- Aircraft cabin simulator
- Personal computer (Intel Pentium Dual Core)
- CCTV (VZOR VMP311)

The specification of the second-hand aircraft passenger seats used in both experiment were as follows:

Product name: Recaro Air Comfort
Model no.: 3010-3
Weight: 29.349 kg
Date of manufacture: July 14, 1981

Next, in order to gather EMG value of the SCM muscle and observe the activity of the participants during the second experiment with the treatment group, different hardware were used. The hardware used during the second experiment were as follows:

- MP150 Biopac system with EMG module (MP150WSW with EMG100C)
- Smart neck support system (SNes)
- Aircraft cabin simulator
- Personal computer (Intel Pentium Dual Core)
- CCTV (VZOR VMP311)

Three smart neck support systems were installed on each aircraft passenger seat inside the aircraft cabin simulator. The computer was used for data logging and video recording. The CCTVs were installed at the front as well as above each participant.

Experimental procedure

Before the experiment with the control group, 15 min of briefing was conducted. Next, the participants were positioned inside the aircraft cabin simulator. After that, the light in the aircraft cabin was dimmed and the participants were advised to rest during the 1-h experiment. The EMG measurement and video recording were conducted on a real-time basis. After 1 h of experiment, the participants were given a questionnaire.

For the experiment with the treatment group, we started the experiment with 45 min of briefing to the participants and the attachment of electrodes on the SCM muscles. After that, we positioned the participants on the economy class aircraft passenger seats. The aircraft passenger seat sitting positions were classified as aisle seat, center seat, and window seat. Next, the light in the aircraft cabin was dimmed and the participants were advised to rest during the 1-h experiment. The EMG signals of the participants were monitored and recorded in parallel with system logging and video recording. The validation experiment setup in the aircraft cabin simulator is shown in Figure 8.6. After the experiment, the EMG electrodes were detached from the participants and a questionnaire was given to each participant. Lastly, debriefing was conducted and each participant was paid with a token of appreciation.

Signal acquisition and processing

The normalized EMG activity was analyzed. Normalization of EMG activity was performed for each participant individually. To measure the MVC of SCM muscle, the participant's head was turned to the maximum head rotation angle.

Data analysis

For the recorded normalized EMG data, the data with the complete cycle were selected for further analysis. The complete cycle is the cycle from (1) SNes detects the participant's head, (2) the support of the participant's head, and (3) the deactivation of SNes when the participant's head is away. The selection of the normalized EMG data is based on the data log information. The data log is recording

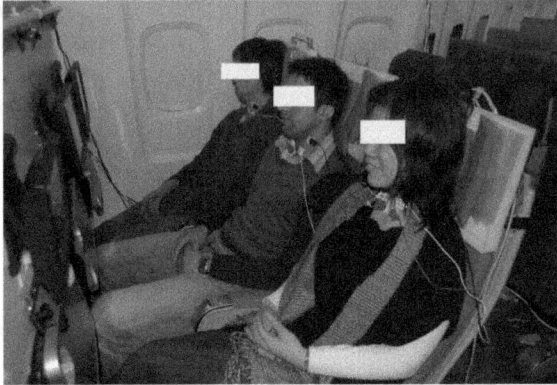

Figure 8.6   The experimental setup of participants for the treatment group in the aircraft cabin simulator

the time when the system is activated and the time when the system is deactivated. The data log with complete cycles of airbag activity will be selected for further analysis. The complete cycle was described as (1) the participant's head is in touch with the airbag; (2) after time *t* the airbag is inflated and supports the participant's neck; and (3) the participant is not in touch with the airbag, the airbag will be deflated. The data with incomplete cycles will be ignored. The selected average normalized EMG value was used for statistical analysis. For the statistical analysis, the time domain was divided into 10 time intervals where 1 time interval represents 1 min. The normalized EMG values were then averaged over 5 sec blocks in each time interval. Hence, each 1 min time interval has twelve 5 sec blocks. The average normalized EMG value was further analyzed with statistical method. A descriptive statistical method was used to analyze the questionnaire about comfort factors as well as to examine differences before support by SNes and after support by SNes.

Limitation
The validation experiment was conducted on SNes inside the aircraft cabin simulator. The experiment was conducted in the static aircraft cabin like environment. Thus, some important factors such as accelerations and air pressure like the real aircraft environment could not be addressed. In addition, the aircraft passenger seat used was a second-hand aircraft seat, which has been used for almost 29 years. Besides, there was no sleeping activity among the participants. For control group, only questionnaire data were available.

8.2.4.3   Results
The results from the questionnaire distinguished between the experiment with the control group and the experiment with the treatment group. The means and standard deviations of the questionnaire scores are shown in Table 8.7. Both groups use

Table 8.7   The questionnaire scores for the two groups (control and treatment)

Group	N	M	SD
Control	30	5.10	1.37
Treatment	30	5.60	1.63

Table 8.8   The comfort factor scores related to the control group and treatment group

No.	Comfort factors	N	Control group M	Control group SD	Treatment group M	Treatment group SD
1	Good neck support	3	3.67	2.31	5.67	3.22
2	Relax	3	5.00	0.00	4.67	1.53
3	Seat cushion firmness	3	5.33	1.16	5.00	2.65
4	Restful	3	4.67	1.16	5.00	1.73
5	No stiffness	3	4.67	0.58	5.33	0.58
6	No sore muscles	3	4.67	1.16	5.33	1.16
7	No fatigue	3	5.67	2.31	7.00	1.00
8	No neck strained	3	5.00	1.73	6.00	2.00
9	Fit	3	6.33	0.58	5.67	0.58
10	Comfortable	3	6.00	1.00	6.33	1.53
	Total		5.10	1.37	5.60	1.63

the mean score across the 10 questions. The mean scores from the statistical results showed that the mean scores for the treatment group (M = 5.60, SD = 1.63) is higher than for the control group (M = 5.10, SD = 1.37).

The means and standard deviations of the comfort factor scores are shown in Table 8.8. We found that the comfort factors, such as "good neck support" (control group: M = 3.67, SD = 2.31; treatment group: M = 5.67, SD = 3.22), "restful" (control group: M = 4.67, SD = 1.16; treatment group: M = 5.00, SD = 1.73), "no stiffness" (control group: M = 4.67, SD = 0.58; treatment group: M = 5.33, SD = 0.58), "no sore muscles" (control group: M = 4.67, SD = 1.16; treatment group: M = 5.3, SD = 1.16), "no fatigue" (control group: M = 5.67, SD = 2.31; treatment group: M = 7.00, SD = 1.00), "no strained" (control group: M = 5.00, SD = 1.73; treatment group: M = 6.00, SD = 2.00) and "comfortable" (control group: M = 6.00, SD = 1.00; treatment group: M = 6.33, SD = 1.53) show the increase of mean ratings for comfort in the treatment group. Subsequently, there are three comfort factors that show the decrease of mean ratings, these are "relax" (control group: M = 5.00, SD = 0.00; treatment group: M = 4.67, SD = 1.53), "seat cushion firmness" (control group: M = 5.33, SD = 1.16; treatment group: M = 5.00, SD = 2.65), and "fit" (control group: M = 6.00, SD = 1.00; treatment group: M = 5.67,

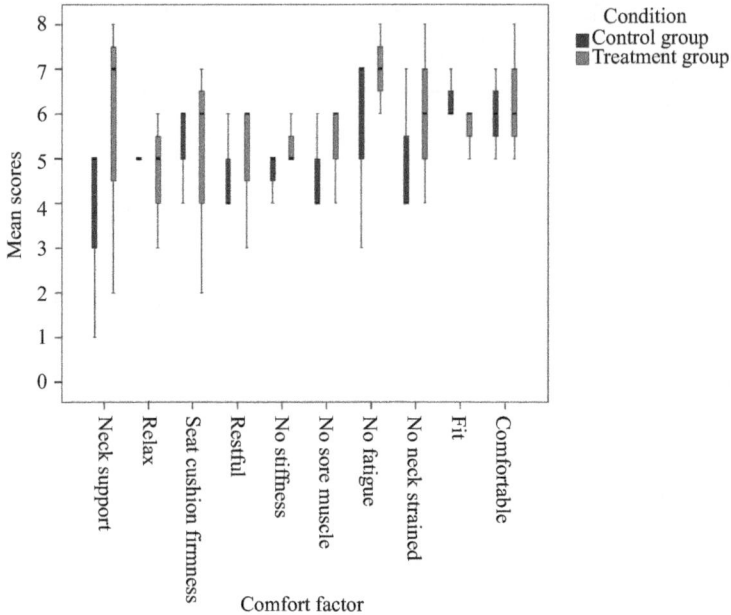

Figure 8.7   The box plot of comfort factors for the control group and the treatment group

Table 8.9   The normalized EMG values for the two test conditions

Test condition	N	M	SD
Before supported by SNes	30	3.03	2.31
After supported by SNes	30	2.82	2.13

SD = 0.58). The mean ratings on the comfort experiences for the experiment with control group and experiment with treatment group are shown in Figure 8.7.

After the experiment with the treatment group, the results from EMG measurements were selected and analyzed. The mean scores of the normalized EMG value after supported by SNes (M = 2.82, SD = 2.13) are lower than the mean scores of the normalized EMG value for before supported by SNes (M = 3.03, SD = 2.31). The means and standard deviations of the normalized EMG value for the two test conditions are shown in Table 8.9. The mean scores of the normalized EMG value after supported by SNes are also lower than the mean scores of the normalized EMG value before supported by SNes. The mean scores for each participant are shown in Table 8.10. The mean scores of the normalized EMG value for the participants in relation with neck support activity are shown in Figure 8.8.

Therefore, H_0 can be rejected and H_1 is selected for hypothesis 2.

Table 8.10   The normalized EMG values for each participant separately

Test condition	N	P1		P2		P3	
		M	**SD**	**M**	**SD**	**M**	**SD**
Before supported by SNes	30	4.93	1.39	3.56	2.81	1.41	0.35
After supported by SNes	30	4.38	1.21	3.37	2.68	1.37	0.35

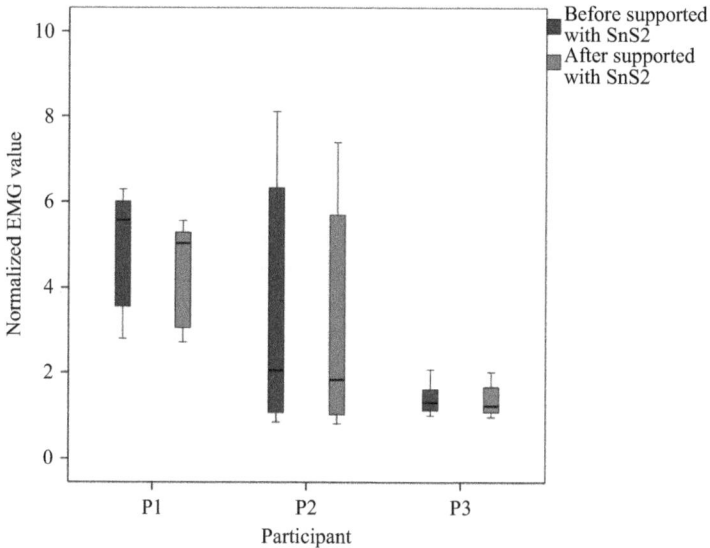

Figure 8.8   The box plot of normalized EMG value for the participants in relation to both neck conditions (before supported by SnS2 and after supported by SnS2)

8.3   Discussion and conclusion

This experiment validated the developed SNes. The major findings from the validation experiment were:

- The mean ratings of a sitting participant in experience on the seat with SNes demonstrate more comfort than without SNes.
- The mean ratings of a sitting participant SCM EMG value supported by SNes are lower than without support condition.

The questionnaire was used for the experiment with the control group as well as the treatment group. The participants evaluated the SNes based on their experience during the experiment. The mean scores of comfort factors for the treatment group are higher than for the control group. The result shows that the seat enhanced with

SNes is able to improve the subjective comfort experience while sitting. Out of ten comfort factors, there were seven comfort factors that showed the increased of mean ratings such as "good neck support," "restful," "no stiffness," "no sore muscles," "no fatigue," "no neck strained," and "comfortable." Three comfort factors presented lower mean ratings, i.e., "relax," "seat cushion firmness," and "fit." The developed SNes prototype demonstrated comfort improvement in seven comfort factors and decrease of comfort experience in three comfort factors.

For the second result, we tested the SCM participants with EMG measurement to validate the SNes objectively. The result from the experiment showed that the SNes is able to reduce the SCM muscle stress. The developed SNes is able to adapt to the participant's neck posture automatically and provides the necessary neck support to reduce the SCM muscle stress.

The EMG measurements of the SCM muscle demonstrated that the developed SNes provides support to the participant's neck as well as reduces the SCM muscle stress. The experiment was conducted in the aircraft cabin simulator and tested in the same environment for both experiments. The result from the questionnaire proved that the participants feel subjectively more comfortable with a seat equipped with SNes. For the experiment with the treatment group, the SCM EMG measurement showed that the SCM EMG value was reduced objectively when it is supported by SNes. The EMG value is lower when both SCM muscles are supported by SNes. The result from the validation experiment is in parallel with the findings in the calibration experiment. It can be proved that the developed SNes is able to improve the comfort experience and to reduce the SCM muscle stress.

References

[1]   Brundrett, G., 2001. Comfort and health in commercial aircraft: a literature review. The Journal of the Royal Society for the Promotion of Health, 121(1): 29–37.

[2]   World Health Organization, 2007. Travel by air: health considerations. World Health Organization. http://whqlibdoc.who.int/publications/2005/9241580364_chap2.pdf.

[3]   Runkle, V.A., 1994. Benchmarking seat comfort. SAE Technical Paper, No. 940217.

[4]   Quigley, C., D. Southall, M. Freer, A. Moody and M. Porter, 2001. Anthropometric study to update minimum aircraft seating standards. EC1270, ICE Ergonomics Ltd.

[5]   Hinninghofen, H., P. Enck, 2006. Passenger well-being in airplanes. Auton Neurosci, 129(1–2): 80–85.

[6]   Helander, M.G., 2003. Forget about ergonomics in chair design? Focus on aesthetics and comfort! Ergonomics, 46(43/14): 1306–1319.

[7]   De Looze, M.P., L.F.M. Kuijt and J.V. Eversand Dieen, 2003. Sitting comfort and discomfort and the relationship with objective measures. Ergonomics, 46(10): 985–997.

[8] Helander, M.G. and L. Zhang, 1997. Field studies of comfort and discomfort in sitting. Ergonomics, 20(9):865–915.

[9] Shen, W. and A. Vertiz, 1997. Redefining seat comfort. SAE Technical Paper, no. 970597.

[10] Viano, D.C. and D.V. Andrzejak, 1992. Research Issues on the Bio-mechanics of Seating Discomfort: An Overview with Focus on Issues of the Elderly and Low-Back Pain. SAE Technical Paper, no. 920130.

[11] Zhang, L., M.G. Helander and C.G. Drury, 1996. Identifying factors of comfort and discomfort in sitting. Human Factors, 38(3): 377–389.

[12] Kolich, M., 2008. Review: A conceptual framework proposed to formalize the scientific investigation of automobile seat comfort. Applied Ergonomics, 39(1): 15–27.

[13] Usoh, M., E. Catena, S. Arman and M. Slater, 2000. Using presence questionnaires in reality. Presecence-Teleoperators and Virtual Environments, 9(5): 497–503.

[14] Liu, H., C.F. Tan, J. Hu, and M. Rauterberg, 2010. Towards high level of presence: combining static infrastructure with dynamic services. Proceedings of International Conference on Electronics and Information Engineering, Kyoto, Japan, pp. V2-535–V2-539.

[15] Witmer, B.G., M.J. Singer, 1998. Measuring presence in virtual environments: a presence questionnaire. Presence, 7(3): 225–240.

Chapter 9

Brain signal classification using normalisation

James Henshaw[1], Wei Liu[2], and Daniela M. Romano[3]

9.1 Introduction to brain signal classification

This chapter introduces methods of brain signal classification and explores situations where it may be improved through the use of normalisation. Brain signal classification is where one makes inferences about the cognitive state of a user based upon the analysis of their brain signal activity, whilst normalisation refers to methods of reducing certain differences between the interpretations of these cognitive states in order to improve accuracy. Brain signal classification is used in a variety of contexts, including: brain–computer interfaces (BCIs), where the user's brain activity is used to interact with external devices, such as computer games or assistive devices; medical applications, which allow diagnoses to be made using machine-learning techniques; and neurofeedback devices, which provide real-time representations of the user's brain activity.

This chapter focuses on BCI brain signal classification. BCI classification is a multistep process (Figure 9.1), which includes:

- **Brain signal acquisition:** This refers to the brain imaging method used to acquire the brain signal, such as electroencephalography (EEG), functional magnetic resonance imaging (fMRI), or near-infrared spectroscopy (NIRS).
- **Preprocessing:** During the preprocessing step, various signal processing methods such as digital filtering and artefact removal methods are applied in order to improve signal quality.
- **Feature extraction:** During this step useful features in the signal associated with the user's cognitive state are extracted.
- **Classification:** This involves using the extracted features to make predictions about the user's current cognitive state. This can involve machine-learning techniques or other detection algorithms.
- **Device control:** This step, commonly known as 'translation', involves converting the classifier outputs into a form usable by the external device, thereby allowing direct communication between the user and the device.

[1]Division of Neuroscience and Experimental Psychology, University of Manchester, United Kingdom
[2]University of Sheffield, Department of Electronic and Electrical Engineering, Sheffield, United Kingdom
[3]University College London, Department of Information Studies, London, United Kingdom

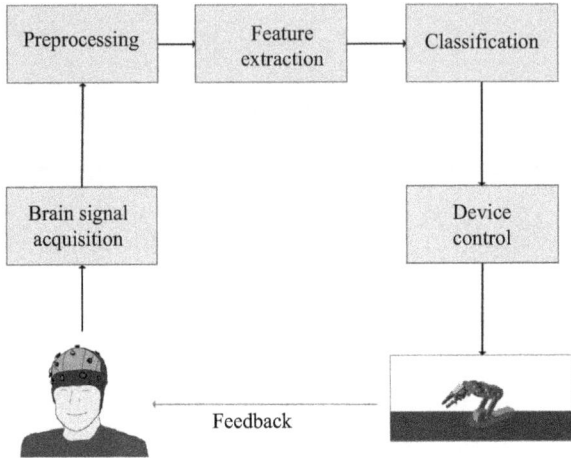

Figure 9.1   BCI brain signal classification process

- **Feedback:** Real-time feedback is essential in order to maximise the user's performance, as it allows them to make adjustments to their strategies where appropriate.

Specifically, this chapter will focus on accurately classifying the steady-state visually evoked potential (SSVEP) response, the brain's natural response to a repetitive visual stimulus (RVS), which is described in Section 9.1.1.

9.1.1   The SSVEP response

The SSVEP neural response is an involuntary response that occurs when the user fixes their gaze on an RVS, such as a flashing light with a fixed flicker rate, and causes a group of neurons to output a signal matching the stimulus frequency that continues for the duration of the gaze. Elicited SSVEP responses have been detected ranging from 1 to 90 Hz [1], and are best detected by electrodes placed over the occipital and parietal lobes [2]. SSVEP–BCIs have several major advantages over other BCI types, such as their high signal-to-noise ratio (SNR), short training times, and high classification accuracies. As a result, they have been used as part of many different BCI applications, including: BCI-controlled wheelchairs [3,4], BCI-controlled exoskeletons [5,6], and BCI-controlled robotic humanoids [7]. The SSVEP response has a wave-like spatial structure [8] and can be detected using a number of methods, which are outlined in the following sections.

9.1.2   Normalisation

BCI performance is generally measured in terms of misclassification rate or information transfer rate (ITR), which assesses the BCI's speed based on both its accuracy and available number of commands. As noted in [9], an uneven distribution in classification accuracy between classes leads to a skewed performance – users are able to perform some actions easily and may not be able to perform others accurately. This can lead to an increased number of false positives in the selected class. Whilst this reduces BCI performance overall, it is not always reflected in the results, as the ITR equation does not take this mismatch into account [9], and the user may attempt to avoid classes that are performing badly.

This problem is a major issue in SSVEP–BCIs as low-frequency SSVEPs tend to have more power than high-frequency SSVEPs, so regardless of the detection method used, there is always a natural mismatch between classes. We can solve this problem by using *normalisation*, a method where a transform is applied that minimises these differences, making it easier to correctly classify these signals. As we shall see, there are a number of different approaches for SSVEP detection and classification, as well as a number of different corresponding normalisation methods. This chapter reviews work conducted into SSVEP normalisation and performs direct comparisons of normalisation methods that exist for the major SSVEP detection methods, allowing researchers to effectively choose which approach to take.

9.2 SSVEP detection methods

9.2.1 Correlation-based classification

Several BCI classification methods exist that use the correlation between the EEG signal and predefined templates to classify EEG trials. The most popular of these methods is canonical correlation analysis (CCA) [10], which has also been further extended into several different methods, including filter bank CCA [11] and multiset CCA [12]. The main advantages of CCA for SSVEP classification are that it requires no calibration data, and produces results with a high classification accuracy.

Implementing CCA for SSVEP classification has several requirements: the multichannel EEG signal is separated into trials, and a set of sine wave templates of the same length as the trial (in samples) are created. These templates are matrices where each row contains a sine wave. These sine waves increase in multiples of the stimulus frequency as the row number increases. As an example, if we wished to create a sine wave template for 7.5 Hz with two harmonics, we would create a three-row matrix containing sine waves of 7.5, 15, and 22.5 Hz. It is important to select stimulus frequencies carefully in order to avoid harmonic interference, which occurs when the harmonics from two or more classes are equal. For example, using a 6- and 12-Hz RVS together would cause a higher probability of misclassification as the 6-Hz RVS would trigger both a 6- and 12-Hz SSVEP response. Sine wave templates are created for all the possible target stimulus frequencies, and each channel of the EEG trial is centred around zero by removing the mean, usually using a bandpass filter. When bandpass filtering, the passband range must include all target stimulus frequencies and their harmonics, meaning the sampling rate must be at least two times greater than this. CCA works by taking two multidimensional variables and finding the underlying correlation between them. This technique can be used with EEG data to perform unsupervised SSVEP detection [12–16]. Taking two multidimensional variables X and Y with weighted linear combinations $x = X^T W_X$ and $y = Y^T W_Y$, the weight vectors W_X and W_Y which maximise the correlation between x and y are found using CCA. Solving the following optimisation problem accomplishes this:

$$\max_{W_X,W_Y} \rho(x,y) = \frac{E[xy]}{\sqrt{E[xx]E[yy]}} = \frac{E\left[W_X^T X Y^T W_Y\right]}{\sqrt{E\left[W_X^T X X^T W_X\right]E\left[W_Y^T Y Y^T W_Y\right]}},$$

where $E[x]$ is the expected value of x, and ρ is the correlation value, which is maximised with respect to weight vectors W_X and W_Y, thereby calculating the canonical correlation between X and Y.

During SSVEP detection, $X \in R^{C \times S}$ is the multidimensional EEG signal with C channels and S samples. $Y_f \in R^{2N_h \times S}$ is the set of multidimensional reference signals based on stimulus frequency f, with $2N_h$ individual sine waves and S samples, where N_h is the number of harmonics. The sine waves are assembled into a matrix [15]:

$$Y_f = \begin{bmatrix} \sin(2\pi f t) \\ \cos(2\pi f t) \\ \cdots \\ \sin(2\pi N_h f t) \\ \cos(2\pi N_h f t) \end{bmatrix},$$

where t is the time in seconds. This action can be performed on MATLAB® using the *canoncorr()* function. By performing CCA on X and Y for all f, the stimulation frequency with the maximal canonical correlation value can be identified, which is selected as the estimated SSVEP frequency.

9.2.2   Power-based classification

Transforming the EEG signal from the temporal domain into the frequency domain (by way of the discrete Fourier transform (DFT)) allows access to a number of frequency domain feature extraction methods. Power spectral density (PSD) features are the most commonly used, and while they have lost popularity to CCA-based methods in recent years, they are still regularly used in SSVEP–BCIs. However, a comparison study of SSVEP–BCI methods found CCA to be around twice as effective as PSD when using a small (1 s) time window of data [17]. PSD feature extraction is a relatively straightforward, three-step process:

1. The multichannel EEG signal is separated into trials and transformed into the frequency domain using the DFT, which is calculated using a fast Fourier transform (FFT) algorithm. For each trial the EEG signal is transformed into an array of FFT coefficients at each available frequency.
2. The FFT coefficients at each of the target frequencies (or as close as possible) are extracted and squared to create PSD features [9].
3. At this point, some dimensionality reduction may be required, as feature vectors/matrices will be of the size $C \times N$, where C is the number of EEG channels and N is the number of stimulus frequencies. A variety of methods can be used, including channel selection, channel averaging, or combining channels based on some pre-determined criteria.

The end result is a feature vector with a PSD feature at each stimulus frequency for each trial. These features can then be translated through a variety of methods such as autoregressive, or machine-learning methods. Machine-learning methods, which we will focus on, involve training a classifier to predict future outputs based on labelled training (calibration) data, a process known as supervised learning; or categorising and predicting future inputs without the use of training data, known as unsupervised learning. Many of the popular supervised methods from BCI research, such as support vector machines (SVM) and linear discriminant analysis (LDA), are designed for two-class classification, where features extracted from both frequencies are plotted against one another in order to plot a hyperplane that separates class one from class two, and can be used to predict future inputs based upon the feature's location in two-dimensional space. However, this can be extended to multi-class classification either through: one-versus-one classification, where a single classifier is trained and evaluated for every possible class combination, and the winning class is decided based on a voting criteria; or one-versus-rest (OVR) classification, where a classifier is trained for each class, against data from all other classes.

9.3   Previous work

The majority of previous work conducted into SSVEP normalisation has used PSD features. Additionally, the normalisation aspect is often a secondary factor, used as part of the study design rather than as a topic of investigation. Nakanishi *et al.* [16] devised an unsupervised normalisation method for CCA that uses information from background frequencies to reduce the disparities between SSVEPs from different frequencies. Their method calculates the CCA correlation coefficients for background EEG activity within neighbouring frequency bands, and summed them before dividing the CCA correlation coefficient at the target frequency by this, creating a ratio value similar to SNR. Testing the technique on an offline EEG dataset ($n = 13$) for eight frequencies (8–15 Hz, $\Delta f = 1$ Hz), this method was found to significantly increase accuracy when compared to standard CCA (84.89% vs 80.08%), and improved detection accuracy for the higher frequency SSVEPs more when compared to the lower frequency SSVEPs. Castillo *et al.* [18] devised a similar method in their study ($n = 19$), where they used PSD features to create a ratio, this time using signal amplitude and 'error', where error is the absolute difference between the peak frequency in the power spectrum and the amplitude at the target frequency. The authors reported an increase in accuracy compared to standard PSD (90.42% vs 84.13%).

The remaining featured studies used normalisation as part of the study design and therefore do not include a comparison to standard CCA or PSD. Sakurada *et al.* [19] applied normalisation while investigating the classification of high-frequency SSVEPs. In their online study, which used a three-class BCI with PSD features ($n = 12$), a baseline was calculated for each class by taking the average spectrum power at the target frequency during the 2-s pre-trial fixation period. From these data, a 'normalised amplitude' (NA) was created, by first calculating the SNR between the stimulus frequency and its pre-trial fixation baseline, and then subtracting from this the SNRs of the opposing classes (which were calculated in an identical manner). If a class's NA exceeded a predetermined threshold (1) while the opposing NAs all failed to exceed a predetermined threshold (0.5), then that class was selected as the output. This normalisation method was found to work effectively, with most participants showing accuracies over 80%. Finally, Diez *et al.* [20] performed a small-scale offline BCI study ($n = 5$) where participants gazed at four RVS (13–16 Hz, $\Delta f = 1$ Hz), with results scaled against a baseline calculated during a 60-s resting period prior to the RVS display portion of the experiment. These methods were found to perform adequately, with average accuracies above 73% in each of the investigated conditions, and were applied in further work [21].

9.4   Comparison of normalisation methods

In our own work we took 17 participants and set up an offline SSVEP experiment that allowed us to conduct multiple types of analyses on the data. During the experiment, participants viewed an RVS containing eight frequencies (6.66, 7.5, 8.57, 10, 12, 15, 20, and 30 Hz) arranged in a 3×3 structure (Figure 9.2), whilst 30 min of neural activity was recorded using a 20-channel Enobio EEG system with NaCl electrodes, producing a total of 30 trials per class. Data were downsampled to 250 Hz and bandpass filtered between 1 and 49 Hz, using a zero-phase Butterworth filter with 2 s of padding on each side of the time window. Further analysis was conducted to compare various CCA-based and PSD-based normalisation methods. Due to the high SNR of the SSVEP response, no artefact removal

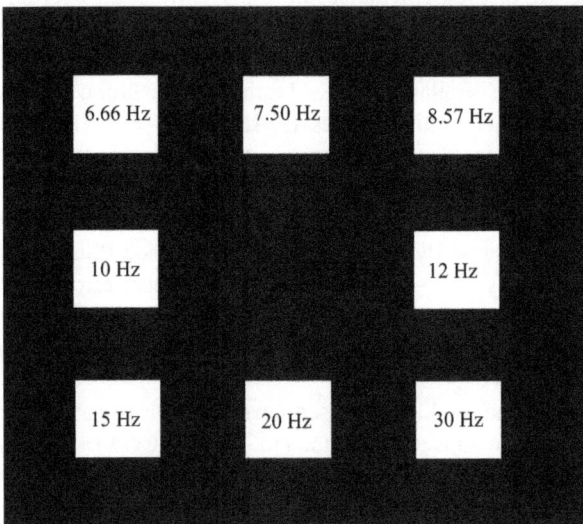

Figure 9.2   RVS stimulator layout

methods were applied. For both the CCA and PSD analysis, three conditions were used: Low frequency (6.66, 7.5, 8.57, and 12 Hz), medium frequency (8.57, 12, 15, and 20 Hz), and wide-range frequency (6.66, 8.57, 12, and 30 Hz). These were selected based on the fact that the harmonics would not interfere with each other, and to see the effects of normalisation in different conditions.

9.4.1 Comparison: CCA-based normalisation

Three CCA-based methods were compared: Standard CCA and CCA with two proposed normalisation methods [22]. The CCA-based normalisation methods we proposed used the pre-trial fixation period to calculate a correlation baseline for normalisation, termed 'baseline ρ', which was calculated using:

$$baseline\ \rho = \frac{1}{K}\sum_{i=1}^{K}\rho(w_i, Y_f)$$

where K denotes the number of time windows used and w_i denotes the ith time window of data. In this study overlapping 1-s time windows offset from -1 to -0.2 s pre-trial ($\Delta t = 0.2$ s) were used to calculate baseline ρ before averaging. Feature extraction was performed using 1-s of EEG data, taken 1 s after stimulus onset. Three CCA-based methods were compared:

1. **Standard CCA** (Figure 9.3), which is just CCA with no normalisation methods applied.

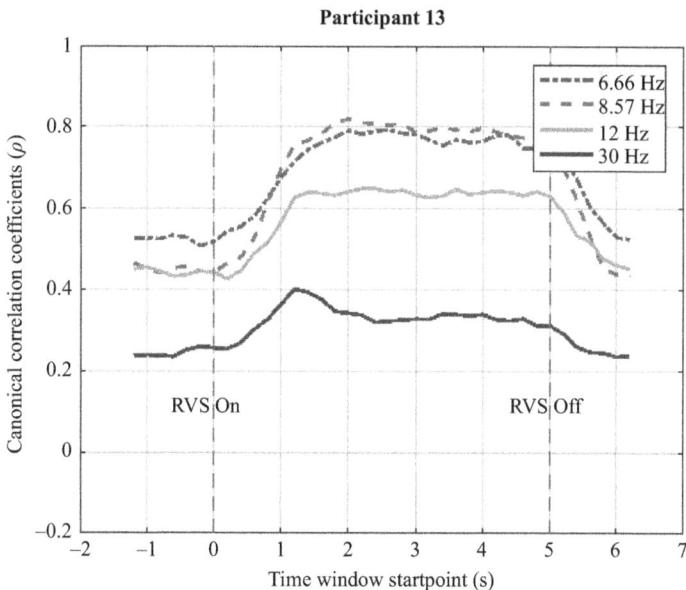

Figure 9.3 Standard CCA canonical correlation coefficients

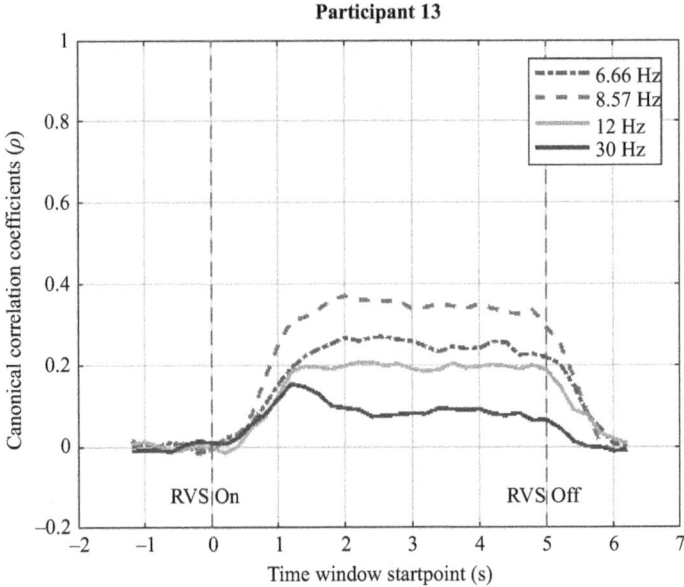

Figure 9.4   BC-CCA canonical correlation coefficients

2. **Baseline-corrected CCA (BC-CCA)** (Figure 9.4), which subtracts the pre-fixation baseline ρ from the standard CCA, using:

$$BC\text{-}CCA = \rho(x, Y_f) - baseline\ \rho$$

where $\rho(x, Y_f)$ gives the canonical correlation between a single trial x and a single sine wave template Y_f.

3. **Scaled CCA** (Figure 9.5), which divides the pre-fixation baseline ρ from the standard CCA, using:

$$scaled\ CCA = \frac{\rho(x, Y_f)}{baseline\ \rho}.$$

Figures 9.3–9.5 show the CCA coefficients from the wide-range frequency condition for a single participant, plotted at 0.2-s intervals and averaged across 30 trials for standard CCA, BC-CCA, and scaled CCA, respectively. Three analyses were run, which were four-class classifications from either the low-frequency, medium frequency, or wide-range frequency conditions (Table 9.1). Each group of classes were analysed using each normalisation method (Figure 9.6).

Overall, in the low-frequency condition, Standard CCA gave a slight improvement to both normalisation methods (+0.49%); however, both BC-CCA and scaled CCA outperformed it in the other conditions. BC-CCA was found to outperform standard CCA by 7.26% in the medium frequency condition, and 9.22% in the wide-range frequency condition (Table 9.2).

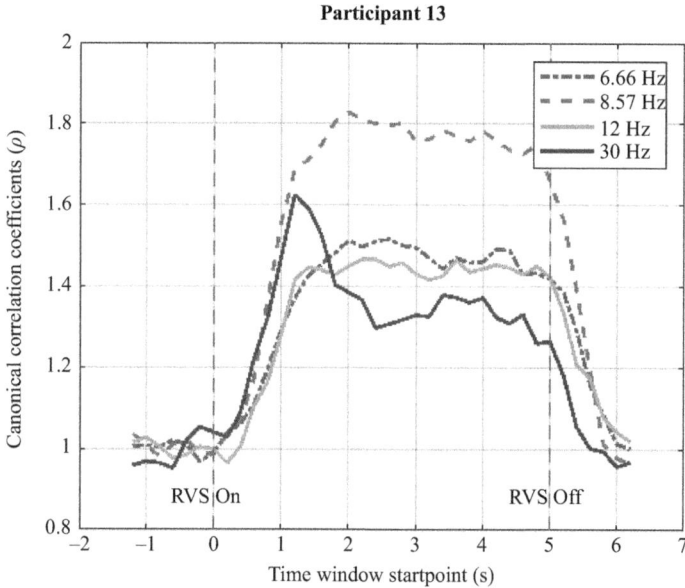

Figure 9.5   Scaled CCA canonical correlation coefficients

Table 9.1   *Different frequency conditions*

Condition	Freq. 1	Freq. 2	Freq. 3	Freq. 4	Range
Low	6.66 Hz	7.5 Hz	8.57 Hz	12 Hz	5.34 Hz
Medium	8.57 Hz	12 Hz	15 Hz	20 Hz	11.43 Hz
Wide range	6.66 Hz	8.57 Hz	12 Hz	30 Hz	23.43 Hz

9.4.2   Comparison: PSD-based normalisation

PSD-based normalisation was carried out using near-identical settings to the CCA normalisation. Feature extraction was performed similarly, however, instead of baseline ρ a baseline of the PSD coefficients was used. Three feature extraction methods were used:

1. **Standard PSD** (Figure 9.7), which uses the PSD coefficients without applying any normalisation methods.
2. **Baseline-corrected PSD (BC-PSD)** (Figure 9.8), which subtracts the pre-fixation baseline standard PSD coefficients at the target time, using:

$$BC\text{-}PSD = PSD - baseline\ PSD$$

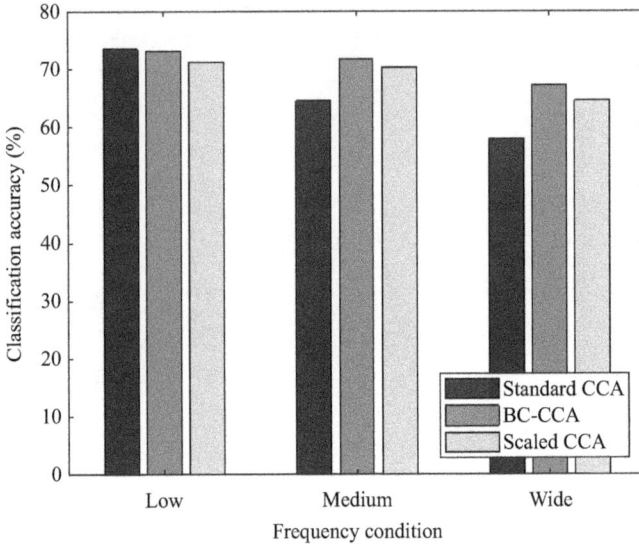

Figure 9.6   Mean accuracy across conditions

Table 9.2   CCA normalisation: mean accuracy across conditions

Condition	Standard CCA (%)	BC-CCA (%)	Scaled CCA (%)
Low	73.48	72.99	71.13
Medium	64.46	71.72	70.20
Wide range	57.84	67.06	64.41

3. **Scaled PSD** (Figure 9.9), which divides the pre-fixation baseline PSD from the standard PSD coefficients, using:

$$Scaled\ PSD = \frac{PSD}{Baseline\ PSD}$$

Similarly to the CCA analysis, data were downsampled to 250 Hz and separated into groups: low frequency, medium frequency, and high frequency. PSD coefficients for each class were found using a 1-s time window ($n = 1{,}024$) using the Hamming window to calculate the FFT coefficients. The squared absolute value of the FFT coefficients was then taken to find the PSD coefficients at any given point. Baseline PSD was found by averaging the PSD coefficients from the pre-fixation period from -1 to -0.2 s ($\Delta t = 0.2$) before stimulus onset. This time, feature extraction was performed using 3 s of data, originating 1 s after stimulus

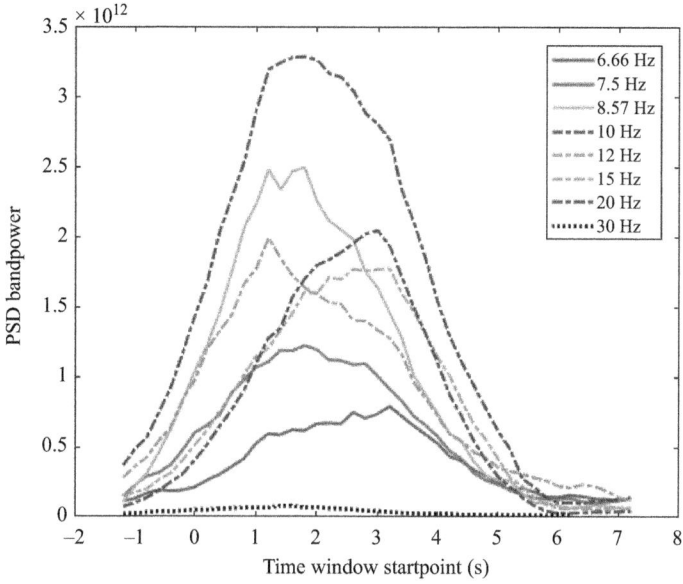

Figure 9.7   Standard PSD

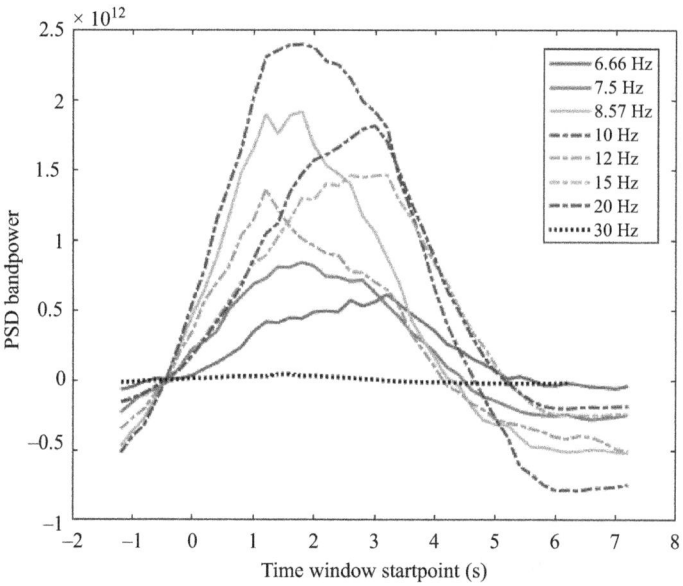

Figure 9.8   BC-PSD

onset. Classification was performed using SVM multi-class OVR classifier. Due to the requirement for training data, k-fold 10×10 cross-validation accuracy was used.

Classification using PSD features extracted from a longer time window length than CCA produced a lower overall accuracy (Figure 9.10), with the highest accuracies found in the medium frequency class (Table 9.3).

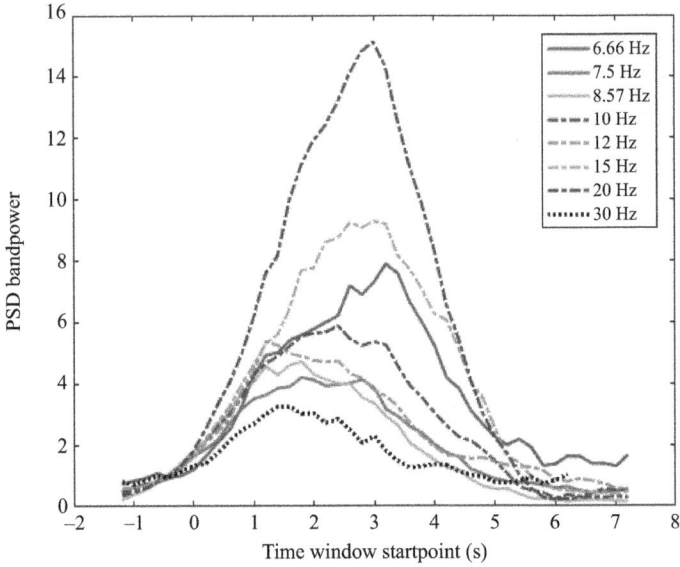

Figure 9.9   Scaled PSD

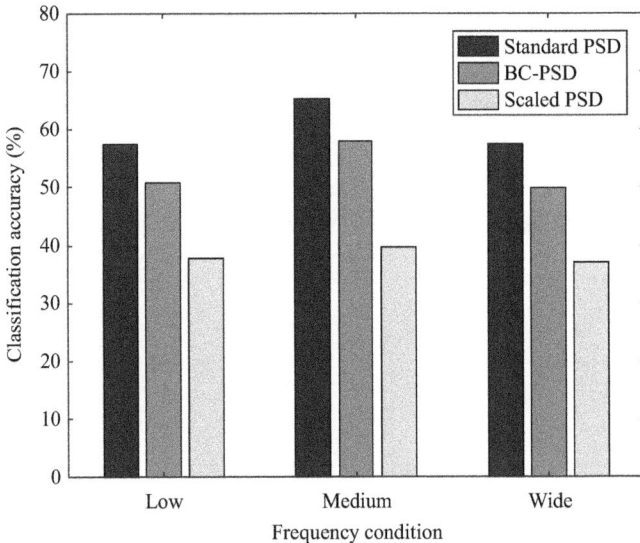

Figure 9.10   PSD feature accuracy (10 × 10 cross-validation)

Table 9.3 *PSD normalisation: mean accuracy across conditions*

Condition	Standard PSD (%)	BC-PSD (%)	Scaled PSD (%)
Low	57.34	50.82	37.79
Medium	65.26	57.85	39.58
Wide range	57.50	49.93	37.04

9.5 Discussion

Normalisation was found to be effective for CCA-based SSVEP BCIs, with its effectiveness increasing as the distance between stimulus frequencies increased. CCA-based normalisation was found to be the most effective, with BC-CCA improving upon standard CCA by 7.26% in the medium frequency condition, and by 9.22% in the wide-range condition, whilst scaled CCA improved accuracy by 5.74% and 6.57% in those conditions, respectively. CCA-based normalisation appears to reduce the difference in CCA conditions, making it more likely for weaker high-frequency SSVEP responses such as those at 20 and 30 Hz to avoid misclassification. As shown in the averaged plot of standard CCA coefficients (Figure 9.3), the 30-Hz peak generally falls beneath the resting baseline of other lower frequencies, making the chance of a false-negative misclassification very high. A slight decrease in accuracy against standard CCA was found in the low-frequency condition for both BC-CCA (−0.49%) and scaled CCA (−2.35%). CCA normalisation effectiveness increases as the range between frequencies increases, suggesting that the normalisation worked as expected.

The same normalisation strategies were not found to be effective in PSD-based BCIs. As with the CCA-based methods, scaled PSD was found to be the weaker of the two normalisation methods across all three conditions. BC-PSD performance was weaker than standard PSD in the low, medium, and wide-range frequency conditions (−6.51%, −7.42%, and −7.57%, respectively). Additionally, as expected PSD-based methods were much less effective than CCA-based methods in all conditions.

This work highlights the improvements that can be made with correctly applied normalisation methods, and using a direct comparison further highlights the difference in effectiveness between CCA- and PSD-based SSVEP detection. It is possible that the reason the baseline-corrected normalisation method outperformed the scaled normalisation method so consistently is that the baseline-corrected methods retain the shape of the coefficients over time, which is particularly important in CCA where the original CCA method is already effective. Scaled methods effectively apply a penalty based upon the baseline activity; SSVEPs with a low baseline activity are increased exponentially the closer this baseline is to zero.

9.6 Summary

Normalisation is a powerful and under-utilised method for improving performance in applications using brain signal classification. Review of studies applying normalisation demonstrated the value of normalisation and the variety of effective methods that can be used to apply it. Novel normalisation methods inspired by these approaches were devised and tested for SSVEP classification using CCA and PSD features. Of these, CCA-based normalisation was found to be the most effective methods, with BC-CCA making the greatest improvement to Standard CCA.

References

[1]   C. S. Herrmann. Human EEG responses to 1–100 Hz flicker: Resonance phenomena in visual cortex and their potential correlation to cognitive phenomena. *Experimental Brain Research*, 137(3–4):346–353, 2001.

[2]   G R Burkitt, R B Silberstein, P J Cadusch, and A W Wood. Steady-state visual evoked potentials and travelling waves. *Clinical Neurophysiology: Official Journal of the International Federation of Clinical Neurophysiology*, 111(2):246–258, 2000.

[3]   Sandra Mara Torres Müller and Teodiano Freire Bastos-filho. Brain-computer interface based on visual evoked potentials to command autonomous robotic wheelchair. *Journal of Medical and Biological Engineering*, 30(6):407–416, 2010.

[4]   Gerolf Vanacker, José Del R. Millán, Eileen Lew, *et al.* Context-based filtering for assisted brain-actuated wheelchair driving. *Computational Intelligence and Neuroscience*, 2007:1–12, 2007.

[5]   Andrew J. McDaid, Song Xing, and Sheng Q. Xie. Brain Controlled Robotic Exoskeleton for Neurorehabilitation. In *2013 IEEE/ASME International Conference on Advanced Intelligent Mechatronics: Mechatronics for Human Wellbeing, AIM 2013*, pp. 1039–1044, 2013.

[6]   Takeshi Sakurada, Toshihiro Kawase, Kouji Takano, Tomoaki Komatsu, and Kenji Kansaku. A BMI-based occupational therapy assist suit: Asynchronous control by SSVEP. *Frontiers in Neuroscience*, 7(7):1–10, 2013.

[7]   Christian J Bell, Pradeep Shenoy, Rawichote Chalodhorn, and Rajesh P N Rao. Control of a humanoid robot by a noninvasive brain-computer interface in humans. *Journal of Neural Engineering*, 5(2):214–220, 2008.

[8]   Samuel Garrett Thorpe, Paul L Nunez, and Ramesh Srinivasan. Identification of wave-like spatial structure in the SSVEP: Comparison of simultaneous EEG and MEG. *Statististics in Medicine*, 26:3911–3926, 2007.

[9]   E. C. Lalor, S. P. Kelly, C. Finucane, *et al.* Steady-state VEP-based brain-computer interface control in an immersive 3D gaming environment. *Eurasip Journal on Applied Signal Processing*, 2005(19):3156–3164, 2005.

[10]   Wei Liu, Danilo P. Mandic, and Andrzej Cichocki. Analysis and online realization of the CCA approach for blind source separation. *IEEE Transactions on Neural Networks*, 18(5):1505–1510, 2007.

[11]   Xiaogang Chen, Yijun Wang, Shangkai Gao, Tzyy-Ping Jung, and Xiaorong Gao. Filter bank canonical correlation analysis for implementing a high-speed SSVEP-based braincomputer interface. *Journal of Neural Engineering*, 12(4):46008, 2015.

[12] Yu Zhang, Guoxu Zhou, Jing Jin, Xingyu Wang, and Andrzej Cichocki. Frequency recognition in SSVEP-based BCI using multiset canonical correlation analysis. *International Journal of Neural Systems*, 24(4):1450013, 2014.

[13] Guangyu Bin, Xiaorong Gao, Zheng Yan, Bo Hong, and Shangkai Gao. An online multi-channel SSVEP-based brain-computer interface using a canonical correlation analysis method. *Journal of Neural Engineering*, 6(4):046002, 2009.

[14] Sarah N Carvalho, Thiago B S Costa, Luisa F S Uribe, *et al.* Comparative analysis of strategies for feature extraction and classification in SSVEP BCIs. *Biomedical Signal Processing and Control*, 21:34–42, 2015.

[15] Zhonglin Lin, Changshui Zhang, Wei Wu, and Xiaorong Gao. Frequency recognition based on canonical correlation analysis for SSVEP-based BCIs. *IEEE Transactions on Biomedical Engineering*, 53(12):315–323, 2006.

[16] Masaki Nakanishi, Yijun Wang, Yu-te Wang, Yasue Mitsukura, and Tzyy Jung. Enhancing Unsupervised Canonical Correlation Analysis-Based Frequency Detection of SSVEPs by Incorporating Background EEG. In *36th Annual International Conference of the IEEE Engineering in Medicine and Biology Society*, pp. 3053–3056, 2014.

[17] Richard M G Tello, Sandra M T Muller, Teodiano Bastos-Filho, and Andre Ferreira. A Comparison of Techniques and Technologies for SSVEP Classification. In *Biosignals and Biorobotics Conference (2014): Biosignals and Robotics for Better and Safer Living (BRC), 5th ISSNIP-IEEE*, number MAY, pp. 1–6, 2014.

[18] Javier Castillo, Sandra Muller, Eduardo Caicedo, and Teodiano Bastos. Feature Extraction Techniques Based on Power Spectrum for a SSVEP-BCI. In *2014 IEEE 23rd International Symposium on Industrial Electronics (ISIE)*, pp. 1051–1055, 2014.

[19] Takeshi Sakurada, Toshihiro Kawase, Tomoaki Komatsu, and Kenji Kansaku. Use of high-frequency visual stimuli above the critical flicker frequency in a SSVEP-based BMI. *Clinical Neurophysiology*, 126(10): 1972–1978, 2015.

[20] Pablo F. Diez, Vicente Mut, Eric Laciar, and Enrique Avila. A comparison of monopolar and bipolar EEG recordings for SSVEP detection. *2010 Annual International Conference of the IEEE Engineering in Medicine and Biology Society*, EMBC'10, pp. 5803–5806, 2010.

[21] Pablo F. Diez, Vicente A. Mut, Eric Laciar, and Enrique M. Avila Perona. Mobile robot navigation with a self-paced brain-computer interface based on high frequency SSVEP. *Robotica*, 32(November 2013):695–709, 2014.

[22] James Henshaw, Wei Liu, and Daniela M Romano. Improving SSVEP-BCI Performance Using Pre-Improving SSVEP-BCI Performance Using Pre-Trial Normalization Methods. In *Cognitive Infocommunications (CogInfoCom), 2017 8th IEEE Conference on*, October, pp. 247–252, 2017.

Chapter 10

The biometric brain dermatoglyphic neural architecture (DNA): brain power at your fingertips

Damera Vijayalakshmi[1]

10.1 Introduction

The brain is largely a mystery to us even to this date in spite of remarkable progress in science and technology. It consists of over 100 billion neurons and works like a giant telephone exchange and the neurotransmitter chemicals help to transfer electrical signals from one neuron to the next. In spite of advancement in research, knowledge regarding several brain functions such as memory, sight, and smell still leave us with gaps in linkages in our information. The changes in consciousness, intelligence and creativity have changed the pattern of electrical and chemical signals.

Our human brain and its neurons form such a complex network and establish such an interesting phenomenon as the universe that no matter how much we progress in the science of the brain and mind through recent studies, we still are left with a lot of unknown miraculous things to be discovered. The proficiency to understand and develop the indispensable studies of neuroscience has already started to gain ground. Numerous scientists have put their heads together to get a universal applicability of how the brain functions, be it how it feels emotions, how we utilise our brain's capacity to transforms the future (which includes the concept of time), how consciousness works and how the brain integrates information (Figure 10.1).

10.1.1 Brain and physiology of fingerprints

Fingerprints have been proven to be a revelation of the psychology of a person and the understanding of the functioning and behaviour of the brain. Researchers have made tremendous progress with the information gained through the genotypic make up of an individual. The fingerprints are an index of a person's uniqueness based on the study of epidermal ridges on the skin on the fingers and toes. There appears to be a connect between fingerprints and the sulci or cortical grooves in the brain hemispheres. Nerve endings are shown to be connected to special brain lobe locations from limb terminals. The fingerprint minutiae are points of reference that unravel the uniqueness of the brain. The brain and finger print growth starts from

[1]Pragathi College of Education, Adikavi Nannayya University, India

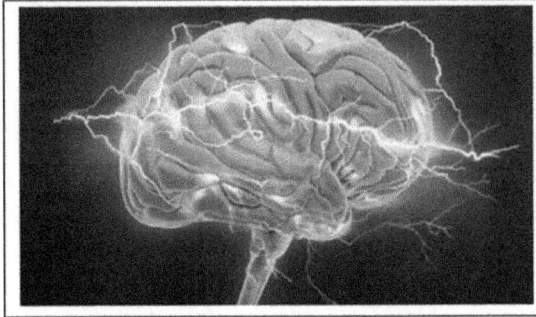

Figure 10.1   Complexity of the brain

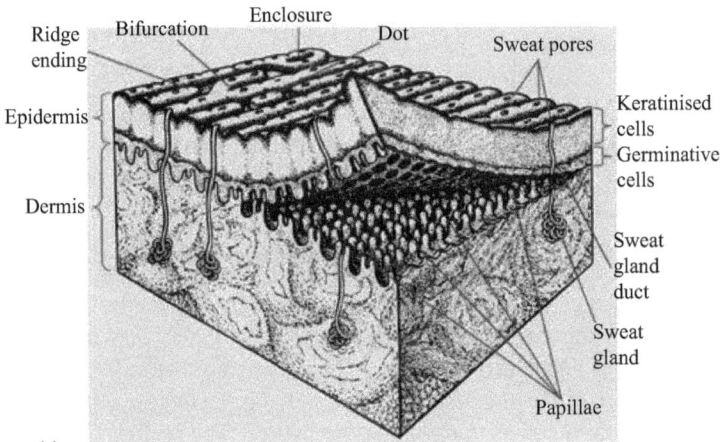

(a)

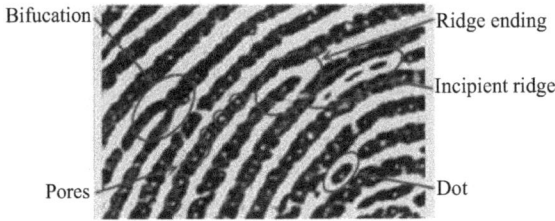

(b)

Figure 10.2   Structure of the skin

the 13th to 18th week of gestation [1] and have shown to be connected to localise brain functionality, learning style and socio-cognitive behaviour. The skin consists of three anatomical layers of dermal tissue cells called epidermis, dermis and hypodermis (Figure 10.2). The ridges surface or volar cells, as they are primarily called, have morphology that suits their functionality. A layer of dermal papillae

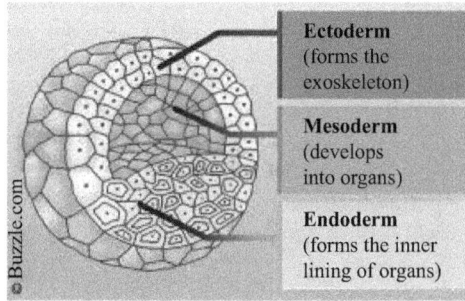

Figure 10.3 Layers of the cell

exists between the epidermis and dermis, which forms the patterned ridges. The pores on the ridges secrete sweat and cause the finger pads to leave latent fingerprints invisible to our eye.

10.1.1.1 Fingerprint and embryogenesis

The fingerprints and the brain are connected through the epidermal growth factor (EGF) and neural growth factor (NGF). It is important to know that the fingerprint patterns are linked to the brain's cortical folds. The development of a single cell into a complete complex organism is called embryogenesis. The development of a single cell into a complete complex organism is called embryogenesis. The embryo is a single cell from which all life forms originate. Later on the zygote fuses the male and the female gamete cells, sperm and ovum. These cells develop into three distinct layers of cells called ectoderm, mesoderm and endoderm, which is the outer, inner and inner layer, respectively (Figure 10.3). Outstanding research in this area was carried out by Dr Rita Levi-Montalcini and Dr Stanley Cohen, which won them the Nobel in Physiology and Biochemistry in 1986. The Canadian neurobiologist Wilder Penfield has also supportive evidence in this field with his research on connections between fingerprints and the several locations of human brain.

10.1.1.2 No brain—no fingerprints

Anencephaly is the absence of the prime brain portions such as the skull and scalp, which occurs because of the neural tube defect (Figure 10.4). It happens because of the failure in complete and proper development of cephalic end of the neural tube. In such cases of a foetus born there is a deformity with no forebrain, which governs all thinking abilities and organ coordination functions. Evidence correlates this relation between brain and fingerprints.

10.2 Connections of brain to fingers

The different lobes of human brain are physiologically connected to different fingers of both the hands (Figure 10.5). Several studies reveal this connection of brain locations to fingers. The left half of the cerebral hemisphere is shown to be related

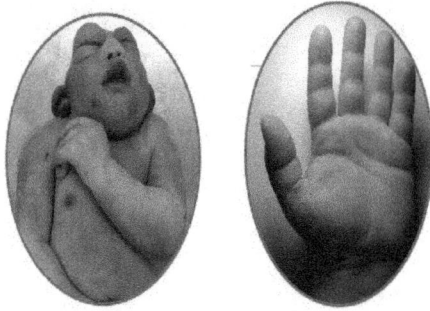

Figure 10.4   No brain—no fingerprints

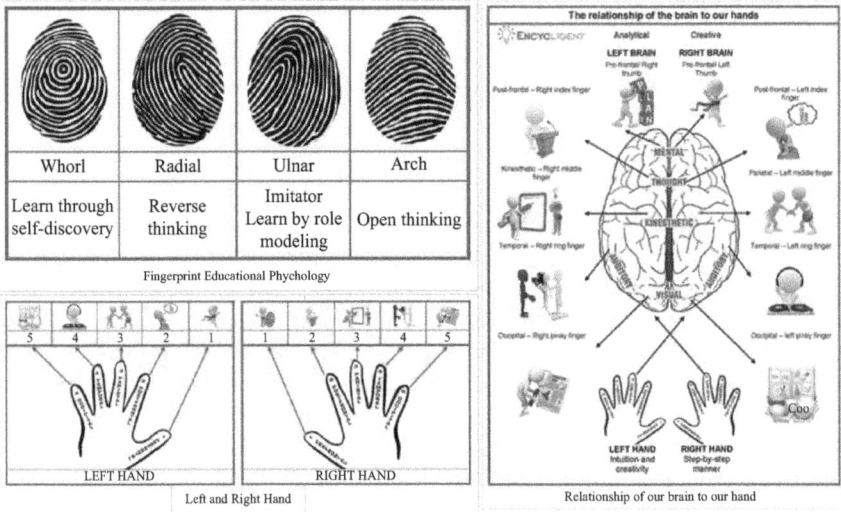

Figure 10.5   Finger connection to the brain

to the fingers of the right hand and the convergent left half of brain is connected to the fingers of the right hand.

Looking at the lobes, every lobe area is responsible for its surrounding areas. The coordination is seen between the thumb to the superior frontal lobe, the index finger to the inferior frontal lobe, the middle finger to the parietal lobe, the ring finger to the temporal lobe and the little finger to the occipital lobe, which is located at the hind part of the brain.

10.2.1   Ridges patterns on the fingers

The fingerprint patterns can broadly be categorised as Loops, Whorls and Arches. Generally Loops are observed in 70% of the people, Whorls are seen in 20–25% of cases and Arches can be seen in only 5–10%. These broad categories can be further be generally be categorised in Arches as Arches and Tented Arches, in Loops as Ulnar Loops and Radial Loops and in Whorls as Spiral, Target, Elongated, Imploding and Composite and Accidental.

Studies show that genetic factors, chance and environmental factors all contribute to the type and pattern occurrence of a finger. Monozygotic or identical twins also do not reveal identical patterns. Fingerprints tell us the uniqueness, the kind of personality a person may have, their preferred learning style, etc., and many more parameters of the functioning of the brain function.

10.2.1.1 Arch

People with arch patterns on any finger show qualities of a rigid and practical approach towards the corresponding brain functionality of those tasks (Figure 10.6). They display qualities of dedication, loyalty, responsibility, caution and reserve. They tend to be unconventional and are actively rebellious, especially rebellious to convention. They show qualities of stubborn nature and are said to be self-repressive and self-defensive. They are unable to articulate their feelings and are undemonstrative with their expressions of emotions. Other qualities of a person with arch pattern are that they are practical, skilful, and have skilled pair of hands and their ability to repair and make allow them to be skilled towards trade and profession. Having an affinity towards traditional music has also been noticed among people with arch patterns. They are also introverted and not very open-minded though: they love socialising with people. Looking at the specific brain functionalities corresponding to each finger reveals more useful information. Arch on the left thumb reveals insecurity in interpersonal relationships, along with high priority for discipline and punctuality. Arches on right thumb indicate patience and firmness for organisation and managerial aspects in personal as well as professional life. The index fingers display a practical approach. While the left middle finger displays the fine art and rhythm perception and the right middle finger deals with finger dexterity, movement and brain coordination. The left ring finger represents part of the brain responsible for understanding and creating music and the right ring finger is connected to areas of the lobe governing memory and linguistic abilities of an individual. Such people have great craftsmanship in particular music form they pursue in career. They show an intense artistic interest

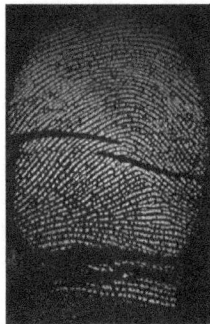

Figure 10.6   Arch

in simple art forms such as dance. An arch on the little finger indicates higher intellect in creativity of abstract domains such as medicine or science though there is no documentation available on the little finger.

10.2.1.2   Tented arch

A straight upright ridge at the core of a simple arch pattern is a tented arch (Figure 10.7). The ridges are pushed upwards towards the tip of the finger. The pattern has similar characteristics of an arch pattern, but they show inconsistency in their performance in tasks related to the specific related intelligence. They lack steadiness and end up displaying nervous behaviour. Such people come under the effect of easy emotional manipulation by others. The tented arches are said to be skewed towards intensity, fanaticism and zealousness. They are prone to be rash, energetic, impulsive and creative. They also are said to easily go out of balance as they are emotional and volatile. They have also been found to have a special liking and attachment to musical tune notes and have a natural liking to them. They are also seen to easily adapt to new environment and situations. They do not feel challenged when changing jobs. They prefer to keep people happy and also have a faith in themselves and prefer to choose what to do and cannot be manipulated easily. They are resistant to new thought process and, hence to convince them, they need logic. They strictly adhere to rules and regulations. Although they do not tend to take much interest in art work of others, they themselves follow artistic trends. Such people want stability in relationships and career because they are emotionally dependent upon close family relatives. Though not very introvert, they love spending time with themselves, reading books and novels, and going to movies. They detest risk taking and crave for stability in personal and professional life and hence are good at administrative assignments.

10.2.1.3   Loops

Approximately 65% of the world population have loop pattern on their fingerprints, which is said to be the most commonly occurring pattern. These ridges flow from one side of the fingertip, loop around the centre of finger pad and loop back to the same direction where they originated. These loops are of two types: they can run either towards or away from the thumb. The loops opening away from thumb is an

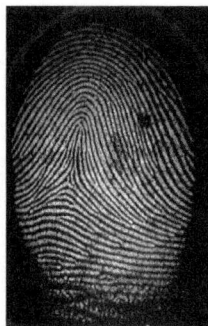

Figure 10.7   Tented arch

ulnar loop and the one opening towards the thumb is a radial loop, and this can be due to the location of the radial and ulnar bone. These loop-patterned people exhibit qualities of flexibility, adaptability and are highly responsive to new ideas. They blend in the crowd and work as a team. They are imaginative, receptive, gullible, lack concentration and are easily distracted. They also exhibit qualities of adaptability and adaptation. They are said to be compassionate and humanitarian. Specifically they are outstanding performers with respect to perception and imagination. They are straightforward and have little or no patience for long sessions of conversation or teaching. Individuals with loops on all their fingers survive the most unfavourable conditions, in spite of being unstable, vacillating and inconsistent. Such people hate to be cornered and can retaliate if not given due importance. More than six loops signify easy going affectionate nature, conformists, receptive and gullible. They believe that the journey is more important than the destinations and have all-round capability.

Ulnar loop

Ulnar loops indicate characteristics of sociability, flexibility and adaptability (Figure 10.8). Their personality is associated with the sulci folds giving people ability to extract ideas from others, manipulate it their way and publish. They also have the ability to identify, pick and emulate qualities of others in themselves. Their openness to new ideas, artistic nature and the wide range of interests make them open to varied interests, are mild in nature and have the ability to take active participation in any conversation.

Radial loop

People with radial loops on their finger tips are egocentric, forceful and domineering (Figure 10.9). They pursue their goals enthusiastically and improvise based on their own requirements. They have the ability to improvise a great deal. They can readily idealise and conceptualise. The radial loop on the index finger shows dominance and egocentric nature. They are thus in an extreme sense of openness but sometime lose sense of their personality. They exhibit qualities of insecurity and instability; they are also hyper responsive and keep vacillating

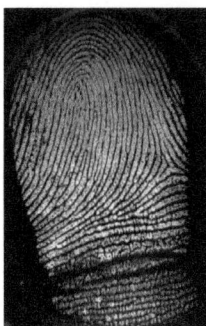

Figure 10.8   Loop

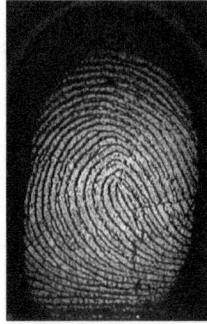

Figure 10.9   Radial loop

between priorities. A radial loop on the index finger reveals an individualistic person who prefers to acquire knowledge on his or her own initiative. They find it hard to have an open mind and are resistant to change. They also do not plan a course of action needed to be taken but can lead a team effectively. Radials are adventurous, dynamic and love to embrace change. They are passionate about newness and change that stability is not a characteristic they enjoy.

10.2.1.4   Whorl

Whorl pattern indicates a person who is a non-conformist and one who has higher inner concentration. They are highly talented and too individualistic and thus resist being influenced by others. Strength, character and intelligence is their trade mark. They display fixed attitudes and are a law unto themselves. They appear to be conventional and law abiding till it suits them. They enjoy challenges and detest mundane routine duties. They prefer complex research and unconventional methods of execution of ideas. Whorls tend to be practical and are found to be quick in action especially at times of emergency. They tend to be preoccupied and prefer to be alienated from others. They are a law unto themselves and prefer to be isolated and reject society.

Spiral whorl

Circular patterns are a trademark of a spiral whorl, which has two deltas at both corners (Figure 10.10). They have vibrant surging kind of personality with fantastic grasping ability. They grasp ideas easily and understand the concepts in whatever information learnt. These people easily get affected by emotional manipulation of others, which spirals them into emotionality. However when they decide upon one goal in life, they are very determined towards achieving it and spiral upwards towards goal accomplishment. Their efforts and hard work display a strong sense of self-consciousness and immense will power to win a competitive situation. Such people are self-motivated and self-driven towards their ideas with passion. Such people need to be directed to act accordingly and utilise this innate potentiality existing within them. They are said to be self-motivated and dislike interference from others.

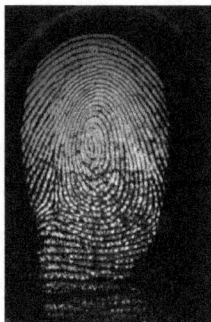

Figure 10.10   Spiral whorl

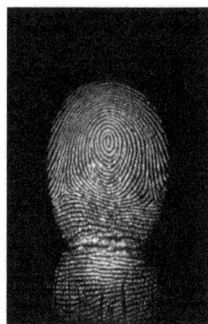

Figure 10.11   Whorl target

Concentric whorl (target)

The whorl target pattern is characterised by having concentric circles of ridge formations (Figure 10.11). These whorl patterns have strong expression of inner determination and hence have focused minds and hence show persistence and discipline towards achieving goals even when set early in their lives. They are self-conscious about their image in society and would encourage their image to be in good public standing. These people tend to be focussed and work hard aggressively towards achievement of their goals. In this attempt to achieve targets they consciously focus on only completion of a task set by themselves that they perceive nothing else but focussed and prioritised goal. The target whorl on the left thumb indicates their strong rules for others, and their inability to relent on others mistakes make them appear to lack compassion, mercy and humanity. On the other hand, when there is a whorl target on right thumb they are clear and focussed for themselves and very precise about their requirements and also display symptoms of straight forwardness. Having a clear vision makes them straight forward and always tend to be self-focused and put themselves before others. Their crystal clarity of thought makes them voice their opinion in frankness, which actually hurt people easily and thus drive people away from themselves.

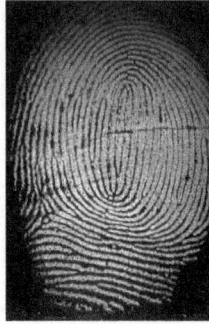

Figure 10.12   Elongated whorl

Elongated whorl

Elongated whorl pattern is characterised by a long oval whorl flanked by two triradii on either sides (Figure 10.12). They exhibit similar tendencies of whorl but in addition are highly focussed towards achieving targets set by them. As they take up assignments genuinely they tend to be quite aggressive and obstinate towards achieving them. Although they are of very decent nature, they are quite sincere towards their outlook towards others. Because of their incredible ability to grasp concepts and look at the situation holistically they are able to look at micro level management and display qualities of multi-tasking. Hence they plan and understand goals and priorities and execute them in a step-by-step systematic manner. Being deductive reasoning people they use a balance of logic and emotionality and are adept at administrative and managerial operations, which involve analysis and evaluation. Being logical they are not only good at analytical reasoning but also good with algorithm and calculations. But their emotionality, on the other hand, is also a challenge because they get emotionally connected and so it is easy to manipulate such people. They are unable to adjust to any issues related to emotionality and hence are vulnerable and are sensitive to flashbacks and memories. They rewind the past memories and sink in their emotions due to intense sensitivity. Hence balancing the logical and emotional aspect of thoughts is a challenge.

Imploding whorl

Imploding whorl is a Tai-Chi pattern at the centre or the core, surrounded by multiple circular layers of ridges, which indeed is considered to be of a rare origin (Figure 10.13). Though the pattern exhibits qualities of symmetry they have opposing orientations and hence are said to have duality in their thought process. They can thus work parallelly on two tasks, which are different in nature, and still have the ability to complete it successfully. Because of this duality of thought process they prefer to work alone rather than brain storm with others in group. The duality also acts as a block in decision making and hence fails to act fast in some situations. They are hence not suitable for situations that deal with crises and emergency management. Being systemic thinkers, imploding whorls form strategies that are too worldly, practical, objective and materialistic and do not display any qualities of idealism and hence rarely share value systems and priorities, which

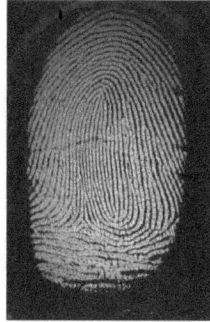

Figure 10.13   Imploding whorl

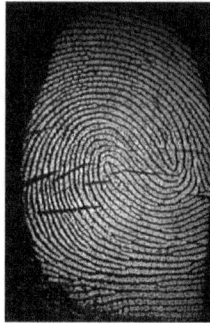

Figure 10.14   Double loop

show a deep understanding and appreciation of life. Due to this lack of openness to new ideas they do not bother about other's thoughts and perceptions.

Composite whorl/double loop

Double loop or the composite whorl looks like the yin yang pattern wherein the individual has a tendency towards duality of thought (Figure 10.14). It is considered to be a rare pattern and can mostly be seen on the thumb and index finger. Because of the ability of these people to be able to look at the holistic picture and look at all angles they are good at counselling and guiding and facilitating people along with a natural capability to judge others in an objective and neutral manner. Such individuals exhibit traits of the abstract and spiritual dimensions. They also like to be at the helm of affairs and love to be stars or sources of attraction by the public. These people may not be conventional by following routine, but they are spiritual as they are said to have their third eye open wider than others. They have a holistic approach and develop a sense of spiritual well-being, and for them inner conscious holds a higher place, showing a true realisation of universe. Their dilemma is, on the one hand, knowing everything and, on the other hand, procrastinating on important aspects of life. Experts have categorised them to come under the perview of schizophrenia and split personality disorder. This is so because they fluctuate in decision making and have self-doubt and invariably jump to conclusions. They have a strong sense of higher psychic abilities and are very eager to gain more knowledge on several aspects of life. Because of their integrative cognitive ability they are eager to gain knowledge on everything they can lay their hands on. And it can also be noticed that they cannot be good at communication with others but yet reveal personal expressions to only chosen few. They are practical and objective when it comes to maintaining interpersonal correspondences. The double loop on the thumb reveals a good ability in personal judgement—the index finger relates to the ability to judge—the middle finger signifies decision making related to career while the little finger suggests a bisexual orientation.

Peacock's eye whorl

The whorl peacock is also a rare pattern found on people's fingers, which signifies a whorl located in the loop (Figure 10.15). The whorl in the shape of a peacock's eye is located in the loop, which shows it somewhat looks like the pattern on a peacock's tail feathers. In this pattern the core consists of more than one spiral triradius, which is lined by a straight line at one of the corners. This pattern is said to welcome good luck and they are said to exhibit a strong sense of discernment and judgemental ability. Such people are competitive and surpass others when the need arises. They possess superior perceptive skills along with outstanding leadership qualities and are also considered to be dominant and influential. They are predominantly found on the ring and little fingers, which works around the capacity to memorise as well as communicative abilities. They are also strong with memory power as well as communicative and observing abilities. They also have the ability to grasp visual pictures and patterns along with auditory pitch and tone perception. Looking at the patterns of whorls in the loop there can be a qualitative difference noted among whorl peacocks. The target-centric whorls within the loop signify a sharper sense of understanding along with the ability to be good with people skills and a very creative frame of mind. They are focussed, highly competitive, professional, self-driven and yet stubborn in their receptivity to other's suggestions.

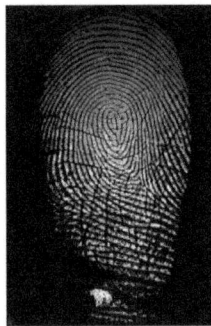

Figure 10.15   Whorl peacock

The spiral whorl in the loop signifies a more emotional passionate, intuitive and creative mindset.

They do not follow trends followed by others and look for a novel unique path. Hence they too exhibit qualities of creativity and passion.

Accidental whorl/variant

Accidental whorls are a combination of two or more patterns and are difficult to be categorised under any one pattern (Figure 10.16). It is a variance from the conventional pattern. As these patterns are unconventional and cannot be grouped under any head, so also are their characteristics where they display traits of two or more patterns. Their expressions vary and so also do their communication patterns, which may cause conflicts. Communication needs to be monitored and guidance should be given by parents to streamline their functionality in more socially appropriate ways.

10.2.2   Fingerprints and human behaviour

Human behaviour has been the target of psychologists for many years where numerous studies were undertaken to understand, categorise and compartmentalise human thoughts, words and deeds. Terms such as personality, behaviour and intelligence have all remained and still remain abstract words because of the different perspectives about their composition and description among various psychologists. The studies on connection between fingerprints and behaviour have also been underway from the days of Galton. As it is not a pure science but a behavioural science, it is difficult to be precise and clearly define. Every person performs a task based on requirement, but how they complete it and the internal process involved in execution of the task varies from person to person. In order to combine both and look at its impact on behaviour has been the task of many a researcher. The fingerprints are said to be the blueprints of one's self. It has proven to be the only way to reach closest to unravelling the mysteries of the mind. In order to understand psychological functions there is a need to understand how the brain processes information. How an individual uses his or her potentiality is

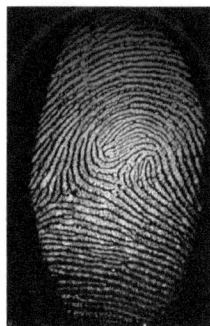

Figure 10.16   Accidental whorl

crucial in this world of competition and achievement. Unless an individual is aware of his or her inborn strengths it is impossible for him or her to understand how to utilise his or her capabilities. Hence hidden talents and potentialities can be well understood through the fingerprints alone. A person is endowed with potentialities by birth from genes and environment in the womb. Once a child is aware of his or her potentialities then professional guidance and direction can be given. Parents, teachers, employers, etc., need an in-depth knowledge to bring about productivity and efficiency in institutions and organisations.

10.3   Dermatoglyphics

In 1892 the scientific study of fingerprints was started by Sir Francis Galton, who was one of the most original biologists of that time. Dr Harold Cummins is considered to be the father of American fingerprint analysis and coined the term "Dermatoglyphics". Its first usage was said to be carried out by the Chinese way back in the 16th century. It was then a common practice in the sale of land holdings to take the impression of the fingerprints as an acknowledgement of the deed. In those days prints of the palm and soles were recorded as a safeguard against the impersonation of children in ancient China. Galton's contributions entitled 'Finger Prints' published in 1892 and 'Finger Prints Dictionaries' published in 1895, Cummins and Midlo's [2] published book entitled 'Finger Prints, Palms and Soles: An Introduction to Dermatoglyphics', etc., were all authentic studies on fingerprints and psychology. The four finger patterns (Arch, Loop, Whorl and Composite) are distinguished by Henry and is still considered to be the most basic patterns in the field of Dermatoglyphics.

10.3.1   Dermatoglyphics and intelligence

Dermatoglyphics is a science that analyses finger ridges or carvings and gives an insight into the intellectual capacities of an individual, and has been a recent development in this field (Figure 10.17). The dermal ridges give us an insight into emotional quotient and multiple intelligences. Though there has been a controversy on coming to a common consensus regarding this concept, there is no doubt that it has given deep insights into many people and their functionality. Psychologist Howard Gardener came up with eight different types of intelligences, and research shows that every individual will display a minimum of at least three to four types of intelligences when the dermal ridges on an individual's finger is analysed. There was seen to exist a bilateral symmetry of the cerebrum and the symmetrical limbs. As is well known the left part of the limb controls the right half of the brain and vice versa.

The neocortex has been proven to be the reason for humans to be conscious beings. Only human beings can reflect and retrospect on past happenings to bring about new perceptions of old situations. Hence all eight intelligences can be correlated and linked directly to several parts of brain functioning. The unique pattern

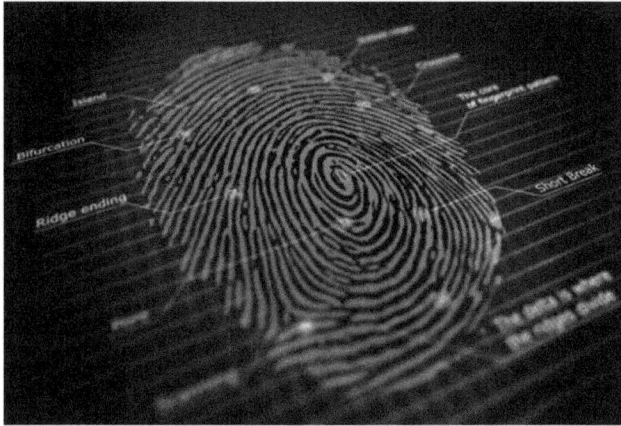

Figure 10.17   Dermatoglyphic analysis

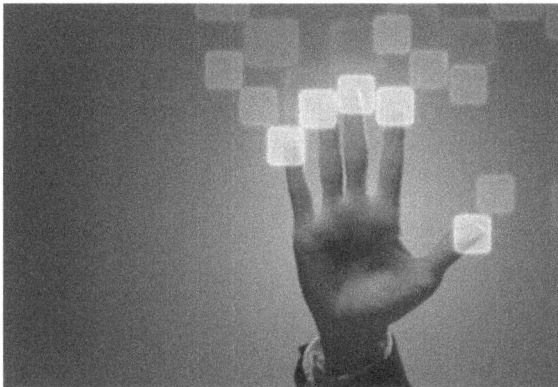

Figure 10.18   Personal identification

of grooves or sulci developed in prenatal stage goes hand in hand with other groove dermal developments.

10.3.2   Dermatoglyphics and personal identification

Personal identification has always been the need of the hour for various reasons (Figure 10.18). Dermatoglyphics in now able to provide us accurate and precise information regarding identification. Polimeni found that Dermatoglyphics serves as a helpful tool for investigators in determining personal identification details. Recently it has been proven that fingerprint evidence is the best form of personal identification yet devised. With millions of comparisons and subsequent identifications it has been proven worldwide without any error by Leadbetter in 2005. Dermatoglyphic analysis today is a well-known, accepted and established

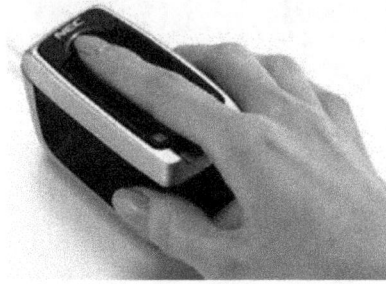

Figure 10.19   Biometric assessment

diagnostic and research tool in medicine and provides important insights into the inheritance and embryologic development of many clinical disorders.

10.3.3   Dermatoglyphics and biometric assessment

Dermatoglyphics, which is the study of dermal ridges as well as the biometric evaluation of a person's intelligence, has triggered new application concepts based on its applicability (Figure 10.19). The novel and dynamic tool of finger-print analysis is the Biometric testing. It is the assessment of the individual's fingerprints to map his/her brain functioning. Harold Cummins in 1926 proposed the term "Dermatoglyphics" for the study of fingerprints at the American Morphological Society. Noel Jaquin, in 1958, researched and proposed that each fingerprint pattern corresponds to a specific type of personality. Professor Roger W. Sperry and his co-researchers were awarded the Nobel Prize in Biomedicine for their research work on the left- and right brain functions as well as the dual-brain theory. At this time Lin Ruei procured the U.S. Patent for Dermatoglyphics. Once formed fingerprints are said to be static and do not change with age—so an individual will have the same fingerprints throughout his or her life. The Biometric technique has thus proven to be the best approach, as the results are a pure measure of innate abilities, not tampered by environmental conditions. The Biometric test offers an elaborate report that identifies several parameters, such as innate intelligences, behavioural patterns and tendencies. This makes the Biometric test an invaluable tool for correctly analysing and identifying a candidate's true personality. A person may easily deceive an interviewer, but it is impossible for fingerprints to lie.

All ten fingers are scanned and based on the valleys and ridges on the fingers together form unique patterns on the skin of palms, fingers, soles and toes. Dermatoglyphics as a science has huge potential with numerous applications in various fields such as biology, medicine, genetics and evolution and is the most widely used method for personal identification.

This biometric application of Dermatoglyphics is wide and varied. Dermatoglyphics is like a map that leads one to understand one's own potential and talents. Everyone inherits innate intelligence and genetics from their parents.

If there is no opportunity for further development then there is no way for one to develop a full range of intelligence of memory, understanding, reasoning, analysis, integration and application. Dermatoglyphics helps us analyse the distribution and cells in the left- and right brain of the cell, and predict where the potential lies. Early intervention and diagnostics can further help develop the strengths and improve our weakness, so that the left- and right brain may grow in a more balanced and blended manner.

10.3.4 Biometric dermatoglyphic neural architecture (DNA) report

The unique fingerprint recognition technology has been the most pervasive, oldest, simplest to install and the lowest cost biometric technology. It has held the largest market size worldwide and has been widely adopted by many industries as well as schools. The Dermatoglyphic report assesses and evaluates the personality of an individual and gives insight into one's potentialities and areas of challenges. As has been well established and widely accepted, the biometric assessment holds a superior place to that of psychometric tests. The biometric test is highly comprehensive, based on a scientific platform and correctly reveals hidden inborn personality traits. The scientific nature and the ease of assessment and applicability has made this unique report commendable.

10.3.5 Dermatoglyphics and left–right brain dominance

The cerebral hemispheres of the human brain has been known to be symmetrical and the operations and functions vary for both (Figure 10.20). The left hemisphere relates to the logical abilities, while the right brain deals with emotions, passion, creation and intuition, which are all controlled by the neural circuitry of the right hemisphere. Along with these hemispheres the brain consists of lobes that are also differentiated based on their functionality.

The left hemisphere dominance depicts people who look deeper into a situation and are prone to have more perceptions and need to look at the comprehension of a situation before they analyse the bigger picture and look for options and solutions. The left brain typically follows a sequential analysis and is very systematic in logical interpretation of any information. Strong left brain dominance indicates strength in language, mathematics, abstraction and reasoning, which is the creation of symbolic information. Here memory is stored in language format and step-by-step reasoning is utilised. The left brain dominance shows qualities of planning, logic, abstract thinking, detailed and scientific frame of thought. These people are detached, liberal, rational, organised and sequential. They are objective, have a convergent type of analysis and do a lot of research before getting to action. They love to follow plans and structure.

The right hemisphere dominance shows more of an intuitive and impulsive bend of mind. The right brain operates on a more holistic functioning and depends on multisensory input to get clarity over the holistic picture. They utilise visual spatial skills along with the auditory cues, which is stored in memory. They tend

Left- and Right Brain Dominance

Left brain	Right brain
• Sequential analysis	• Holistic functioning
• Systematic	• Multisensory input
• Logical interpretation of information	• Holistic picture
• Production of symbolic information (language, mathematics, abstraction, reasoning)	• Visual spatial skills (dancing & gymnastics)
	• Memory is stored in auditory
• Memory is stored in language format	• Spatial & visual modalities
• Step-by-step reasoning	• Emotional
• Planned	• Mystical
• Logical	• Musical
• Mathematical	• Creative
• Digital	• Intuition
• Abstract	• Analogic
• Precise	• Imaginative
• Analytical	• Heuristic
• Linear	• Empathetic
• Detached	• Figurative
• Liberal	• Irregular
• Rational	• Concrete
• Organised	• Relational
• Detailed	• Nonlinear
• Scientific	• Intuitive, multiple
• Sequential	• Subjective
• Objective	• Divergent
• Convergent	• **Group or hands on activity**
• **Follow plans & structure**	
• Analysis	• Shared learning
• Research	• Group discussion
• Realistic projects	• Role play
• Worksheets	• Experiments

Figure 10.20   Left versus right brain

to be more emotional, mystical, musical, creative, intuitive and analogic. Their imaginative and heuristic approach makes them more empathetic, figurative, irregular, concrete, intuitive, subjective and divergent. They enjoy hands-on activity, shared learning, group discussion and role plays. They love to experiment and see what happens. They hence have the natural tendency to look at the larger picture and are very random and subjective in thinking capabilities. Personality qualities of a right brain are adventurous and carefree nature, dependent on feelings and fantasies and are very proficient at synthesising concepts and ideas. They are found to possess qualities of spatial perception, impulsiveness, spontaneity and risk-bearing activities.

10.3.6   Connection of brain locations to fingers

Research has proven that different lobes of human brain are connected to the different fingers of both the hands. There is an opposite connection between the limb and the brain. The functional coordination between each side of the brain with the opposite hands and more specifically to each of those fingers is studied. Genetics and developmental biology give further clarity regarding these connections. The thumb is connected to the prefrontal lobe, while the index finger is connected to the frontal lobe. The three other fingers are related to the inputs to brain. They connect middle finger to the parietal lobe, the ring finger to the temporal lobe and the little finger to the occipital lobe. Each lobe area is responsible for specific functions. Each finger on the left and right fingers perform specific yet different aspects of their functionality.

10.3.7   Ridges on the fingers connected to Neocortex

Developmental biologists have researched on the brain and fingerprint connection and have evidence that the ridges and the brain functions are genetic and prenatal (Figure 10.21). The ridges develop in the mother's womb during 13th to 18th week of pregnancy and are largely influenced genetically. Research in medical science has proven that the ridge growth takes place in synchronisation with Neocortex. The Neocortex, which is a learning system, is primarily the brain's centre of intelligence and its structural makeup has direct influence on an individual's ability to perceive, learn and react to an input. This innate potentiality to comprehend inputs from the environment is influenced by experiences that an individual perceives even as early as the foetal brain development in the womb. Sex differences, mother's thoughts and real-life experiences all shape the intelligences and functionality of personality. The dynamic structure of Neocortex changes dramatically over lifetime and quite interestingly fingerprints do not alter. Neurobiologists claim

BRAIN FUNCTIONS CONNECTED TO THE TEN FINGERS		
Leadership capabilities, objective driven, like to socialise and are spontaneous.	Executive Function	Management capability of an individual and planning, decisiveness, logical rationalisation and ability to self-reflect.
Imagination, idea formation, visualisation, 3D, self-expectations and self-confidence.	Thinking Function	Calculated analysis, logical rationalisation and vocabulary control.
Muscle flexibility, control over body movement, and integrate sensory information and form eye body coordination and artistic ability.	Kinaesthetic Function	Manual dexterity, finger control and action sequencing.
Music appreciation, ability to perceive tone, pitch, rhythm, emotion, feeling, tone, sensitivity & sensibility.	Auditory Function	Language understanding, phonics, hearing identification and auditory memory.
Graphical imagery and to visually perceive images. Perception of images and to be sensitive to visual cues.	Visual Function	Visual identification capability, their reading ability, observation, concentration & sensibility in reading.

Figure 10.21   Left- and right hand connected to brain functioning

that there is a link between fingerprint ridges and cerebral cortex and hence intelligence is bound to reflect fingerprint patterns. The Integrated Automated Fingerprint Identification System (IAFIS) maintained by the Federal Bureau of Investigation (FBI) has a huge database for research.

10.3.8   Dermatoglyphics and brain lobes functionality

Behaviour is the index of the mind. Mind involves processing of the brain and its transformation to action called behaviour. Hence let us understand how the brain processes information. The brain consists of five lobes. Each lobe plays a specific role in the processing of information from the senses to the brain and the commands the brain sends out based on this information. So these lobes represent input, process and output. Three lobes constitute inputs, one lobe processes and one lobe sends the output in the form of action or behaviour. Let us look at this in detail.

10.3.8.1   The thumb and the prefrontal lobe (higher cognitive functions)

The prefrontal lobe reveals personality characteristics, impulse control, judgement, creativity, leadership and discipline. Impulsive tendencies (spot decisions), inhibited tendencies (plenty of options but unable to decide) or balanced actions can be observed. Overall it assists in planning, management, communication, coordinating and controlling our behaviour and emotions. It also regulates our creative ability, leadership qualities, intuition and visualisation.

10.3.8.2   The index finger and the frontal lobe (thinking and imagination)

The functionality of this lobe is to perform analyses and visualise the logic behind the information received. Logical thinking, abstract thinking, creativity, visualisation, language, concepts and ideas formation are all a function and characteristic of this lobe. This is the path to understanding.

10.3.8.3   The middle finger and the parietal lobe (kinaesthetic ability)

The middle brain region is associated with processing tactile sensory information such as pressure, touch and pain. The somatosensory cortex processes the body's senses. It is responsible for movement differentiation, physical movements, operation understanding, bodily mobility, rhythmic movement, muscle coordination and physical appreciation. The parietal lobe dominance thus involves actions as an input for information. These people can only learn after doing or performing a task, gain experience and then know differently. Spatial awareness, sensory integration of information and learning by doing assimilates the kinaesthetic source of information and reaches the brain. Simply put learning by doing.

10.3.8.4   The ring finger and the temporal lobe (auditory perception)

The temporal lobe is located after the parietal lobe and is connected to the primary auditory cortex, which is responsible for listening, understanding, interpretation of sound and language. The hippocampus is also located in the temporal lobe, which is why this portion of the brain is also heavily associated with the formation of memories. The left part controls phonics differentiation, language understanding and sound identification ability and the right part controls auditory and music appreciation ability. The temporal lobe dominance involves listening as an input for information. These people form opinions, judgements and act based on what they hear. Processing auditory information, differentiating sound, pitch and rhythm, understanding speech by listening assimilates the auditory source of information and reaches the brain. Simply put learning by listening.

10.3.8.5   The little finger and the occipital lobe (visual perception)

This is located at the hind part of the brain and is associated with interpreting visual stimuli and information. The primary visual cortex, which receives and interprets information from the retinas of the eyes, is located in the occipital lobe. The left part controls visual Identification, observation and reading comprehension and the right part controls visual and image appreciation ability. The occipital lobe involves seeing as an input for learning. These people only believe what they see. Processing visual information about objects, colours, motion, distance, words, signs and symbols by seeing captures the visual source of information and reaches the brain. Simply put learning by seeing.

10.3.9   Dermatoglyphics and learning styles

Learning styles of a person relate to the unique style a person has with which he or she can acquire information. There can be a dominance of auditory, kinaesthetic or visual or there can be a combination of these three (Figure 10.22). Each one of us has a unique combination of learning styles. How we receive information differs from person to person. Information reaches the brain to be processed based on the inputs and the learning style influences such information received. According to Barbe *et al.* [3], there are three primary learning modalities. A person can have more than one, naturally or imbibed over the course of time. They may also get altered with age. These are as follows: Visual (picture, shape, sculpture, paintings), kinaesthetic (gestures, body movement, object manipulation, positioning) and auditory (listening, rhythms, tone, chants). When the percentage of dominance is prioritised the three ranks get categorised into one of the six styles of learning. The hierarchy of learning styles can be seen in six forms – VAK, VKA, KVA, KAV, AVK and AKV. This helps one to become aware of the strength of the input that is needed to reach the brain. Individuals generally use primary learning style and use secondary learning style to reconcile (Figure 10.23).

The visual learner has an excellent grasp of direction and space, graphics, graphs, charts and spellings. The visual learner prefers to see and learn. The auditory learner has a strong auditory and listening capability. He/she is discussion driven. The auditory learner prefers to hear and learn. The kinaesthetic learner prefers physical hands-on and practical activities to learn and understand. They prefer to do and learn. It is not of more importance what a student is learning, but it makes difference how smartly one learns.

The 'finger–brain lobe connection' hypothesis (unlikely true!)

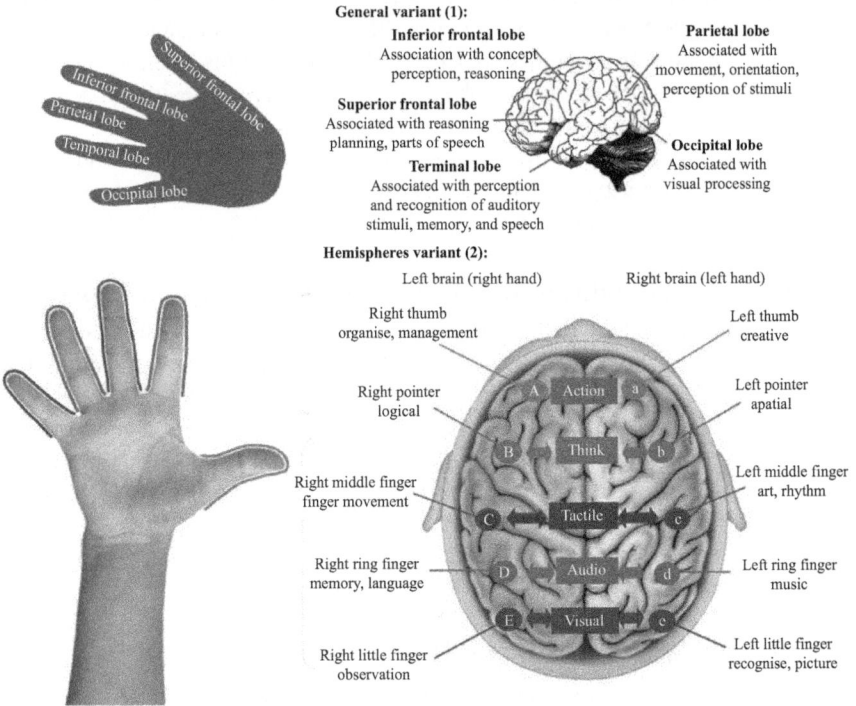

General variant (1):

Inferior frontal lobe
Association with concept
perception, reasoning

Superior frontal lobe
Associated with reasoning
planning, parts of speech

Terminal lobe
Associated with perception
and recognition of auditory
stimuli, memory, and speech

Parietal lobe
Associated with
movement, orientation,
perception of stimuli

Occipital lobe
Associated with
visual processing

Hemispheres variant (2):

Left brain (right hand)   Right brain (left hand)

Right thumb
organise, management

Right pointer
logical

Right middle finger
finger movement

Right ring finger
memory, language

Right little finger
observation

Left thumb
creative

Left pointer
apatial

Left middle finger
art, rhythm

Left ring finger
music

Left little finger
recognise, picture

A Action a
B Think b
C Tactile c
D Audio d
E Visual e

Figure 10.22   Fingers connected to left- and right brain

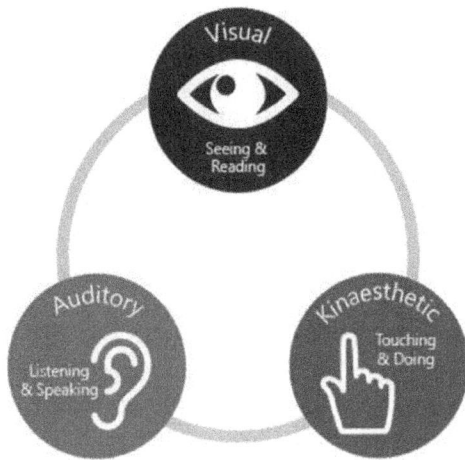

Visual
Seeing &
Reading

Auditory
Listening
& Speaking

Kinaesthetic
Touching
& Doing

Figure 10.23   VAK learning styles

Visually stimulation learning refers to a person's intent on receiving signals via visual cues. He/she is stimulated by pictures and colours. Auditory stimulation learning receives inputs by learning when imparted through lectures, discussions, speeches or talks. Their ability to comprehend pitch, tone or voice modulation enables them to draw inner meaning into a simple conversation. The tactile stimulation learning happens when a person performs or implements an idea or theory through some experimental or practical model. They acquire information by carrying out an activity or task and involve lots of gestures, hand and body movement and touching of materials. They learn best through hands-on training or workshop programmes. They are unable to sit still for long durations. The final one is the kinaesthetic type of learning mechanism. Psychological experts have found that these kind of learners indulge in some physical activity while concentrating on academic lessons. It may be roaming around in a place, bouncing balls, etc. They are also found to take keen interest in activities involving acting, sports, etc. Everyone utilises all three learning styles, but they have a preference based on the dominant style in them, which is the major contribution to effective learning. To learn any new job, concept or task we use a combination of visual input, auditory knowledge and by doing that which aids the learning process.

10.3.10 The DNA assessment and multiple intelligence

Intelligence is a complex term and has been debated over by a galaxy of psychologists who attributed several traits to be inclusive of it, for example, Robert Stenberg's Triarchic theory of intelligence, A. R. Luria's PASS theory of intelligence and Piaget's theory of cognitive development, etc. Generally however intelligence is the ability to learn, conceptualise and derive meaning from pre-perceived consciousness from society or self and then applying reason or logic (Figure 10.24). Other cognitive abilities that may follow include ability to solve a problem, make decisions, retain memory and using some set protocols of communication. Humans are exclusively known to communicate in verbal language. To think and reflect upon makes human a creation unique in their own terms. Moving away from the conventional ways of measuring intelligence Howard Gardner came up with a new theory of eight multiple intelligences that show our uniqueness and

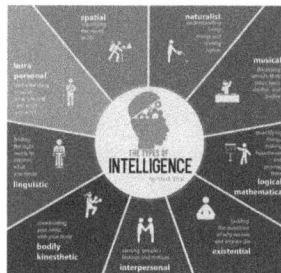

Figure 10.24   Multiple intelligences correlated to fingerprints

speciality, which needs to be utilised to help us choose our career and make life choices for progress and thus paving the way to success. He proposed that humans possess abilities that are general and specific; multiple intelligence shows the proportions of these abilities in a person. This path-breaking research done claimed that conventional idea of evaluating a person based on his/her intelligence quotient, which according to him, was based only on logical–computational and linguistic ability, and to some extent, assessment of spatial intelligence was not enough to quantify the skills of a person in a holistic way. According to him, intelligence was something defined as "a bio psychological potential to process information that can be activated in a cultural setting to solve problems or create products that are of value in a culture".

Dermatoglyphics has been studied in connection with Gardner's theory, which reveals multiple intelligences that focus primarily on eight types of intelligence, namely – logical–mathematical, verbal–linguistic, visual–spatial, bodily–kinaesthetic, interpersonal, intrapersonal, naturalistic and musical.

The Visual–Spatial Intelligence dominance reveals the ability to be able to process 3D space, spatial relations, visual processing, build things, eye for detail and a person who senses changes. The ability to process space makes such intelligent people good drivers, architects, designers, pilots, etc. They enjoy solving puzzles, taking apart an object part by part and study it in detail, and also love to study maps and charts. Visual/spatial ability is the ability to perceive and mentally manipulate a form or object, and to perceive and create tension, balance and composition in a visual or spatial display. Core capacities include mental imagery, spatial reasoning, image manipulation, graphic and artistic skills and an active imagination make them excel as sailors, pilots, sculptors, painters and architects. Strength in this ability makes them crave for mazes or jigsaw puzzles, drawing or day dreaming, etc. These people tend to see things in one's mind in planning to create a product or solve a problem.

The Verbal–Linguistic Intelligence dominance denotes the ability to understand body language, verbal and nonverbal communication. It also shows a good verbal memory (remember everything said before) and comprehension of language (understand the mood of a person); the visual aspect of writing, the ability to talk, explain and understand what is said by others shows the ability to be a communicator and an orator. It indicates the ability to use language to excite, please, convince, stimulate or convey information. It involves ease in speaking a language, and also being perceptive to the flavour, order and rhythm of words. It is the capability of expressing what is on the mind and to understand other people. This ability is required for success in various professions such as writer, orator, speaker, lawyer, etc. Young adults with this kind of intelligence enjoy writing, reading, telling stories and doing crossword puzzles. Learning is through the spoken and written word. This intelligence is considered an asset in the traditional classroom, which involve traditional assessments of intelligence and achievement.

The Logical–Math Intelligence dominance indicates the ability in solving problems, abstract thinking, the ability to deal with numbers and solve complex visual spatial problems. They are also good in designing strategies to deal with situations. They have the mathematical/logical ability to calculate, quantify, consider propositions and hypotheses, explore patterns, categories, carry out complete mathematical operations and relationships by manipulating objects or symbols, and also to experiment in a controlled, orderly manner. Such people perceive relationships and connections and are able to use abstract, symbolic thought, sequential reasoning skills with inductive and deductive thinking patterns. Mathematicians, scientists, detectives all display strength in this intelligence. Because of the innate interest in seeing patterns, categories and relationships they are able to perform effectively in arithmetic problems, strategy games and experiments. Since they utilise reasoning and problem solving they are also found to excel in the traditional classroom, where students were asked to adapt to logically sequenced delivery of instruction.

The Body–Kinaesthetic Intelligence dominance shows excellence in fine motor movements, having the ability to spatial orientation and sensory integration, balance, rhythm and ability to read body language. They are thus graceful and balanced with good hand–eye coordination. They have good ability to use their body in movement and communication. They are good sportsperson and have a natural flair for sports and games. They have the bodily kinaesthetic ability to use fine and gross motor skills in sports, performing arts, or arts and crafts production and are called body smart. It involves a sense of timing and the perfection of skills through mind–body union. Using the body to solve problems, to create products and to convey ideas and emotions make them good athletes, dancers, surgeons and craftspeople. They are also called "overly active" learners and understand only through concrete experience.

The Musical Intelligence dominance indicates the ability to differentiate voice tone, pitch modulation, process recognition and perception of auditory stimuli. Having a good auditory capacity and understanding what is the mood based on the tone of a person is the inherent capacity of musical dominant ability. Love for music, quality sound and perceptivity to auditory input is an inherent inborn talent. This capacity makes a person enjoy musical expression, melody, sound and music. People vary in their interests for auditory input. Some prefer talks while some music. People with this musical/rhythmic ability enjoy, perform or compose a musical piece as they have sensitivity to pitch and rhythm of sounds. They have a knack to discern pitch, rhythm, timbre and tone, and this enables them to recognise, create, reproduce and reflect on music, as demonstrated by composers, conductors, musicians, vocalist and sensitive listeners. Interestingly, an affective connection between music and the emotions; and mathematical and musical intelligence share common thinking processes wherein identification of patterns happens through all the senses.

The Intrapersonal Intelligence reveals judgement, reasoning, self-reflection, confidence, original, planning, motivation and emotional behaviour. They exhibit good thinking and process information in the brain in a systematic, planned manner. They are self-motivated and self-driven and aware of their own strengths and weaknesses thus making them independent thinkers and have the potential to be a good psychologist. Intrapersonal ability is the ability to gain access to understand one's inner feelings, dreams and ideas. Knowledge turned inward entails the ability to understand one's own emotions, goals and intentions. Such people tend to pose deep questions about human existence, the meaning of life, the purpose of birth, the purpose of one's existence, the meaning of death and the purpose of living etc.

The Interpersonal Intelligence dominance displays social behaviour, motivation, emotions, memory formation, language comprehension and mentorship. A strong interpersonal intelligence indicates that connecting to people and interacting with them, understanding, influencing and being influenced makes them a good leader with people's skills and a passion to guide and help others. Interpersonal ability is to understand other people, to notice their goals, motivations, intentions and to work effectively with them along with an ability to empathise with others, observe and understand others' moods, feelings and temperament. Teachers, social workers, actors and politicians – all exhibit interpersonal intelligence wherein they display effective verbal and non-verbal communication, the ability to note distinction among others, sensitivity to moods and temperaments of others and the ability to entertain the people's perspectives. This intelligence is useful in business and promotes collaboration and working cooperatively with others.

The Naturalistic Intelligence strength indicates the affinity to nature, the ability at visual identification and spatial relationship; they also have an affinity and respect for people and all living beings. This intelligence shows love and respect for outdoors and are sensitive to life and accept and respect life and all living things. They are nature lovers and have the qualities to become a doctor, an agriculturist, etc., who respect life in its true sense. Evaluating the family occupation gives clarity to choose the direction of the gene inclination towards medicine or agriculture. Naturalist ability to recognise flora and fauna, communion with the natural world and the human ability to discriminate among living things as well as sensitivity to other features of the natural world such as clouds and rock configurations. Our evolutionary life from hunters, gatherers and farmers to botanists and chefs reflect this genetic disposition. Learning is through classification, categories and hierarchies. The naturalist intelligence picks up on subtle differences in meaning. It is not simply the study of nature; it can be used in all areas of study.

Processing of information corresponding to different intelligences might prove to be similar for many people but some of them are more customised. The genetic makeup as well as experiences from environment contributes to the uniqueness and exclusivity.

10.4   Dermatoglyphics and its applications

Dermatoglyphics is a science of the fingerprint analysis which has a vast applicability sphere. It can be applied to almost any field and has proven to be very accurate in prediction of behaviour. It has evolved from a multi-disciplinary approach due to an integration of various topics like embryology, anthropology, genetics, medicine, biology, dermatology, psychology etc. It has been proved that it can serve as a diagnostic tool as it has a genetic base and is a part of inherent innate nature by birth. This innate potential is again a genetic disposition and is a lifetime potential inherent in any person. The secret lies in unravelling it, understanding its potential and using it to maximise achievement and also to enhance the happiness quotient. The distribution of cells in the brain and dominance can be understood through this science of fingerprint analysis and hence a valuable tool for day to day effective functioning. Since our brain stays with us for life it acts as a predictor of capability and achievement which paves the way for career and relationship expertise.

10.4.1 Dermatoglyphics as genetic markers

Dermatoglyphic patterns, such as fingerprints, are potential genetic markers for a number of behavioural syndromes. It reveals behavioural and psychological traits that are inborn and inherent and hence a valuable tool to reckon with. Psychologists like Iacono and many more have become increasingly interested in the search for genetic markers to be able to guide, control and transform behavioural tendencies. The dermatoglyphic patterns on the fingers commonly referred to as fingerprints are said to be phenotypic characteristics. There has been no dearth of studies to prove that these dermal patterns are strongly determined by genetic factors as indicators of genetically based syndromes. Studies have shown their relationship to a number of disorders known to be due to chromosomal or genetic sources. Specific fingerprint pattern distributions have been associated with Down's Syndrome, Turner's Syndrome, Klinefelter's Syndrome, de Lange's Syndrome, Rubinstein–Taybi's Syndrome and several others. Psychosis has also been seen to have originated through specific finger ridge patterns.

10.4.2 Early detection as indicator for prevention of schizophrenia

As psychotic tendencies have been proven to be genetic and this can be identified by fingerprint patterns, early detection and intervention strategies for schizophrenia are receiving increasingly more attention. The degree of asymmetry of the fingerprints is indicators of early abnormal developmental processes. The dynamic interaction between genetic factors and insults during embryonic development has augmented the development of psychotic disorders such as schizophrenia. These psychotic tendencies are thus considered as a neurodevelopmental disorder which might occur before the end of the second gestational trimester. Diverse abnormalities in schizophrenia like the distortion of the corpus callosum and asymmetry of brain, have been recognised on computed tomography and magnetic resonance imaging scans. Since Dermatoglyphics, the epidermal ridges and patterns of the hand are established by the end of the second trimester and have been considered as markers of prenatal brain injury. The rationale behind this hypothesis is that epidermal ridges share ectodermal origins with the central nervous system. The epidermal ridges start to develop in the 11th gestational week and their critical stage of differentiation occurs in foetal months 3–4, coinciding with a critical phase of brain development. Though the morphology of the epidermal ridges is genetically determined, it can also be influenced by environmental factors in the womb such as a viral infection, radiation or alcohol and drug abuse, which can disturb the harmonious flow of the brain development. Once formed however the epidermal ridges remain unchanged and hence the ectoderm use unusual dermatoglyphic patterns to characterise disturbances to brain development. Experimental research has proven the direct link between epidermal ridges and schizophrenia using different features to characterise the configuration of epidermal ridges, and hence, the association between Dermatoglyphics and cerebral structural measures in patients with schizophrenia is valuable. The altered prenatal neurodevelopment formed at the second trimester of prenatal development has been etiologically relevant to the development of schizophrenia and the unusual dermatoglyphic patterns, which have been hypothesised to be proxy markers of altered early development in psychosis.

10.4.3   Dermatoglyphics and medical conditions

Down's Syndrome, Klinefelter's Syndrome, cerebral palsy, schizophrenia, congenital diabetes, cardiac diseases, etc., are all medical conditions that have been correlated to fingerprint pattern and are considered congenital defects. Dr Stanley Cohen, under the supervision of Dr Rita Levi Montalcini, has also undertaken revolutionary research in the field of bot neurology and embryology. Their studies revealed the functional loci of both EGF and NGF which are related and regulated by amino acid sequence of transforming protein.

10.4.4   Dermatoglyphics and diseases

Li *et al.* were the first to build a hereditary model of left and right asymmetry in humans, which can be used to determine whether a person is the father of another using the of inter digital areas of Dermatoglyphics patterns. Another method has also been developed using palm prints to assess parental identification, which seems to be more reliable. These studies reveal that though the connection and association has been proven and that there is an association, more studies could reveal further complexities in this regard.

10.4.5   Dermatoglyphics and sports

Olympic gold medals can be an everyday happening if people are identified at an early age and nurtured based on their potentialities. Sportsmanship and Dermatoglyphics have been seen to be correlated. Selection of candidates needs to be done based on this reliable external genetic markers for selection of individuals with high level sportsmanship. Studies on genetic markers and sportsman ship reveal that they are correlated.

10.4.6   Dermatoglyphics and applications to daily life

- Personal growth:
  - o   Helps strengthen interpersonal communication and interaction skills,
  - o   Know how to appreciate people, improve relations between the sexes,
  - o   Enhance emotional quotient and adversity quotient,

○ Discover one's unique gift,
○ Improve career and
○ Enhance the sense of the value of life and happiness.

- Education:
  ○ Helps multiple intelligence assessment for children,
  ○ Parent–child communication and education,
  ○ Target at talents,
  ○ Personalised education,
  ○ Identified one's gifted area,
  ○ Select a major that best fits one's desired career path and
  ○ Define the most appropriate way of teaching and learning.

- Enterprises:
  ○ Helps in recruitment,
  ○ Assessment of job competency and execution style,
  ○ Plan education and training,
  ○ Explore the potential of employee,
  ○ Leadership,
  ○ Interpersonal communication and interaction, and
  ○ Consolidation of human resources.

References

[1] Mandeep Singh, Oindri Majumdar. Dermatoglyphics: Blueprints of Human Cognition on Fingerprints. Punjab, India: Thapar University. 2015.
[2] Harold Cummins, Charles Midlo. Finger Prints, Palms and Soles. An Introduction to Dermatoglyphics. Philadelphia: The Blakiston Company. p. 11; 1943.
[3] Walter Burke Barbe, Raymond H. Swassing, Michael N. Milone, Jr. Teaching through Modality Strengths: Concepts and Practices. Columbus, Ohio: Zaner-Blosner. ISBN 978-0-88309-100-5.

Further reading

[1] Alter Milton. Dermatoglyphic analysis as a diagnostic tool. *Medicine*. 46(1); 35–56: 1967.
[2] Archana Singh, Rakesh Gupta, SHH Zaidi, Arun Singh. Dermatoglyphics: A brief review. *International Journal of Advanced & Integrated Medical Sciences*. 1(3); 111–115: 2016.
[3] Cheah, P. Y., *et al.* The Drosophila l (2) 35Ba/nocA gene encodes a putative Zn finger protein involved in the development of the embryonic brain and the adult ocellar structures. *Molecular and Cellular Biology*. 14(2); 1487–1499: 1994.
[4] Cummins H, Midloo C. Finger Prints, Palms and Soles. An Introduction to Dermatoglyphics. New York: Dovar Pub. INC; 1961.

[5]   David Eagleman. 10 unsolved mysteries of the brain. What we know—and don't know—about how we think. *Discover*. 2007.

[6]   Maria Luisa A. Valdez, Thaakor Pathak. Assessment of dermatoglyphics multiple intelligence test (DMIT) reports: Implication to career guidance program enhancement of academic institutions. *Asia Pacific Journal of Multidisciplinary Research*. 2(2): 24–31: 2014.

[7]   Abhimanyu MP, Bottiger W, Singh GD. An exploratory study about client satisfaction in Dermatoglyphics multiple intelligence test. *International Journal of Applied Research*. 2(3); 802–806: 2016.

[8]   Edward Campbell. Fingerprints and Behaviour: A Textbook on Fingerprints and Behavioural Correspondences (Volume 1). Amida Biometrics, LLC, 2012.

[9]   Encyclopedia Britannica. Primate-Mammal: Sensory reception and the brain. Dermatoglyphic pattern study. *APMC Journal*. Available at: https://www.britannica.com/animal/primate-mammal/Sensory-reception-and-the-brain.

[10] F. H. Rauscher, G. L. Shaw, and C. N. Ky, Music and spatial task performance. *Nature*. 365;611: 1993.

[11] Galton F. Finger Prints: The Classic. Dover Publications, 2004. 216; p. 1892.

[12] Gardner H. Frames of Mind: The Theory of Multiple Intelligences. New York: Basic Books; 1983.

[13] Gardner, H. Ch. 8. The Eight One: Naturalistic Intelligence. How Are Kids Smart: Multiple Intelligences in the Classroom— Administrators' Version. Morris, M (ed). 1995. ISBN 1-887943-03-X [16].

[14] Gardner, H., Hatch, T. Multiple intelligences go to school: Educational implications of the theory of multiple intelligences. *Educational Researcher*. 18(8);4: 1989.

[15] Gardner, Howard E. Intelligence Reframed: Multiple Int. Perseus Books Group, 2000.

[16] Gardner, Howard. Heteroglossia: A global perspective. *Interdisciplinary Journal of Theory of Postpedagogical Studies*. 1984.

[17] Gardner, Howard. Frames of Mind: The Theory of Multiple Intelligences. New York: Basic Books, 1993.

[18] Hall, Lynn S. Dermatoglyphic analysis of total finger ridge count in female monozygotic twins discordant for sexual orientation. *Journal of Sex Research*. 2000.

[19] http://csjournals.com/IJCSC/PDF6-2/24.%20Oindri.pdf

[20] http://midbrainevs.com/content/brain-and-finger-how-it-connects

[21] http://www.wofs.com/index.php/miscellaneous-mainmenu-38/443-fortune-a-personality-traits-fromthe-tips-of-your-fingers

[22] https://brainmagic.in/benefits-of-dermatoglyphics-multiple-intelligence-test/

[23] Huitt, William, J. Hummel. Piaget's Theory of Cognitive Development. Educational Psychology Interactive, Valdosta, GA: Valdosta State University. 2003.

[24] Kelso, JA Scott. Dynamic Patterns: The Self-organization of Brain and Behavior. Cambridge, MA: MIT press, 1997.

[25] Kincheloe, Joe L. Multiple Intelligences Reconsidered. Peter Lang. p. 159: 2004 ISBN 978-0-8204-7098-6.

[26] Leite, Walter L., Svinicki, Marilla, Shi, Yuying. Attempted Validation of the Scores of the VARK: Learning Styles Inventory with Multitrait–Multimethod Confirmatory Factor Analysis Models. *Educational and Psychological Measurement.* 70(2); 323–339: 2009.

[27] M. I. Posner, M. K. Rothbart. Research on attention networks as a model for the integration of psychological science. *Annual Review of Psychology.* 58; 1–23: 2007.

[28] John J. Mulvihill, David W. Smith. The genesis of dermatoglyphics. *The Journal of Pediatrics.* 75(4); 579–589: 1969; *Asia Pacific Journal of Multidisciplinary Research.* 2(2); 2014.

[29] Alice V. Maceo. Anatomy and Physiology of Adult Friction Ridge Skin. Fingerprint Sourcebook. 2011.

[30] Davide Maltoni, *et al.* Handbook of Fingerprint Recognition. Springer Science & Business Media, 2009.

[31] Mandeep Singh. Introduction to Biomedical Instrumentation. PHI Learning Pvt Ltd, 2010.

[32] Multiple intelligences, related personality and learning types and behaviour. Available at http://dermatoglyphics.org/

[33] Rohit P Prabhu, C N Ravikumar. A novel extended biometric approach for human character recognition using fingerprints. *International Journal of Computer Applications.* 77(1): 2013. (0975–8887).

[34] Jack A. Naglieri, James C. Kaufman. Understanding intelligence, giftedness and creativity using the PASS theory. *Roeper Review.* 2006.

[35] Narayanan Srinivasan. Cognitive neuroscience of creativity: EEG based approaches. *Methods.* 42(1); 109–116: 2007.

[36] Norris M. Durham, Chris C. Plato, editors. Trends in Dermatoglyphic Research. Dordrecht/Boston/London: Kluwer Academic Publishers. p. 4: 1990.

[37] Wilder Penfield, Edwin Boldrey. Somatic motor and sensory representation in the cerebral cortex of man as studied by electrical stimulation. *Brain.* 60(4): 1937.

[38] Wilder Penfield, Theodore Rasmussen. The cerebral cortex of man: A clinical study of localization of function. *JAMA.* 144(16); 1412: 1950.

[39] Penrose LS, Ohara PT. The development of the epidermal ridges. *Journal of Medical Genetics.* 10(3); 201–208: 1973.

[40] Nalini K. Ratha, Ruud M. Bolle. Effect of Controlled Image Acquisition of Fingerprint Matching. *Proceedings of the Fourteenth International Conference on Pattern Recognition IEEE,* 1998.

[41] Robert A. Rohm, "Who Do You Think You Are Anyway?", Personality Insights Incorporated, 1997.

[42] Francis Galton. Fingerprints. London: MacMillan & Co. 1892.

[43] Robert J. Sternberg. Toward a triarchic theory of human intelligence. *Behavioral and Brain Sciences* 7(2);269–316: 1984.

[44]   The Fingerprint Sourcebook, Eric H Holder Jr, Laurie O Robinson, John H Laub, National Institute of Justice.

[45]   The Science of Fingerprints Classification and Uses. United States Department of Justice, Federal Bureau of Investigation. Types of Patterns and Their Interpretation. Chapter II, Page V. Available from http://www.crime-scene-investigator.net/fbiscienceoffingerprints.html#chapter_ii. Accessed on 22-09-2016.

[46]   Tupper, K. W. Entheogens and existential intelligence: The use of plant teachers as cognitive tools. *Canadian Journal of Education*. 27(4); 499–516: (2002).

[47]   Walter McKenzie. Media selection: Mapping technologies to intelligences. *Virginia Society for Technology in Education (VSTE)*. 17(1): 2002.

[48]   Lynn Waterhouse. Multiple intelligences, the Mozart effect, and emotional intelligence: A critical review. *Educational Psychologist*. 41(4);207–225: 2006.

Chapter 11

Electrocardiography: overview, preparation, and technique

Thulasyammal Ramiah Pillai[1], Raach Oussama Khalil[2], and Narendiran Krishnasamy[3]

11.1 Introduction

The electrocardiogram (ECG) is an indispensable diagnostic tool for doctors to treat patients with heart disease by recording the electrical activity of the heart. For over a century, it remains an important process in clinical practice for diagnosis and monitoring abnormalities of the heart [1]. Furthermore, ECG also plays a major role in therapeutic decision making [2] and helps physicians in the accurate placement of central venous catheters (CVC) tip thus avoiding potential complications [3].

There are various imaging techniques for the diagnosis of cardiovascular disease, but the ECG remains the most economic and commonly used tool since it provides information about the electric activity generated by the heart accurately and quickly. The pattern of electrical propagation is not random, but spreads over the structure of the heart in a coordinated manner [4].

Depending on the symptoms displayed by patients and their gravity, the physician may request a particular method to investigate the electric heart activity; 12-lead standard ECG to have an overview of the different sections, 3-lead ECG monitoring in ICU and emergency care, Holter monitor and event recorder for episodic symptoms, cardiac loop recorder and implantable loop recorder that are automated and wireless ECG that can communicate directly with a wireless device.

The wireless ECG is nearly three times more efficient in diagnosing and detecting heart rhythm abnormalities than the other machines available in this field [5]. While, Wen Ling Chang *et al.* suggested that portable ECG device via remote care system may aid in clinical diagnosis, therapeutic interventions, or patient referral for cardiac arrhythmias [6]. However, Vezzosi *et al.* mentioned that the smartphone device is not a substitute for 6-lead ECG or Holter monitoring, but does

[1]School of Computing and IT, Taylor's University, Malaysia
[2]School of Bioscience, Taylor's University, Malaysia
[3]Clinical Skills Unit, School of Medicine, Taylor's University, Malaysia

represent an additional tool in the management of dogs with arrhythmias or monitoring dogs at risk for heart rhythm disturbances [7]. There are numerous arguments regarding the wireless ECG. However, 12-lead ECG test-standard ECG machine cannot be substituted by all these wireless ECG because of the stable and reliable readings of the ECG.

In hospitals, patients are monitored by utilizing 12-lead cardiac monitors to detect the presence of arrhythmia, heart defects, and presence of ischemia and infracts and hypertrophy. In this there is a constant need to be monitored by the physicians. The visual inspection of the monitors is impractical, tedious and the diagnosis may vary among physicians. Leonard Steinfeld had stated that approximately one-third of the current presumably well-trained and certified pediatric cardiologists out in practice had failed to interpret correctly the abnormal ECG results obtained from children before participation in active sports [8] and it is not only limited to pediatricians.

Continuous observation and detection of abnormal ECG signals can be difficult due to a large number of patients in intensive care units and the necessity of 24 h continuous monitoring. In addition to a simple ECG test, a longer recording of ECG signal is obtained using a portable Holter monitor worn by the patients [9]. The cardiologist needs to examine the recordings and diagnose the patients accordingly. The examination of these recordings is a time-consuming process due to the length of the records and the presence of various interferences.

The ECG has always been the basic choice for diagnosing cardiac abnormalities. These abnormalities in heart rate (number of heart beats per minute) and/or its rhythm (regular or irregular), may progress to arrhythmias [10–13]. Furthermore, symptoms of heart diseases are reflected by the nature and details of arrhythmia which can be an irregular single heartbeat (arrhythmic beat), or an irregular group of heartbeats (arrhythmic episode).

Arrhythmias represent a serious threat to the patient recovering from acute myocardial infarction, especially ventricular arrhythmias like ventricular tachycardia (VT) and ventricular fibrillation (VF). In particular, VT and VF are life-threatening conditions that produce significant hemodynamic deterioration [14] and must be diagnosed early. Other arrhythmias like atrial premature contraction (APC), premature ventricular contraction (PVC), and supraventricular tachycardia (SVT) are not as lethal as VF but are important in diagnosing the disorders of the heart.

Arrhythmias can occur in a healthy heart, but they may indicate a serious problem that may lead to stroke or sudden cardiac death [15]. Therefore, automatic arrhythmia detection and classification is critical in clinical cardiology, especially when performed in real time. This can be achieved through the analysis of ECG and its extracted features [15]. Hence, significant amount of research has been focused on the development of algorithms for the arrhythmia diagnosis [16].

Hence, computer programs have been developed to help in this visual analysis by providing condensed printouts. Computer-assisted arrhythmia recognition is critical for the management of cardiac disorders [16]. Several methods for automated arrhythmia detection have been developed [Mahesh, 17]. Two or three types of arrhythmias only can be classified using these techniques and it consumes significantly large processing time. Hence, an advanced Generalized Autoregressive Moving Average (GARMA) model and Generalized Linear Model (GLM) classifier will be utilized to classify the various types of arrhythmias [9,10,16]. This study is designed to cater a large number of patients, to eliminate subjective inaccuracies, to aid the physician in the diagnosis, to reduce the time of diagnosis, to simplify the monitoring task, and to improve diagnostic efficiencies. The current challenge is to establish a reliable method for detection and diagnosis of arrhythmia [16].

11.2 History

In 1855 Kollicker and Mueller found that the leg of the frog when dissecting kicked with each heartbeat. Ludwig and Waller found that the heart's rhythmic electrical stimuli could be monitored from a person's skin in the middle of 1880. They called this device the "capillary electrometer" and it was not suitable for clinical application or even for economic exploitation, but it was very interesting [17].

In the late Nineteenth century (1887) Augustus D Waller recorded electrical activity of the human heart using saline filled tube electrodes [18]. Willem Einthoven and Thomas Lewis are generally regarded as having been the most influential people in the development of ECG. Lewis's 1925 book, "The Mechanism and Graphic Registration of the Heart Beat", has long been accorded the status of a masterpiece in cardiology [19]. In the last years of the nineteenth century, Willem Einthoven studied the animal action potentials using the capillary electrometer. He made several modifications to predict the human ECG correctly using a string galvanometer, which was developed in 1902.

In the 1960s Pipberger pioneered his effort in computerized ECG and extended it to vector cardiographic (VCG) research. In 1967 and 1975 Pipbeger gave recommendations for ECG instrumentation to American heart Institution. In 1969 the Caceres first diagnostic computer was born for ECG. In 1970, Caceres and Dreifus edited a book called "Clinical Electrocardiography and Computers", which contains many important aspects of computer-ECG developments and contribution by both of them [20]. In Table 11.1, we have written the history of ECG in chronological order.

11.3 Overview

The ECG (record) is a graphical recording of the electrical signals generated by the heart. The signals are generated when cardiac muscles depolarize in response to electrical impulses generated by pacemaker cells. Upon depolarization, the muscles contract and pump the blood throughout the body [23]. The ECG is used to interpret the cardiac rhythm, detect the myocardial ischemia and infarction, conduction system abnormalities, pre-excitation, long QT syndromes, atrial abnormalities,

Table 11.1 History of ECG

Date	Activity	Person	Paper
In the late 19th century (1887)	Electrical activity of the human heart was recorded using saline-filled tube electrodes	Augustus D Waller	The history of electrocardiography (Journal of Electrocardiology) (2017) (Luderitz and Luna) [18]
In the early years of the development of ECG	1. Willem Einthoven and Thomas Lewis are generally regarded as having been the most influential in the development of ECG 2. Lewis's 1925 book, The Mechanism and Graphic Registration of the Heart Beat (4), has long been accorded the status of a masterpiece in cardiology (5).	Thomas Lewis	Reappraisal of Thomas Lewis's place in the history of electrocardiography (Xiao and Lawrence) [19]
In the last years of the 19th century	1. Study the animal action potentials using the capillary electrometer 2. He made several modifications to predict the human ECG correctly using a string galvanometer, which was developed in 1902	Willem Einthoven	The history of electrocardiography (Journal of Electrocardiology) (2017) [18]
In the 1960s	Pipberger pioneered his effort in computerized ECG and extended it to vectorcardiographic (VCG) research	Pipberger	Autaharju PM, The birth of computerized electrocardiography Hubrt V. Pipberger 1966 [20]
In 1967 and 1975	Pipbeger gave recommendations for ECG instrumentation to American heart Institution	Pipberger	Autaharju PM, The birth of computerized electrocardiography Hubrt V. Pipberger 1966 [20]
In 1969 In 1970	The Caceres first diagnostic computer was born for ECG Caceres and Dreifus edited a book called "Clinical Electrocardiography and Computers", which contains many important aspects of computer-ECG developments and contribution by both of them	Caceres Caceres and Dreifus	Diagnostic computers [22] Clinical electrocardiography and computers [21]

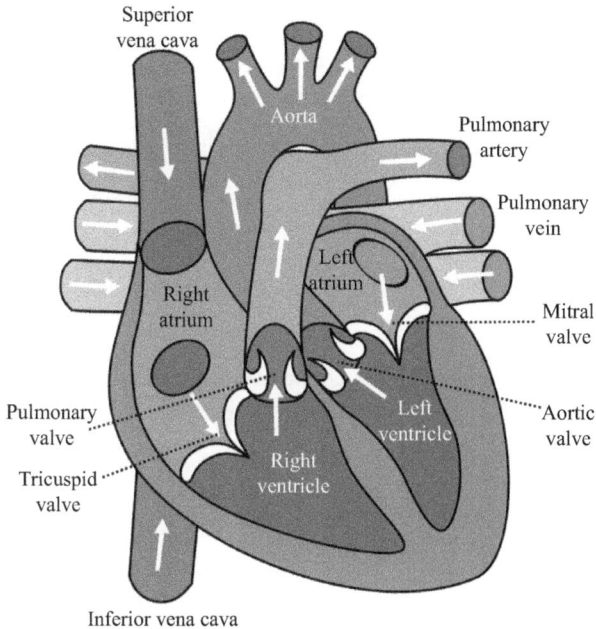

Figure 11.1   A diagrammatic structure of the human heart [25]

ventricular hypertrophy, pericarditis, and other conditions [24]. The performance of an automatic ECG analyzing system depends mostly upon the accurate and reliable detection of the QRS complex [4]. Hence, we will study how this QRS complex was developed. First of all, let us study the structure of the human heart.

The diagrammatic structure of the human heart is shown in Figure 11.1. The heart is made up of four chambers namely; two upper chambers called left and right atrium (auricles) and the two lower chambers are called the left and right ventricles. The oxygen poor blood is received through superior and inferior vena cava and flows into the right atrium. The right atrium contracts and forces blood into the right ventricle. The right ventricle pumps the blood to the lungs. The oxygen-enriched blood is received through pulmonary veins into the left atrium and left ventricle from lungs. The left ventricle pumps the blood to the rest of the body through aorta. These movements developed the QRS complex and it is captured through ECG.

The ECG is obtained by using electrodes attached to the skin across different areas of the heart. A single lead ECG recorder would typically have three electrodes; namely, the positive electrode, the negative electrode, and an indifferent electrode (ground or "right leg" drive electrode). The electrode placed on the left arm will be called as left arm (LA) electrode, the one placed on right arm is called right arm electrode (RA), the electrode placed on left leg is called left leg (LL) electrode, while the electrode placed on right leg is called right leg (RL) electrode. There are six chest electrodes V1, V2, V3, V4, V5, and V6. There are only ten electrodes attached to the skin of a patient.

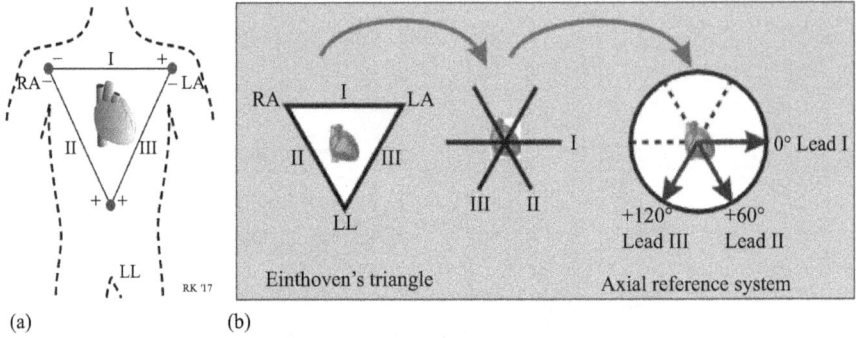

Figure 11.2   (a) Limb leads in the Einthoven's triangle (b)Limb leads are presented in the axial reference system [26]

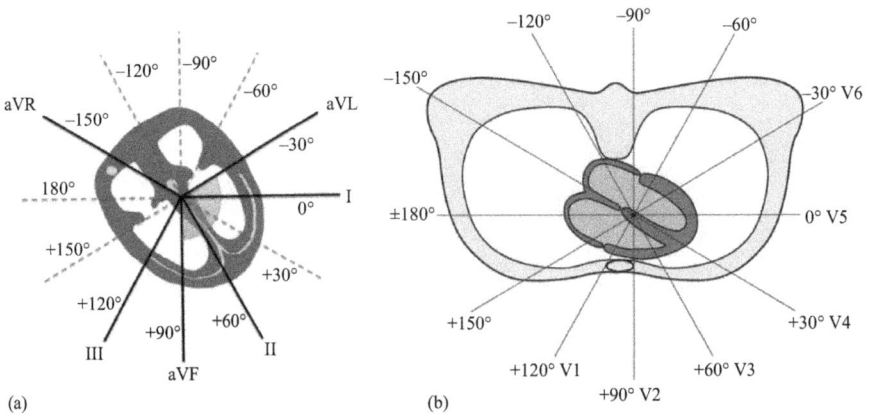

Figure 11.3   (a) Limb leads and augmented leads (b) Position of all the leads [27]

The placement of the electrodes determines the directional viewpoint of the heart. Each viewpoint is called a "lead". The leads I, II, and III are called the limb leads and it is shown in Figure 11.2(a). This triangle is called the Einthoven's triangle. The leads I, II, and III are moved accordingly as in Figure 11.2(b). The leads I, II, and III in first diagram of Figure 11.2(b) are parallel to the leads I, II, and III in second diagram of Figure 11.2(b), respectively. These leads had been presented in the third diagram of Figure 11.2(b), which is called as axial reference system. The axial reference system is also called as the Cabrera system. This axial system presents the extremity leads of the 12-lead ECG, which provides an illustrative logical sequence that helps interpretation of the ECG.

The signals from the limb electrodes can be combined to give augmented leads called aVL, aVR, and aVF. These signals are combined with the leads I, II, and III in Figure 11.3(a). The six chest electrodes V1, V2, V3, V4, V5, and V6 give six views of the heart signals across the front of the chest. These leads are called

Table 11.2 Signal combination of the leads

Lead	Electrode + (real)	Electrode − (real/virtual)	Signal combination	Approximate medical angle	Mathematical angle
I	LA	RA	LA-RA	0°	0°
II	LL	RA	LL-RA	+60°	−60°
III	LL	LA	LL-LA	+120°	−120°
aVL	LA	RA, LL	LA-1/2(RA+LL)	−30°	+30°
aVF	LL	RA, LA	LL-1/2(RA+LA)	+90°	−90°
aVR	RA	LA,LL	RA-1/2(LA+LL)	−150°	+150°
V1	V1	LA, RA, LL	V1-1/3 (LA+RA+LL)	+120°	−120°
V2	V2	LA, RA, LL	V2-1/3 (LA+RA+LL)	+90°	−90°
V3	V3	LA, RA, LL	V3-1/3 (LA+RA+LL)	+60°	−60°
V4	V4	LA, RA, LL	V4-1/3 (LA+RA+LL)	+30°	−30°
V5	V5	LA, RA, LL	V5-1/3 (LA+RA+LL)	0°	0°
V6	V6	LA, RA, LL	V6-1/3 (LA+RA+LL)	−30°	+30°

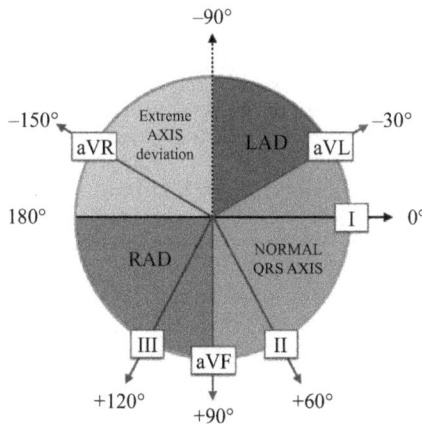

Figure 11.4 Axial reference system and heart condition [28]

precordial leads. The position of these leads are given in Figure 11.3(b). There are 12 leads altogether. The signal combination of these leads is given in Table 11.2. The position of these leads will determine the condition of the heart abnormalities, which can be seen in the axial reference system in Figure 11.4.

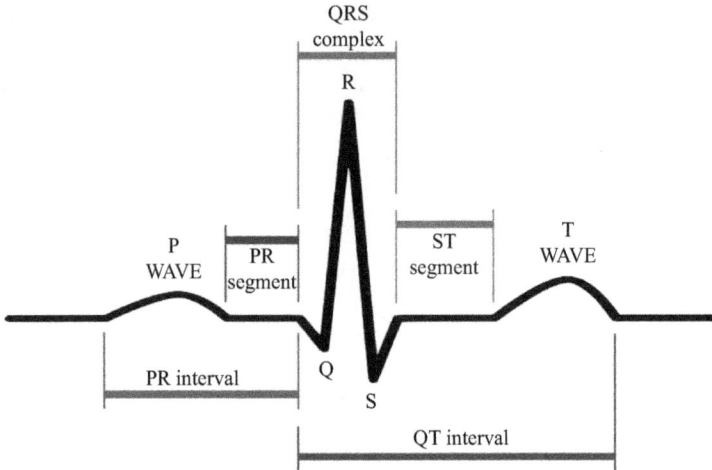

Figure 11.5   Schematic representation of a single cycle of ECG corresponding to one heart beat [29]

Table 11.3   Parts of the ECG and activities

Parts of ECG	Activities
P wave	Depolarization of the atrial myocardium
	Start of atrial contraction that pumps blood to the ventricles
	Activation of the right and left atria
QRS complex	Depolarization of ventricular myocardium
	Start of ventricular contraction that pumps blood to the lungs and the rest of the body
	Depolarization of the activation of right and left ventricles
T wave	Repolarization of the ventricular myocardium
	End of T wave coincides with the end of ventricular contraction
U wave (normal ECG may not show)	Origin is uncertain
	Late depolarization of the ventricular myocardium
	Prominent under abnormal conditions

These signal combinations of the leads formed the ECG recordings.

The ECG signal of a normal heart consists of three parts, such as P wave, QRS complex, and T wave. The parts of the waves are shown in Figure 11.5 and the activities in Table 11.3. The condition of the heart also can be diagnosed using heart rate, PR Interval, QRS complex width, T wave, and some other abnormal waves, which appears only in certain disease conditions.

11.4   Interpreting the ECG: a six-step approach

There are various methods to interpret the ECG. However, we are going to interpret the ECG data using the six-step method. These six steps are

1. Rate and rhythm
2. Axis determination
3. Intervals
4. Morphology
5. STE-Mimics
6. Ischemia, Injury, and Infarct

11.4.1   Interpret ECG using rate and rhythm

11.4.1.1   Methods for calculating heart rate

Heart rate is calculated as the number of times the heart beats per minute (bpm). On an ECG tracing the bpm is usually calculated as the number of QRS complexes.

Method 1: Count large boxes

Regular rhythms can be determined by counting the number of large graph boxes between the two R waves. The bpm is 300 divided by the number of large boxes. This is an approximate heart rate. The ECG example in Figure 11.6 shows six big boxes between the two R waves. The number 300 is divided by six and we obtained the value 50. Hence, this patient's bpm is 50.

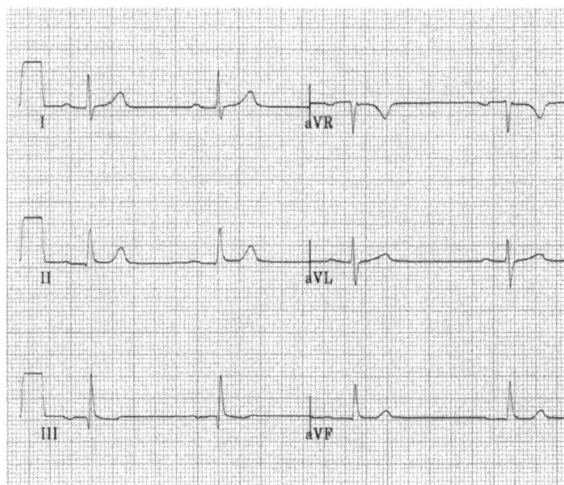

Figure 11.6   Example of ECG [30]

Method 2: Count small boxes

The most accurate way to measure a regular rate is to count the number of small boxes between two R waves. The number of small boxes is divided into 1,500 to calculate bpm. The ECG sample in Figure 11.6 shows 31 small boxes. This 1,500 is divided by 31 and it is equivalent to 48. The patient's bpm is 48.

Method 3: Six-second ECG rhythm strip

The best method for measuring irregular heart rates with varying R–R intervals is to count the number of R waves in a 6-s (sec) strip and multiply by 10. This gives the average number of beats per minute. This can be seen in Figure 11.7.

11.4.1.2   Methods for identifying the rhythm

The ECG provides the most accurate means for identifying cardiac arrhythmias (abnormal rhythms), which can be easily diagnosed by understanding the electrophysiology of the heart. An arrhythmia (abnormalities in heart rhythm) detection algorithm is developed based on three parameters namely, the RR interval, QRS width, and PR interval. The range of these parameters for various classes of disease are listed in Table 11.4.

This has been explained vividly in this section for various arrhythmias.

Sinoatrial node arrhythmias

Sinus rhythms all originate in the sinoatrial (SA) node as in Figure 11.8. The SA node begins the electrical impulse, which spreads outward in wave fashion, stimulating both atria to contract. The electrical impulse spreads through the atria and yields a P wave on the ECG.

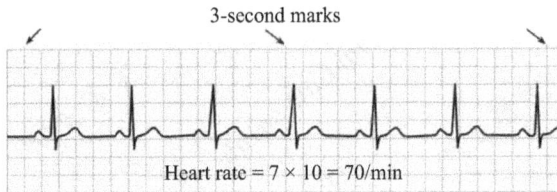

Figure 11.7   A 6-second ECG strip [31]

Table 11.4   Disease classification based on heart rate, PR interval, and QRS width

Types of	Heart rate (bpm)	PR interval (s)	QRS width (s)
Normal sinus rhythm	60–90	0.12–0.21	0.06–0.08
Sinus bradycardia	40–60	0.12–0.21	0.06–0.08
Sinus tachycardia	More than 100	0.12–0.21	0.06–0.08
SVT	More than 150	Usually not possible to measure	0.06–0.08 or more than 0.10
VT	100–250	None	More than 0.10
Bundle branch block	Depends on rate of underlying rhythm	0.12–0.2	More than 0.12

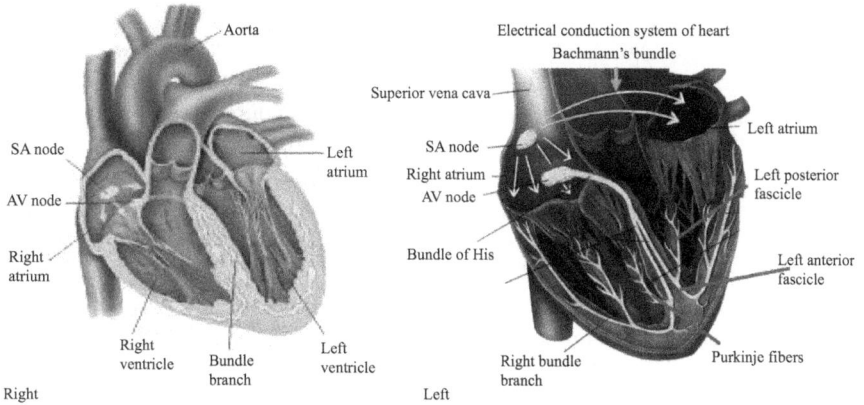

Figure 11.8   Electrical conduction system of heart [32]

Table 11.5   Sinus rhythms based on rate, rhythm, P wave, PR interval, and QRS complex

Sinus rhythm	Rate (bpm)	Rhythm	P wave	PR interval	QRS
NSR	60–100	Regular	Normal	Normal	Normal
SB	Less than 60	Regular	Normal	Normal	Normal
ST	More than 100	Regular	Normal	Normal	Normal
Sinus Arrhythmia	Normal	Irregular	Normal	Normal	Normal
SP	Normal to slow	Irregular	Normal	Normal	Normal
SA block	Normal to slow	Irregular	Normal	Normal	Normal

The ECG features common to all of them are upright P waves, all similar in appearance; normal duration PR intervals, normal QRS complexes if no ventricular conduction disturbances are present. Sinus rhythms are classified as normal sinus rhythm (NSR), sinus bradycardia (SB), sinus tachycardia (ST), sinus arrhythmia, sinus pause (SP), and sinoatrial block (SA block). The categorization of sinus rhythms based on rate, rhythm, P wave, PR interval and QRS complex are given in Table 11.5.

SA node arrhythmias can be determined using the rate and rhythm only. The P wave, PR interval, and QRS complex are normal for SA node arrhythmias.

Atrial arrhythmias
Atrial arrhythmias originate in the atria. The impulse reaches the atrioventricular (AV) node where there is a brief pause, allowing blood to enter the ventricles. Thus the pause produces the short piece of flat baseline after each P wave (PR segment).

The stimulus of depolarization proceeds rapidly down the His bundle into the bundle branches, although depolarization slows within the AV node. The His bundle divides into right and left bundle branches within the interventricular septum. The electrical stimulus is distributed via the terminal Purkinje fibers to the

224 EEG signal processing

ventricular myocardial cells. This is the depolarization of the myocardial cells, which produces a QRS complex on ECG tracing. The QRS complex represents only the depolarization of the myocardial cells of the ventricles.

The common ECG features are P waves, and normal duration QRS complexes if no ventricular conduction disturbances are present. Atrial rhythms to be described are wandering atrial pacemaker (WAP), multifocal atrial tachycardia (MAT), premature atrial contraction (PAC), atrial tachycardia (AT), SVT, paroxysmal supraventricular tachycardia (PSVT), atrial flutter (A-flutter), atrial fibrillation (AF), and Wolff–Parkinson–White (WPW) syndrome. The statistics on rate, rhythm, P wave, PR interval, and QRS complex according to atrial rhythm is given in Table 11.6.

In this case all the parameters vary according to the abnormalities of the heart.

Junctional arrhythmias

The intermodal pathways in the heart merge with the cells of the AV, which include the AV node. The AV junction is the origin of junctional rhythms. The rhythms described are junctional (J), accelerated junctional rhythms (AJR), junctional tachycardia (JT), junctional escape beat (JEB), and premature junctional contraction (PJC). The statistics on rate, rhythm, P wave, PR interval, and QRS complex according to junctional arrhythmias' rhythm is given in Table 11.7.

In junctional arrhythmias all the values of the parameters vary except the QRS complex. QRS complex depends only on the depolarization of the myocardial cells of the ventricles.

Ventricular arrhythmias

All arrhythmias that originate in the ventricles depolarize the ventricles abnormally and at a slower speed. The Purkinje fibers transmit the electrical impulse (depolarization) to the myocardial cells, causing ventricular contraction, and producing a QRS complex on the tracing. The Q wave is the first downward stroke of the QRS complex, and it is followed by the upward R wave. The Q wave is often not present. The upward R wave is followed by a downward S wave. This total QRS complex represents the electrical activity of ventricular depolarization.

The ventricular rhythms are idioventricular (IV), accelerated idioventricular rhythm (AIR), PVC, monomorphic ventricular tachycardia (MVT), polymorphic VT (PVT), torsade de pointes (TDP), VF, pulseless electrical activity (PEA), and asystole (A). The statistics on ventricular rhythms are shown in Table 11.8.

In this case all the parameters differ from the NSR parameters.

AV and bundle branch blocks

AV blocks reflect delay or interruption of impulses through the AV junction due to disease in this region. They are traditionally divided into three categories: first, second, and third degree. They are called as first degree AV block (FDAVB), second degree AV block: Type I (MOBITZ1), second degree AV block: Type II (MOBITZII), and third degree AV block (TDAVB). Another disorder, involving bundle branch conduction through the ventricles, is bundle branch block (BBB). The characteristics of the AV and BBB are given in Table 11.9.

Table 11.6 Atrial arrhythmias based on rate, rhythm, P wave, PR interval, and QRS complex

Atrial rhythm	Rate (bpm)	Rhythm	P wave	PR interval	QRS
WAP	60–100	Irregular	At least three different forms	Variable	Normal
MAT	More than 100	Irregular	At least three different forms	Variable	Normal
PAC	Depends on rate of underlying rhythm	Irregular	Present; may have a different shape	Varies or normal	Normal
AT	150–250	Regular	Normal but differ in shape	May be short in rapid rates	Normal but can be aberrant at times
SVT	150–250	Regular	Frequently buried in preceding T waves and difficult to see	Usually not possible to measure	Normal but may be wide if abnormality conducted through ventricles
PSVT	150–250	Irregular	Frequently buried in preceding T waves and difficult to see	Usually not possible to measure	Normal but may be wide if abnormality conducted through ventricles
A-flutter	Atrial: 250–350 Ventricular: Variable	Atrial: Regular Ventricular: Variable	Flutter waves have a saw-toothed appearance; some may not be visible, being buried in the QRS	Variable	Usually normal but may appear widened if flutter waves are buried in QRS
AF	Atrial: More than 350 Ventricular: Variable	Irregular	No true P waves; chaotic atrial activity	None	Normal
WPW	Depends on rate of underlying rhythm	Regular unless associated with A-fib	Normal unless A fib is present	Short: Less than 0.12	Wide: More than 0.10 Delta wave is present

Table 11.7   Junctional arrhythmias based on rate, rhythm, P wave, PR interval, and QRS complex

Junctional arrhythmias	Rate (bpm)	Rhythm	P wave	PR interval	QRS
J	40–60	Regular	Absent, inverted, buried, or retrograde	None, short, or retrograde	Normal
AJR	61–100	Regular	Absent, inverted, buried, or retrograde	None, short, or retrograde	Normal
JT	101–180	Regular	Absent, inverted, buried, or retrograde	None, short, or retrograde	Normal
JEB	Depends on rate of underlying rhythm	Irregular whenever an escape beat occurs	Absent, inverted, buried, or retrograde	None, short, or retrograde	Normal
PJC	Depends on rate of underlying rhythm	Irregular whenever a PJC occurs	Absent, inverted, buried, or retrograde	None, short, or retrograde	Normal

Table 11.8   Ventricular arrhythmias based on rate, rhythm, P wave, PR interval, and QRS complex

Ventricular arrhythmias	Rate (bpm)	Rhythm	P wave	PR interval	QRS
IV	20–40	Regular	None	None	Wide, bizarre appearance
AIR	41–100	Regular	None	None	Wide, bizarre appearance
PVC	Depends on rate of underlying rhythm	Irregular	None	None	Wide, bizarre appearance
MVT	100–250	Regular	None	None	Wide, bizarre appearance
PVT	100–250	Regular or irregular	None	None	Wide, bizarre appearance
TDP	100–250	Irregular	None	None	Wide, bizarre appearance
VF	Indeterminate	Chaotic	None	None	None
PEA	Reflects underlying rhythm	Reflects underlying rhythm	Reflects underlying rhythm	Reflects underlying rhythm	Reflects underlying rhythm
A	None	None	None	None	None

Table 11.9 AV and BBBs arrhythmias based on rate, rhythm, P wave, PR interval, and QRS complex

AV and BBB	Rate (bpm)	Rhythm	P wave	PR interval	QRS
FDAVB	Depends on rate underlying rhythm	Regular	Normal	Prolonged	Normal
MOBITZI	Depends on rate underlying rhythm	Atrial: Regular Ventricular: Irregular	Normal, more P waves than QRS	Progressively longer until one P wave is blocked and a QRS is dropped	Normal
MOBITZII	Atrial: 60–100 Ventricular: Slower than atrial rate	Atrial: Regular Ventricular: Regular or irregular	Normal, more P waves than QRS	Normal or prolonged but constant	May be normal, but usually wide if the bundle branches are involved
TDAVB	Atrial: 60–100 Ventricular: 40–60	Usually regular but atria and ventricles act independently	Normal; may be superimposed on QRS complexes or T waves	Varies greatly	Normal if ventricles are activated by junctional escape focus; wide if escape focus is ventricular
BBB	Depends on rate underlying rhythm	Regular	Normal	Normal	Wide with or without a notched appearance

11.4.2 Axis determination in axial reference system (methods for determining the QRS axis)

There are two methods to identify the QRS axis in the axial reference system.

Method 1

The condition of the heart can be diagnosed using the ECG as in Figure 11.6. We will use the axial reference system to identify the QRS axis in Figure 11.4. This ECG sample has been taken from google image for reference as an example. The six leads in Figure 11.6 above are examined and it is determined whether it is positive, negative, or equiphasic and it is tabulated in Table 11.10. The medical angle was identified. The intersection of these angles is $-30° < \theta < 30°$. This falls in the region of normal QRS region in the axial reference system as in Figure 11.4.

Method 2

There is another method of checking the region of the QRS axis called axial method. There are five steps to determine the QRS axis and the steps are given with the answers for the above ECG in Figure 11.6. The five steps with the solution are given in Table 11.11. The answers for both the methods namely, Method 1 and Method 2 are similar. The signal is NSR.

Table 11.10   Junctional arrhythmias based on rate, rhythm, P wave, PR interval, and QRS complex

Lead		Medical angle
Lead I	Positive	$-90° < \theta < 90°$
Lead II	Positive	$-30° < \theta < 150°$
Lead III	Positive	$-150° < \theta < 30°$
aVR	Negative	$-60° < \theta < 120°$
aVL	Equiphasic	$-180° < \theta < 180°$
aVF	Positive	$0° < \theta < 180°$
The intersection region		$-30° < \theta < 30°$

Table 11.11   Five steps to determine the QRS axis

Step	Activity	Answer
1	Determine the equiphasic lead	aVL is the equiphasic lead
2	Find that lead on the axial reference system	It is $-30°$ in the axial reference system
3	Find the perpendicular lead to $-30°$	Lead II is the perpendicular lead to $-30°$
4	Determine whether the lead II is positive or negative in Figure 11.6	Lead II is positive in Figure 11.6
5	Find lead II positive in the axial reference system	It is in the normal QRS axis

11.4.3 Methods for determining the interval

There are various methods to measure the PR interval, QRS complex, and QT interval. We are going to show the simplest method where we calculate the number of small boxes and multiply by 0.04 s (40 millisecond).

Methods for calculating PR interval

The PR interval is shown in Figure 11.9 and it is equivalent to 3.5 length of small boxes where it is 0.14 (3.5 × 0.04) s. The PR interval checklist is given in Table 11.12.

Methods for calculating QRS complex

The QRS complex length measurement is shown in Figure 11.10. The length is approximately 2.5 small boxes, which is equivalent to 0.10 s. The standard QRS complex measurement list is given in Table 11.13.

Methods for calculating QT interval

The way how the QT is measured is shown in Figure 11.11. The formula and how to measure the corrected QT (QTc) is given in Figure 11.12. The standard QTc interval also is given in Table 11.14.

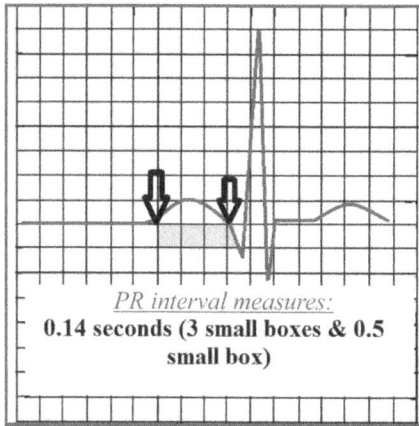

Figure 11.9   PR interval measures [33]

Table 11.12   PR interval

	Seconds	
Normal PR	0.12–0.22	
Prolonged PR	More than 0.22	First degree AV block
Shortened PR	Less than 0.12	Pre-excitation

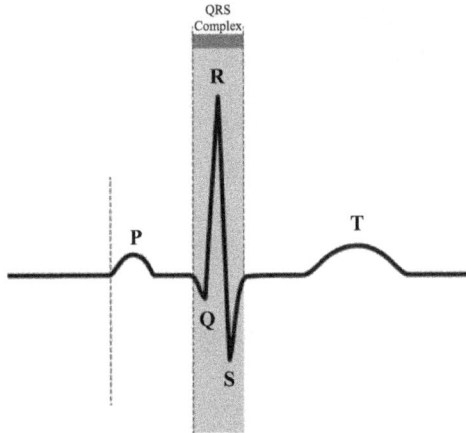

Figure 11.10   QRS complex [34]

Table 11.13   QRS complex measurement

	Seconds	
Normal	0.06–0.10	
Narrow complexes	Less than 0.10	Supraventricular in origin
Broad complexes	More than 0.10	Ventricular in origin
		Due to aberrant supraventricular complexes

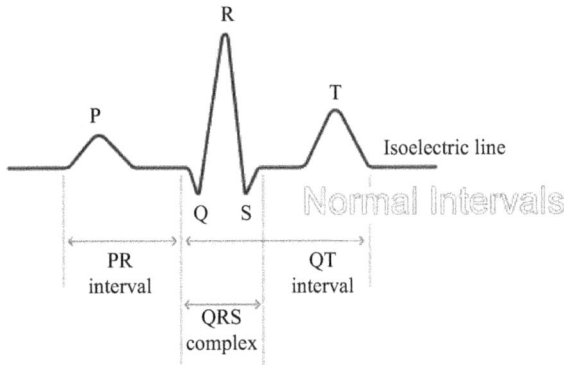

Figure 11.11   PR, QRS, and QT interval [35]

11.4.4   Morphology

The morphology of P, QRS, and T are given in detail in this section.

P morphology

The pictures in Figure 11.13 show how the P wave is formed. It can be seen in lead II of ECG reading of Figure 11.14. RAE is right atrial enlargement, while LAE

A Normal sinus rhythm   B Atrial fibrillation

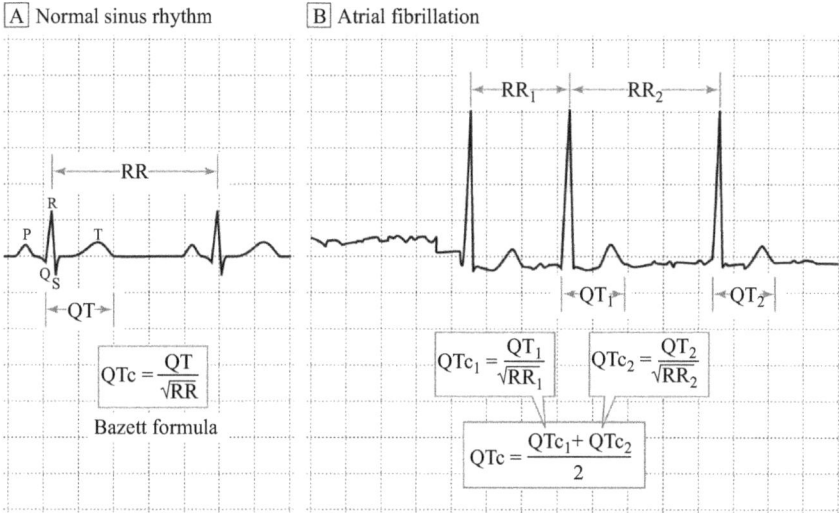

$$QTc = \frac{QT}{\sqrt{RR}}$$

Bazett formula

$$QTc_1 = \frac{QT_1}{\sqrt{RR_1}} \qquad QTc_2 = \frac{QT_2}{\sqrt{RR_2}}$$

$$QTc = \frac{QTc_1 + QTc_2}{2}$$

Figure 11.12   QTc calculation method for NSR and AF [36]

Table 11.14   QTc interval

	Male (ms)	Female (ms)
Normal	Less than 430	Less than 450
Borderline	431–450	451–470
Prolonged	More than 450	More than 470

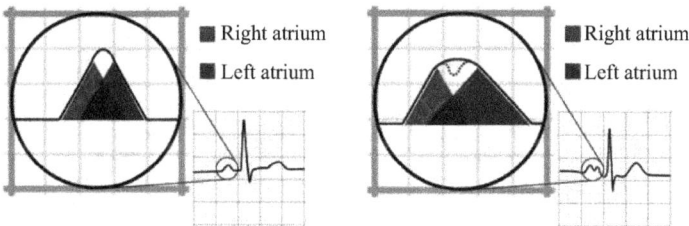

Figure 11.13   P wave formation [37]

is left atrial enlargement. The P morphology can be seen in leads II and VI to detect the ECG abnormalities.

P, QRS, and T morphology

The formation of P, QRS, and T waves are given clearly in Figure 11.15. The positive QRS, negative QRS, and biphasic QRS are shown clearly for NSR in Figure 11.16. In Figure 11.17, we can see the QRS complex in the precordial leads of NSR, left BBB and right BBB.

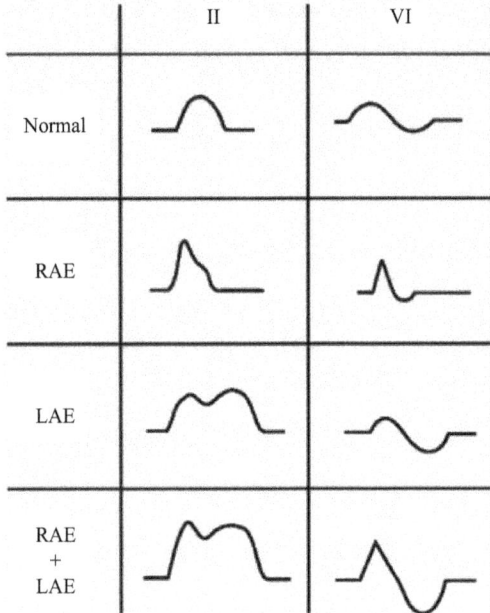

Figure 11.14   P wave in lead II and precordial lead VI [38]

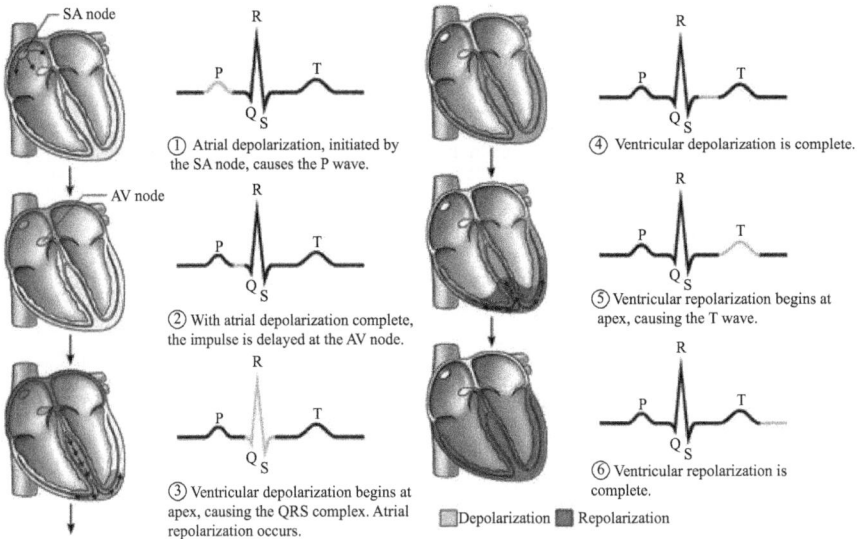

Figure 11.15   P, QRS, and T wave [39]

I	aV$_R$	V$_1$	V$_4$
Positive QRS	Negative QRS		
II	aV$_L$	V$_2$	V$_5$
III	aV$_F$	V$_3$	V$_6$
		Biphasic QRS	

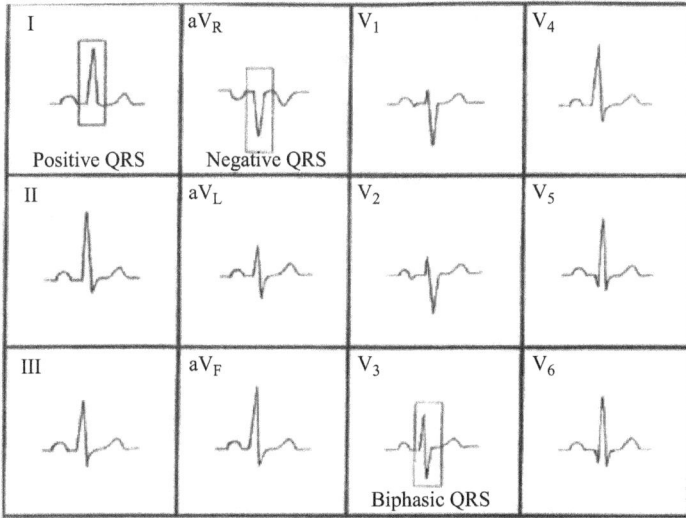

Normal QRS complex morphology

Figure 11.16   Positive QRS, negative QRS, and biphasic QRS [40]

11.4.5   STE-mimics

There are many conditions which will cause ST-segment elevation on the 12-lead ECG. We can have an abnormal repolarization, which can cause ST-segment elevation on the 12-lead ECG. These are also called as "QRS confounders" or "STEMI imposters". It can be seen in Figure 11.18.

11.4.6   Ischemia, injury and infarct

The classical triad of an acute myocardial infarction is ischemia, injury, and infarction. The three "I" is the basis for recognizing and diagnosing the signs of myocardial infarction. Ischemia means literally reduced blood, referring to poor blood supply. T wave inversion is the characteristic sign of Ischemia and may vary from a slightly flattened or depressed wave to deep inversion. Inverted T waves may indicate ischemia in the absence of myocardial infarction. There can be reduced blood supply to the heart without creation of an infarction. Injury indicates the acuteness (recent) of an infarct, and the ST segment elevation denotes injury. The ST segment is that section of baseline between QRS complex and the T wave. Elevation of the ST segment signifies injury. The elevation of the ST segment gives us the evidence that an infarct is acute. These features can be seen in Figures 11.19 and 11.20.

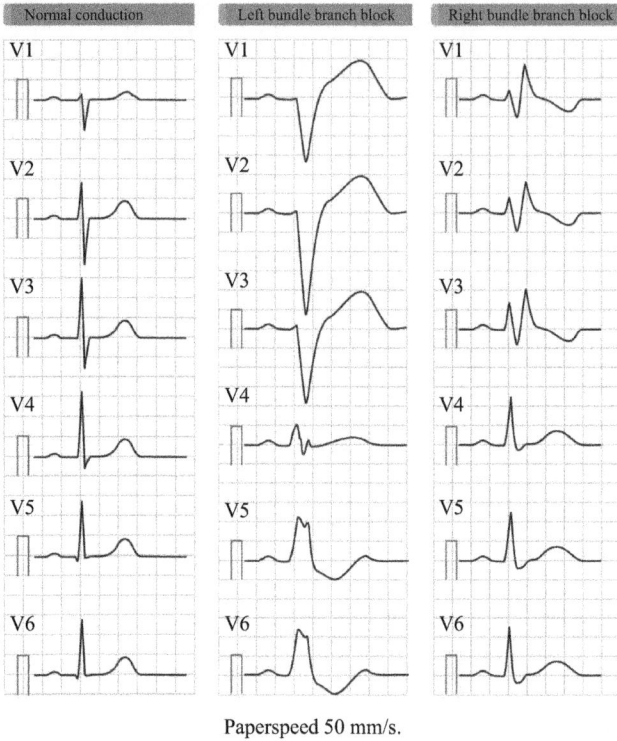

Paperspeed 50 mm/s.

Figure 11.17   NSR, LBBB, and RBBB [41]

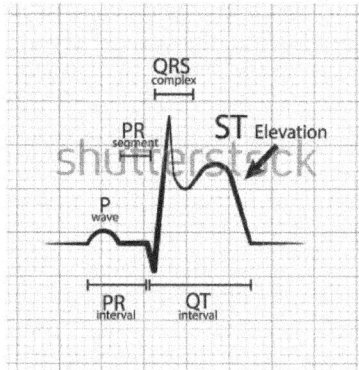

Figure 11.18   ST segment elevation [42]

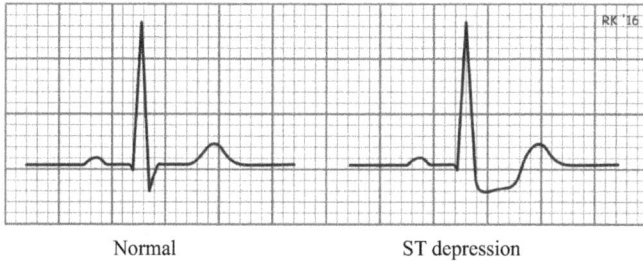

Normal   ST depression

Figure 11.19   ST segment depression compared with normal QRS [43]

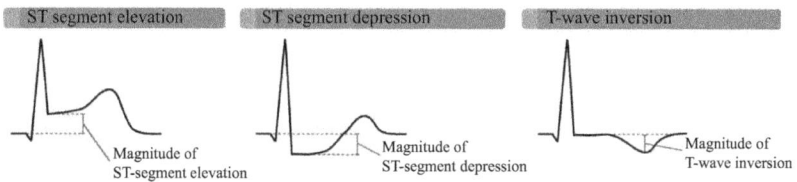

Figure 11.20   ST segment elevation, depression, and T wave inversion [44]

11.5   Computer-assisted ECG interpretation

Computer-assisted arrhythmia recognition is critical for the management of cardiac disorders [45]. Several methods for automated arrhythmia detection have been developed [46]. Generally, these techniques classify two or three arrhythmias or have significantly large processing time. Hence, a method using deep learning will be utilized to classify the various types of arrhythmias. Deep learning is a part of machine learning that uses algorithms inspired by the structure and function of the brain called artificial neural networks. Classic algorithms carry a specific pre-defined task on the presented data, while with deep learning a computer is able to learn from the data itself. Deep learning offers the possibility to treat a large amount of data (many patients, lengthy records) and the performance of the classification to get better with more data processed.

This study is designed to cater a large number of patients, to eliminate subjective inaccuracies, to aid the physician in the diagnosis, to reduce the time of diagnosis, to simplify the monitoring task, and to improve diagnostic efficiencies using the advancement of computing technology.

Patients are monitored using cardiac monitors in hospitals to detect the presence of arrhythmia. This requires continuous monitoring by the physicians. The visual inspection of the monitors is tedious and the diagnosis depends on the physician. Computer programs have been developed to help in this visual analysis by providing condensed printouts. This again requires meticulous study by the physician to identify arrhythmia.

There are five steps that need to be taken to classify the ECG data. The five steps are lead misplacement detection, pre-processing step, feature extraction step, the classification step, and the deep learning step.

11.5.1   Detection of limb lead misplacements

Firstly, the lead misplacement will be determined using various algorithms [46–51]. This stage is crucial to avoid the error in diagnosing heart condition of a patient.

Electrode misplacement can significantly alter the ECG and thus lead to wrong diagnoses. About 40 million ECGs are recorded in the United States each year [52]. It is estimated that 0.4%–4% of all ECGs are taken with misplaced electrodes [53], indicating that hundreds of thousands of ECGs are incorrectly collected each year. Misplaced leads in an ECG can degrade the diagnostic information, increase the number of false alerts, and prompt potentially harmful therapeutic procedures to patients [54]. Hence, many algorithms have been written to overcome these problems.

The reversal between the LA and RA electrodes is the most common electrode placement error, and many ECG recorders have built in logic to recognize this problem [35]. Early algorithms use rule-based criteria to detect the reversal between LA and RA [14]. A few other algorithms have been developed for different types of electrode misplacement [45–71]. Kors and Herpen were the first to use intrinsic relationships between different leads of the ECG as features in detection of cable reversals. They investigated 14 types of misplacement including the 5 types of limb cable reversals and 9 types of precordial cable reversals. Heden *et al.* used various ECG waves and intervals as features.

The Marquette's program suspects LA–RA interchange "if the QRS axis is between 90° and 270° and the P axis is between 90° and 210°" [56]. This program yields accurate results (93.91% sensitivity and 100% specificity) for ECGs with clear P waves; the results are disappointing (39.34% sensitivity and 100% specificity) for ECGs without P waves [57]. The recent review by Batchvarov *et al.* [58] provides a systematic review and comparison of various algorithms. The work of Heden *et al.* [57] and that of Kors and Herpen [51] present the highest classification accuracies. Heden *et al.* were the first to use artificial neural networks for detection of electrode misplacement. When classifying the reversal of LA electrode and RA electrode. They obtained a specificity of 99.95% and sensitivity of 99.11% when the P wave was present and a specificity of 99.92% and sensitivity of 94.5% when the P wave was absent. They also obtained a specificity of 57.6% and sensitivity of 99.97% for the reversal of LA and LL electrodes and a specificity of 71.76% and sensitivity of 99.92% on average for the precordial lead reversals. Kors and Herpen demonstrated specificities ($>=99.5\%$) for all 14 types of misplacement and very good sensitivities ($>=93\%$) for all interchanges except the LA/LL reversal (sensitivity $= 17.9\%$, specificity $= 99.5\%$). Furthermore, Luderitz *et al.* [18] reviewed and compared the algorithm of Heden *et al.* and that of Kors and Herpen using three different databases from Physionet [59]. The work of Xia *et al.* shows that existing algorithms work well on records of high signal quality and without severe distortions, but the performance is less satisfactory on records with noise and arrhythmias.

Xiaopeng developed an algorithm for automatic detection of electrode misplacement and evaluated its performance under consideration of a realistic misplacement rate [60]. The algorithm consists of two discrimination steps. Step 1 determines whether an ECG has been correctly collected. If the prediction of Step 1 is misplacement, Step 2 then determines the type of misplacement. Previous algorithms reported their performances on a database including equal number of misplaced and correct records. Xiaopeng showed that their algorithms may have high false positive rates on misplacement prediction. Resampling was conducted at both the training and test sets for faithful evaluation and for optimal performance. The performance of Step 1 is 99.6% accuracy, 91.7% sensitivity, 99.9% specificity, 98.9% positive predictive value and 99.7% negative predictive value. The overall accuracy of Step 2 is 90.4% [60].

11.5.2   Pre-processing of ECG

Preprocessing stage consists of resampling the ECG data, QRS detection, and noise filtering techniques.

11.5.2.1   Resample the ECG data

The modern ECG signals currently used can be displayed and manipulated in a different range of sampling frequencies (number of readings per second) depending on the usage. It is commonly used and printed at 1,000 Hz. For digital processing and computer interpretation, it can be down-sampled to 200–250 Hz or to 150 Hz for storage as lower sampling frequency signals take less memory.

11.5.2.2   Remove noise from ECG data

These ECG signals are contaminated by various kinds of noise. The various kinds of noise are power line interference (PLI), electrode contact noise, motion artifact, muscle contraction, and baseline wander (BW). There are two categories of noise, which are found in ECG signals; namely, persistent noise and burst noises.

A.   Persistent noises

The persistent noises are correlated in the signal, which comes from all the leads having a similar temporal distribution, but with different intensity level. These noises exhibit a variety of frequency bands. The low frequency range signifies BW, the medium frequency signifies the PLI and the high frequency signals signify the electromyography (EMG) noise [61].

Baseline wander (BW)

BW is commonly seen noise in ECG [62]. BW is caused by respiration, motion of the patients, and ECG instruments, variations in electrode–skin impedance, dirty lead wires/electrodes, and the movement of cables [63]. BW disturbance is especially dominant in exercise ECG, and in ambulatory, and Holter-monitoring. The range of frequency in which BW is dominant is typically less than 1.0 Hz; however, for exercise ECG this range can be wider [12].

Power line interference (PLI)

PLI coupled to signal carrying cables is particularly troublesome in medical equipment. It is seen that the PLI can contaminate the ECG recordings, due to differences in the electrode impedance and stray currents through the patient, cables, or in instruments with a floating input for a higher patient safety [64].

Cables carrying signals from the examination room to the monitoring equipment are prone to electromagnetic interference (EMI) of frequency (50 or 60 Hz) by ubiquitous supply lines. Sometimes the recordings (like ECG or EEG) are totally dominated by this type of noise [43]. Reducing (filtering) such PLI signal is a significant challenge given that the frequency of the power line signal lies within the frequency range of the ECG and EEG signals [65,66]. PLI is a significant source of noise during biopotential measurements. PLI introduces 50 to 60 Hz frequency component in that signal, which is the major cause of corruption of ECG [67].

EMI degrades the signal quality and disturbs the tiny features that may be crucial for monitoring and diagnosis, and it is observed that it can strongly distort biopotentials. Various biomedical signals contain distinct features in the time-domain analysis.

Electromyography noise (EMG)

Contraction of the muscles besides the heart contributes to the EMG noise. When other muscles in the vicinity of the electrodes contract, generation of depolarization and re-polarization waves takes place and these waves are picked up by the ECG. The gravity of the crosstalk depends on the amount of muscular contraction (subject movement), and the quality of the probes. It is well-established fact that the amplitude of the EMG signal is stochastic (random) in nature and is typically modeled by a Gaussian distribution function [68]. The mean of the noise can be assumed to be zero; however, the variance is dependent on the environmental variables and will change depending on the conditions. While the actual statistical model is unknown, it should be noted that the electrical activity of muscles during periods of contraction can generate surface potentials comparable to those from the heart, and could completely drown out the desired signal. EMG noise is common in subjects with uncontrollable tremor, disabled persons, kids, and persons fearing the ECG procedure.

B.   Burst Noises

Burst noise is normally categorized as a white Gaussian noise (WGN). These noises are electrode pop noise, electrode motion artifact, electro surgical noise, and instrumentation noise [63].

Electrode contact noise

Electrode contact noise caused by loose contact, motion artifact and baseline drift due to respiration.

Patient electrode motion artifact

This noise is caused by electrode movement. This electrode movement is caused by the patients' vibration, movement, or respiration.

Instrumentation noise

The instrumentation noise is caused by the ECG machine itself, electrode probes, cables, signal processor, and the analog-to-digital converter.

These noises can cause damage to the feature extraction of the biomedical signals, which lead to misinterpretation of these signals [62]. Hence, we need to eliminate these noises using various methods, which will be discussed.

C. Noise Filtering

The following pre-processing step will be carried out to remove noise due to PLI, respiration, muscles tremors, and spikes. ECG signals are usually non-stationary that consists of trends or noise. There are many types of techniques which were used namely, Finite Impulse Response (FIR) and wavelet transform. The high-pass filter, digital filter, time-variant filter and adaptive filter are usually used to remove BW noise.

Yurong suggested a new framework consisting of three steps to reduce this noise [42]. Firstly, the adaptive notch filter will be used to produce sub-signals of ECG. Secondly, Independent Component Analysis (ICA) will be used to decompose multichannel signals into fundamental components. Finally, adjust the BW obtained from ICA.

The subtraction procedure was utilized to eliminate PLI from the ECG signal [69]. The wavelet transform is considered as the best method for de-noising of ECG as it does not require any reference model and accuracy is also much better [67].

The contaminated electromyogram is cleaned using adaptive subtraction method. This method consists of four steps namely, QRS detection, ECG template will be developed by averaging the ECG complexes; low pass filter will be developed to remove undesirable artifacts and finally do the subtraction [70]. The digital filter technique is suitable for ECG analysis. This digital filter will improve this ECG signal with the help of the Chebyshev Type II filter [71]. Furthermore, some of the methods of how to remove the noise had been tabulated in Table 11.15.

In this study, a FIR filter will be constructed to filter a noisy ECG signal. The ECG signals will be imported to R language from Institut Jantung Negara (IJN) database. The ECG signals will be plotted. We will use the bandpass filter with the order of 14. The pass-band cut-off frequencies are $f_{c1} = 37.5$ Hz and $f_{c2} = 68.75$ Hz, respectively. The Blackman window will be used. The direct realization of FIR filter based on the direct implementation of the expression will be carried out [8]. These are the pre-processing procedures that will be utilized in this study.

ECG signals are usually non-stationary that consists of trends or noise. In this study, a simple Wiener filter will be constructed to filter a noisy ECG signal. The ECG signals will be imported to R language from Institut Jantung Negara (IJN) database. The ECG signals will be plotted. A random WGN will be generated. The characteristic of the noise will be assumed to be $0.9 \, N \, (n - 1) + N \, (n)$. The noise signal will be plotted. This signal will be combined with the original ECG signal to produce a noisy output. The noisy output will be plotted. The autocorrelation characteristic of the noise and the cross correlation of the noise and the signal will be determined to design a Wiener filter. The autocorrelation characteristic of the

Table 11.15   Techniques used for noise filtering and QRS detection

To remove baseline drift Part 1 noise removal Part 2 QRS detection	Part 1 Two stage median filter using window $f_s/2$ and f_s Part 2 (a) Enhancement of peaks by sixth order (b) Determining of window starting point of k1 and end point k2 (c) Determination of maxima point in the range of (k1,k2)	Ashok Kumar, 2014 [4]
To remove noise due to PLI, electromagnetic noise and baseline wandering in the heart beat signal	ECG signal is passed through a 12-tap low pass filter Secondly, ECG is passed through a five-point derivative to obtain the slope of R wave	Sandeep Raj, 2015 [1]
To reduce muscle noise, 60 Hz interference, base line wander and T wave interference	The normalized and centered ECG signal is filtered by a band-pass filter	Salah hamdi, 2018 [72]
The baseline wandering effect is removed	Low pass filter with the cut-off frequency of 0.7 Hz The amplitude of each lead is then normalized and the mean is removed The preprocessed ECG is divided into the learning set consisting of first s_1 samples, the lead selection set with the next s_2 samples and the reconstruction set containing s_3 samples	

noise and cross correlation of the noise and signal will be plotted. Wiener filter matrix will be designed based on the n-th order of the filter. The Wiener filter matrix will be used to evaluate the Wiener filter coefficient. The Wiener filter matrix will be constructed for a Wiener filter of 1st order to evaluate the filter coefficient. The Wiener filter will be convoluted with the noisy signal to obtain the output filtered signal. The filtered signal will be plotted and compared with the original input signal. The error in filter will be evaluated and the whole process will be repeated with 2nd, 3rd, 4th, 5th, and 6th order filter and the results will be compared [73]. These are the pre-processing procedures that will be utilized in this study.

11.5.2.3   Detection of QRS complex

The removal of BW is a usually necessary step achieved by filtering in order to detect properly the R peaks or QRS regions. An accurate detection of R peaks is mandatory for a relevant diagnosis, as these peaks correspond to contraction of the ventricles that will pump the blood to the organs. Disturbances of ventricles activity usually mean a life-threatening condition that requires immediate intervention. These disturbances are reflected in the frequency and intensity of R peaks and/or QRS complexes. Common methods employ algorithm that will magnify R peaks potential on an ECG in order to bring it above the threshold detection; this problem is solved through the use of adaptive threshold [74] as wavelet transformation is commonly used as it accommodates different types of noise simultaneously as nonlinear transformation based. Although recently the common use of machine learning improved detection of features and atypical QRS based on more elaborate classification rules in order to distinguish between true peaks and false positives like hidden Markov model (HMM) [75] or clustering methods like k-nearest neighbor (k-NN) [76].

11.5.3 Feature extraction

The third step is the feature extraction step. Various methods were used to extract the features of the ECG namely combination of the False Nearest Neighbor (FNN) and the ARMA Autoregressive (AR), heart rate variability (HRV) and Discrete Wavelet Transform (DWT), Fast Fourier Transform (FFT), Moving Average (MA), Vector Time-Varying Regressive (TVAR), hybrid model, Autoregressive X (ARX), ARMAX, Autoregressive Autoregressive Exogenous Input (ARARX), ARIMA and stochastic pacing combined with ARMA [77–83].

In the feature extraction stage we propose to employ the GARMA technique to classify normal sinus rhythm (NSR) besides various cardiac arrhythmias. GARMA is a new class of ARMA type models with indices to describe some hidden features of a time series [84,85]. GARMA model is simple and it is suitable for real-time classification at the Intensive Care Unit (ICU) or ambulatory monitoring. GARMA normally is used in financial time series and in forestry but this is the first time it will be used in medical field [85,86]. Hannan–Rissanen Algorithm (HRA), Whittle's Estimate (WE) and Maximum Likelihood Estimate (MLE) will be used to estimate the parameters of GARMA model and the performance of these estimators will be compared. The GARMA coefficients will be categorized according to the various types of arrhythmias using a classifier.

The second step is the feature extraction step. Various methods were used to extract the features of the ECG namely combination of the (FNN) and the ARMA, ARMA, Autoregressive (AR), combination of finite impulse response (FIR) and AR, HRV and DWT, fast Fourier transform (FFT), moving average (MA), vector time-varying regressive (TVAR), hybrid model, Savitzky–Golay filter, autoregressive X (ARX), ARMAX, autoregressive autoregressive exogenuous input (ARARX), ARIMA and stochastic pacing combined with ARMA [77–83].

In order to achieve parsimony we need to include both AR and MA. Thus, we propose to employ the mixed ARMA model with an index called GARMA. The advantage of GARMA is that, it is suitable for the real time classification at the ICU or ambulatory monitoring and it can be used in various applications besides it can analyze and forecast a time series with changing frequency via a direct method as well as it can be adapted for extracting good features from ECG signals, thus enabling the discrimination of certain ECG arrhythmias [87].

11.5.3.1   Estimation methods

The third step is the parameter estimation step. The estimation of the parameters of AR was done using Burg's algorithm [88]. Burg's algorithm usually gives higher likelihoods than the Yule–Walker equations for pure AR models [89]. The innovations algorithm gives slightly higher likelihoods than the HRA algorithm for MA models. However, the Hannan–Rissanen algorithm (HRA) is usually successful for mixed models [73,89]. The Whittle Estimator (WE) is considered as an accurate estimator [73]. The Maximum Likelihood Estimator (MLE) is a popular method of parameter estimation and is an indispensable tool for many statistical techniques [73].

11.5.3.2   Features to be extracted

There are so many features of ECG data need to be considered to analyze the ECG data. The features had been mentioned in the fourth section of this chapter. The features are rate and rhythm, axis of axial reference system, PR interval, QTc interval, QRS complex, morphology of P, QRS, and T waves, ST segment elevation, ischemia, injury, infarct, and the coefficients obtained from the QRS complex using other statistical methods mentioned earlier. The number of features becomes big. However, we can obtain a better accuracy using deep learning with the various ECG characters.

11.5.4   Classification

Finally, the third step is the classification step. Various studies have been focused on the development of algorithm to classify the arrhythmia. There are varieties of classifiers, which are used to categorize arrhythmias, such as GLM, Quadratic discriminant Function (QDF), Multilayer Perception (MLP), Support Vector Machine (SVM), Linear Discriminant Analysis (LDA), k-Nearest Neighbor (k-NN), Logistic Model Tree (LMT) and Artificial Neural Network (ANN) are the types of classifiers used to categorize arrhythmias. GLM relaxes the normality and homoscedasticity assumptions, availability of alternate links and it avoids the retransformation problems [88]. GLMs offer an efficient method of modeling, besides accommodating a relationship between linear predictor and mean [88]. Due to that, GLM will be utilized to classify the arrhythmias using the GARMA coefficients.

Arrhythmia can be categorized into various classes. The following studies have categorized arrhythmia into different number of classes, such as three [90], six [88,91], nine [92], and eleven [93]. The ECG feature detection is to investigate how many different ventricular conduction defect (VCD) categories can be formed. This reduces the number of classification parameters into a small set for a meaningful classification [88]. We are going to consider NSR and the five types of arrhythmias namely APC, PVC, SVT, VT, and VF.

The data set includes around 100 segments each of normal ECGs, APC, PVC, SVT, VT, and VF. These data will be used to classify the various types of arrhythmias accordingly and to test the accuracy of the GARMA and GLM models in the classification of arrhythmias.

We are going to consider the NSR and the above mentioned five types of arrhythmias because of the morbidity and mortality caused by this type of arrhythmia. One of the objectives of the direct ECG feature extraction is to investigate the number of VCD categories. Furthermore, VT and VF are life-threatening cardiac arrhythmias. However, PVC and APC are not so lethal, but they are important for diagnosing heart diseases [89]. In addition, SVT and VT are grouped as ventricular rhythms [92]. APC and SVT will lead to atrial fibrillation and atrial flutter. Whereas, PVC and VF will lead to CA. Due to these reasons, we are classifying these six types of arrhythmias. Furthermore, Quelli *et al.* and Dingfei *et al.* used these same set of six types of arrhythmias in their study [88,91,92].

This study will enhance the knowledge of arrhythmia in the medical field by suggesting a better and efficient way of preventing, diagnosing, and treating the arrhythmias amongst different ethnic groups in Malaysia. This study will introduce an efficient method to accurately categorize various types of arrhythmias. This comprehensive model-study opens up other avenues for future researchers to use some other ECG character extraction methods and different classification techniques. The GARMA modeling and GLM for classification of various types of arrhythmias is an effective method to improve the accuracy for the detection of the arrhythmia patients.

The decision tree approach will be used in this study to classify the various types of arrhythmias. There are several distinct advantages of using decision trees in many classification and prediction applications. The advantages are decision trees implicitly perform variable screening or feature selection, it requires relatively little effort from users for data preparation, nonlinear relationships between parameters do not affect tree performance and it is easy to interpret and explain to executives [94]. In this part, we are going to use deep learning again to obtain a better accuracy.

11.5.5 Deep learning

The study has incorporated the idea of machine learning. The machine learning can be categorized into two categories namely, supervised machine learning and unsupervised machine learning.

The supervised machine learning learn to predict the target values from the labeled data. The supervised learning can be further grouped as classification and regression. The target values of the classification are discrete values, while the target values of regression are continuous values.

The unsupervised machine learning find the useful structure in labeled data or knowledge in unlabeled data. The unsupervised machine learning finds groups of similar instances in the data (clustering) and find unusual patterns (outlier detection). A basic machine learning workflow can be seen in Figure 11.21. We use 70% or 80% of the data collected as the training set and the remainder of the data as the testing set of data. The various machine learning algorithms have been specified in Figure 11.22. Some of the example of case studies are given in Figure 11.23. However, the deep learning has been introduced to improve the accuracy of the predictive model. Hence, the comparison between the machine learning and deep learning has been shown in Figure 11.24.

This study will enhance the knowledge of arrhythmia in the medical field by suggesting a better and efficient way of preventing, diagnosing, and treating the

Machine learning workflow

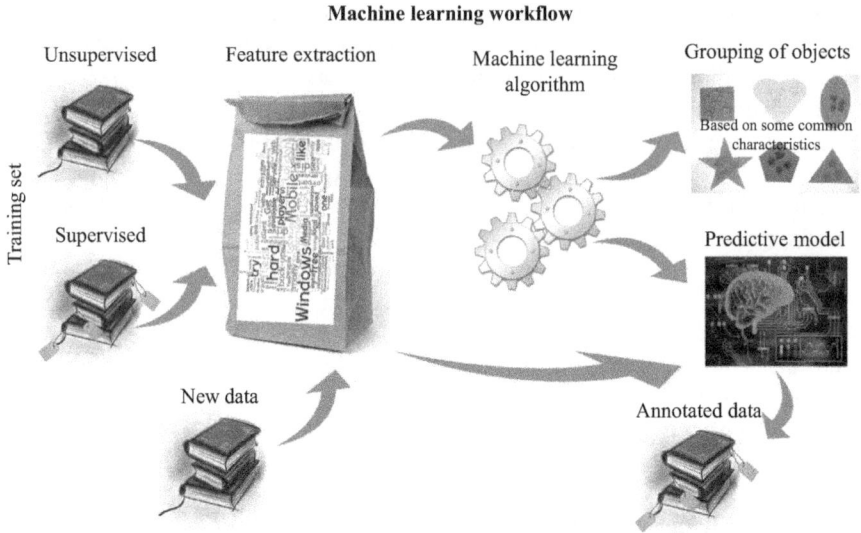

Figure 11.21   Basic machine learning workflow [95]

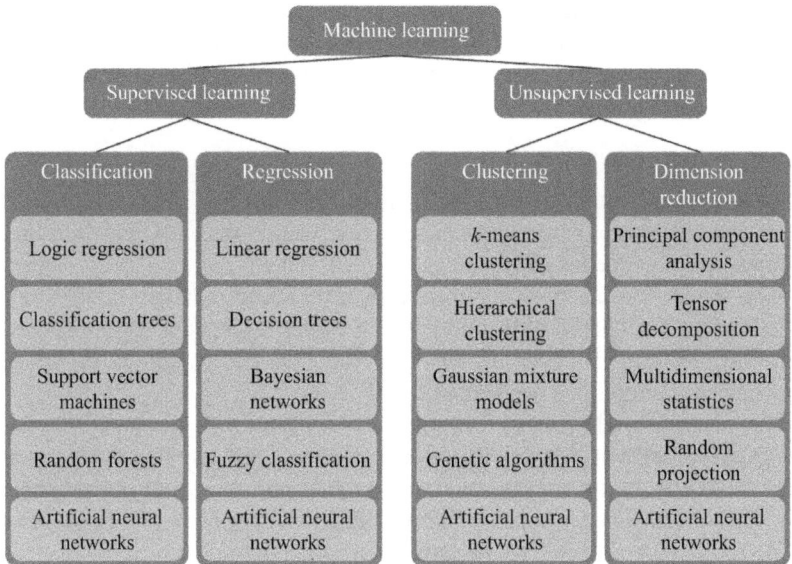

Figure 11.22   Machine learning algorithms [96]

arrhythmias. This study will introduce an efficient method to accurately categorize various types of arrhythmias. This comprehensive model-study opens up other avenues for future researchers to use some other ECG character extraction methods and different classification techniques.

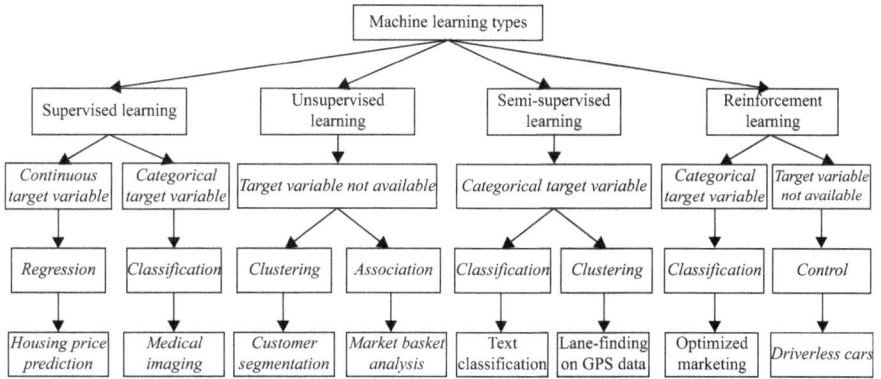

Figure 11.23 Machine learning types and example of case studies [96]

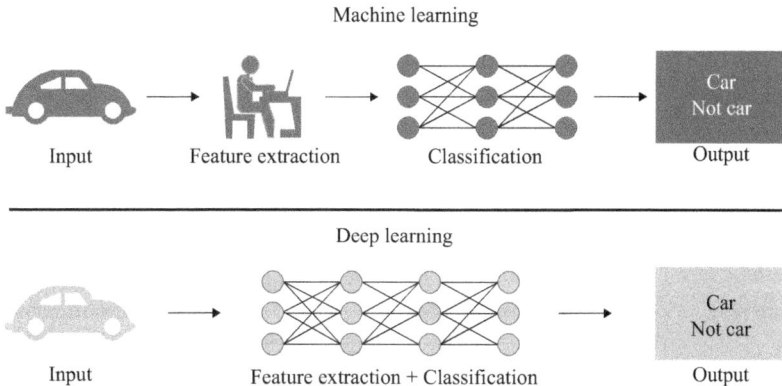

Figure 11.24 Comparison between machine learning and deep learning [97]

11.6 Conclusion

There are few steps in analysis of ECG signals. The steps are namely noise elimination, cardiac cycle detection, extraction of features from ECG points, formulation of characteristic feature set, and finally classification of the ECG.

There are five steps in the analysis of ECG signals. The five steps are preprocessing step, feature extraction step, parameter extraction step, parameter estimation step, and finally the classification step. The various methods that have been proposed for the automatic classification of ECG signals can be seen in Table 11.16. Currently, we are using machine learning techniques only. The interpretation of the ECG data can be done more efficiently, accurately, and fast using deep learning techniques.

[18]   Luderitz B, Luna A, "The history of electrocardiography," Journal of Cardiology 50 (2017) 539.

[19]   Xiao HB, Lawrence C, "Reappraisal of Thomas Lewis's place in the history of electrocardiography" Journal of Electrocardiography Vol 29 No 4 1996.

[20]   Autaharju PM "The birth of computerized electrocardiography: Hubrt V. Pipberger (1920–1993)," Cadiology Journal 14 (2007) 420–421.

[21]   Caceres Cesar A, Dreiffus Leonard S, editors, "Clinical electrocardiography and computers." New York and London: Academic Press (1970).

[22]   Caceres CA. Rikli AH, "Diagnostic computers." Springfield IL: Charles C. Thomas (1969).

[23]   U.R. Acharya, J. S. Suri, J. A. E. Spaan, S. M. Krishnan, "Advances in Cardiac Signal Processing." Springer (2010).

[24]   Bayes De Luna A Basic, "Electrocardiography Normal and Abnormal ECG patterns." Maiden, MA: Wiley Blackwell (2007).

[25]   "Know about the Human Heart and Its Functions", Heart-pulse-diseases, 2018. Online. Available: https://heartpulsediseases.wordpress.com/2016/10/22/human-heart-and-its-functions/. Accessed: 13-Mar-2018.

[26]   "CV Physiology | Terms of Use, Trademarks, and Copyright", Cvphysiology. com, 2018. Online. Available: http://www.cvphysiology.com/Ancillary/terms. Accessed: 13-Mar-2018.

[27]   "Index of /Arrhythmias", Cvphysiology.com, 2018. Online. Available: http://www.cvphysiology.com/Arrhythmias/. Accessed: 13-Mar-2018.

[28]   "ECG: The Cardiac Axis", TED-Ed, 2018. Online. Available: https://ed.ted.com/on/pipUDnkw. Accessed: 13-Mar-2018.

[29]   Browning L, "Cardiac axis diagram with right axis deviation ecg images", http://jppoker.co/wiring/cardiac-axis-diagram.html, 2018. Online. Available: http://jppoker.co/wiring/cardiac-axis-diagram.html. Accessed: 13-Mar-2018.

[30]   "Dextrocardia ECG (Example 1) | LearntheHeart.com", Healio.com, 2018. Online. Available: https://www.healio.com/cardiology/learn-the-heart/ecg-review/ecg-archive/dextrocardia-ecg-example-1. Accessed: 13-Mar-2018.

[31]   "ECG V A Pictorial Primer", Medicine-on-line.com, 2018. Online. Available: http://www.medicine-on-line.com/html/ecg/e0001en_files/07.htm. Accessed: 13-Mar-2018.

[32]   "Heart Valve Disease", Hertsandessexcardiology.co.uk, 2018. Online. Available: http://www.hertsandessexcardiology.co.uk/symptoms-and-diseases/valvular-heart-disease. Accessed: 13-Mar-2018.

[33]   Registerednursern.com, 2018. Online. Available: http://www.registered nursern.com/wp-content/uploads/2015/07/how-to-measure-pr-interval-300x 293.png. Accessed: 13-Mar-2018.

[34]   "maryvincy", maryvincyRN, 2018. Online. Available: https://maryvincy. wordpress.com/author/maryvincy/. Accessed: 13-Mar-2018.

[35]   "Normal Duration Times Function of the Heart Picture to Pin on Pinter-est", Thepinsta.com, 2018. Online. Available: http://www.thepinsta.com/ normal-duration-times-function-of-the-heart_I4tIP5kS*sjRDaX3OO5TyX7J xgj4Cp4Jf3BDyd8086A8vgZyvil%7CCX8M3bJ1SICYvO8VKGZtozjCzE

DjIiCECQ/lxGqi5BC*G0FDCLgxjupRqbsX*JC6gRzLaX92zBHrGtCrixhA
JuJ*BMw0lnZ*iyDdEJtlqjkb%7CXxJBF9JtdbVi%7C97%7Ca5z1WIFwvZ
Y2OveEUfhAUUTIMSyFkKL8C2FtYAWk0NT7BvdGZQ%7CZOJErjnov
WL8VqOtLuTu1XL%7CtM5Q*k/. Accessed: 13-Mar-2018.

[36] "Heart Equation Calculator", Loveinsurance.club, 2018. Online. Available: https://loveinsurance.club/quotes/heart-equation-calculator.html. Accessed: 13-Mar-2018.

[37] "Enlarged P Wave ECG Pictures to Pin on Pinterest – ThePinsta", Thepinsta. com, 2018. Online. Available: http://www.thepinsta.com/enlarged-p-wave-ecg_aR0g7sQ8n*eM98GEnrpSH9k9gU4CtKOr%7CuIuCh6TGec/. Accessed: 13-Mar-2018.

[38] "Nursing stuff", Pinterest, 2018. Online. Available: https://www.pinterest.com/pin/274297433526962621/. Accessed: 13-Mar-2018.

[39] "The cardiac cycle and ECG – online presentation", En.ppt-online.org, 2018. Online. Available: https://en.ppt-online.org/279892. Accessed: 13-Mar-2018.

[40] "ECG skills enhancement", Slideshare.net, 2018. Online. Available: https://www.slideshare.net/jillirenemd/ecg-skills-enhançement. Accessed: 13-Mar-2018.

[41] "Right bundle branch block (RBBB): ECG, criteria, definitions, causes & management – ECG learning", ECG learning, 2018. Online. Available: https://ecgwaves.com/right-bundle-branch-block-rbbb-ecg-criteria/. Accessed: 13-Mar-2018.

[42] "ECG of ST elevation myocardial infarction (STEMI) and detail of ECG (P wave, PR segment, PR interval, QRS complex, QT interval, ST elevate, T wave) Acute coronary syndrome, angina pectoris", Shutterstock.com, 2018. Online. Available: https://www.shutterstock.com/image-vector/ecg-st-elevation-myocardial-infarction-stemi-403308256. Accessed: 13-Mar-2018.

[43] Public domain

[44] Ved V, "Difference between Usual Machine Learning and Deep Learning Explained!", d4datascience.wordpress.com, 2018. Online. Available: https://d4datascience.wordpress.com/2016/03/31/difference-between-usual-machine-learning-and-deep-learning-explained/. Accessed: 13-Mar-2018.

[45] Surawicz B, Knilans TK, Misplacement of leads and electrocardiographic artifacts, in: Surawicz B, Knilans TK eds, *Chow's Electrocardiography in Clinical Practice*, WB Saunders, Philadelphia, (2001) 569–582.

[46] Zielinski J, "Negative P wave in lead I due to right atrial enlargement and displacement of the heart in the chest," Pneumonologie 153 (1976) 197–201.

[47] Issa ZF, Miller JM, Zipes DP, "Clinical Arrhythmology and Electro-physiology: A Companion to Braunwald's Heart Disease." WB Saunders, Philadelphia (2012) page 131.

[48] Heden B, Ohlsson M, Holst H, *et al.* "Detection of frequently overlooked electrocardiographic lead reversals using artificial neural networks," American Journal of Cardiology 78 (1996) 600–604.

[49] Abdollah H, Milliken JA, "Recognition of electrocardiographic left arm/left leg lead reversal," American Journal of Cardiology 80 (1997) 1247–1249.

[50]   Ho KKL, Ho SK, "Use of the sinus P wave in diagnosing electrocardio-graphic limb lead misplacement not involving the right leg (ground) electrode," Journal of Electrocardiology 34 (2001) 161–171.

[51]   Kors JA, Herpen G, "Accurate automatic detection of electrode interchange in the electrocardiogram," American Journal of Cardiology 88 (2001) 396–399.

[52]   Criley JM, Nelson WP, "Virtual tools for teaching electrocardiographic rhythm analysis," Journal of Electrocardiology 39 (2006) 113–119.

[53]   Rudiger A, Hellermann JP, Mukherjeec R, Follath F, Turina J, "Electrocardiographic artifacts due to electrode misplacement and their frequency in different clinical settings," American Journal of Emergency Medicine 25 (2007) 174–178.

[54]   Rajaganeshan R, Ludlam CL, Francis DP, Parasramka SV, Sutton R (2008) "Accuracy in ECG lead placement among technicians, nurses, general physicians and cardiologists," International Journal of Clinical Practice 62 (2008) 65–70.

[55]   Haisty WK, Pahlm O, Edenbrandt L, Recognition of electrocardiographic electrode misplacements involving the ground (right leg) electrode, American Journal of Cardiology 71 (1993) 1490–1495.

[56]   Marquette Electronics, Physicians guide to Marquette electronics resting ECG analysis, Milwaukee (1988).

[57]   Heden B, "Electrocardiographic lead reversal," American Journal of Cardiology 87 (2001) 126–127.

[58]   Batchvarov VN, Malik M, Camm AJ, "Incorrect electrode cable connection during electrocardiographic recording," Europace 9 (2007) 1081–1090.

[59]   Xia H, Garcia G, Zhao X, Automatic detection of ECG electrode misplacement: A tale of two algorithms, Physiological Measurement 33 (2012) 1549–1561.

[60]   Xiaopeng Zhao, Henian Xia, Irfan Asif, Dale C Wortham and Elena G Tolkacheva (2014) "Resampling for reliable evaluation and improved performance in automatic detection of electrode misplacements in ECG: Studies based on limb-lead misplacements," Journal of Biomedical Technology and Research 1(1) (2014) 6000103.

[61]   Turner DD, Knuteson RO, A principal component analysis noise filter value-added procedure to remove uncorrelated noise from atmospheric emitted radiance interferometer (AERI) observations Pacific Northwest National Laboratory USA (2006).

[62]   Luo Y, Hargraves RH, Belle A, *et al.*, "A hierarchical method for removal of baseine drift from biomedical signal: Application in ECG analysis," The Scientific World Journal Volume (2013) 1–10 Article ID 896056, https://doi.org/10.1155/2013/896056.

[63]   Limaye H, Deshmukh2 V.V, "ECG noise sources and various noise removal techniques: A survey," International Journal of Application or Innovation in Engineering & Management (IJAIEM) 5 (2) (2016) 86–92.

[64]   Levkov C, Mihov G, Ivanov R, Daskalov I, Christov II, Dotsinsky I, "Removal of power-line interference from the ECG: A review of the subtraction procedure," Biomedical Engineering Online 4 (2005) 50.

[65]   Sörnmo L, Laguna P, Bioelectrical signal processing in cardiac and neurological applications, Boston, MA: Elsevier Academic Press (2005).

[66] Rangayyan RM, Biomedical signal analysis: a case-study approach, IEEE Press Series on Biomedical Engineering (2002) 145–146.

[67] Thalkar S, Upasani D, "Various techniques for removal of power line interference from ECG signal," International Journal of Scientific & Engineering Research 4(12) 2013 12–23.

[68] Tikkanen P, "Characterization and application of analysis methods for ECG and time interval variablity data," PhD. Dissertation, University of Oulu, Oulu Finland (1999).

[69] Levkov C, Mihov G, Ivanov R, Daskalov I, Christov I, Dotsinsky I, "Removal of power-line interference from the ECG: a review of the subtraction procedure," Biomedical Engineering Online 4:1 (2005) 50.

[70] Abbaspour S, Fallah A, "Removing ECG artifact from the surface EMG signal using adaptive subtraction technique," Journal of Biomedical and Physics Engineering 4:1 (2014) 33–38.

[71] Jagtap SK, Uplane MD, "A real time approach:ECG noise reduction in Chebyshev Type II digital filter," International Journal of Computer Applications 49(9) (2012) 52–59.

[72] Hamdi S, Ben abdallah A, Bedoui MH, "A robust QRS complex detection using regular grammar and deterministic automata," Biomedical Signal Processing and Control 40 (2018) 263–274.

[73] Brockwell PJ, Davis RA, "Introduction to time series and forecasting." 2nd edition, Springer, New York (2002).

[74] Sahoo S, Biswal P, Das T, Sabut S, "De-noising of ECG signal and QRS detection using Hilbert transform and adaptive thresholding," Procedia Technology 25 (2016) 68–75.

[75] Akhbari M, Shamsollahi MB, Sayadi O, Armoundas AA, Jutten C, "ECG segmentation and fiducial point extraction using multi hidden Markov model," Computers in Biology and Medicine 79 (2016) 21–29.

[76] Saini I, Singh D, Khosla A, "QRS detection using K-Nearest Neighbor algorithm (KNN) and evaluation on standard ECG databases," Journal of Advanced Research 4(4) (2013) 331–344.

[77] Aguila JJ., Arias E., Artigao MM, Miralles JJ, "A prediction of electrocardiography signals by combining ARMA model with nonlinear analysis methods," Recent Researches in Applied Computer and Applied Computational Science (2011) 31–37.

[78] Goshvarpour MS, Goshvarpour A, "Spectral and time based assessment of meditative heart rate signals," International Journal of Image, Graphics and Signal Processing 4 (2013) 1–10.

[79] Liu J, Jamshidi M, Pourbabak S, "Modeling cardiovascular dynamics using a parallel structure with auto-regressive-regressive and neuro-fuzzy inference," IC-MED 2(1) (2008) 55–66.

[80] Krebs MD, Tingley RD, Zeskind JE, Kang JM, Holmboe ME, Davis CE, "Autoregressive modeling of analytical sensor data can yield classifiers in the predictor coefficient parameter space," Bioinformatics 21(8) (2005) 1325–1331.

[81] Boardman FS, Schlindwein A, Rocha AP, Leite A, "A study on the optimum order of autoregressive models for heart rate variability," Physiological Measurement 23 (2002) 325–336.

[82] Boskovic, M, Despotovic, Bajic D, "Predictive ECG coding using linear time-invariant models," Archives of Oncology 12(3) (2004) 152–158.

[83] Lemay M, Lange ED, Kucera JP, "Uncovering the dynamics of cardiac systems using stochastic pacing and frequency domain analyses," PLOS Computational Biology 8(3) (2012) e1002399

[84] Pillai RP, Shitan M, Peiris S, "Time series properties of the class of first order autoregressive processes with generalized moving average errors," Journal of Statistics: Advances in Theory and Applications 40(13) (2009) 2259–2275.

[85] Pillai RP, Shitan M, "Application of GARMA (1, 1; 1, δ) model to GDP in Malaysia: An illustrative example," Journal of Global Business and Economics 3(1) (2011) 138–145.

[86] Pillai RP, Shitan M, "An application of generalized ARMA (GARMA) time series modelling of forest area of Malaysia," International Journal of Modern Physics: Conference Series 9 (2012) 390–397.

[87] Ieda M, Kanazawa H, Kimura K, *et al.*, "Sema3a maintains normal heart rhythm through sympathetic innervation patterning," Natural Medicine 13(5) (2007) 604–612.

[88] Ge D, Srinivasan N, Krishnan SM, "Cardiac arrhythmia classification using autoregressive modeling," Biomedical Engineering Online 1 (2002) 5.

[89] Venables WN, Dichmont CM, "GLMs, GAMs and GLMMs: An overview of theory for applications in fisheries research," Fisheries Research 70 (2004) 319–337.

[90] Vuksanovic V, Alhamdi M, "AR-based method for ECG classification and patient recognition," International Journal of Biometrics and Bioinformatics 7(2) (2013) 74–92.

[91] Quelli B, Elhadadi H, Aissaoui Bouikhalene B, "Diagnosis using QDF based algorithm," International Journal of advanced research in Computer Science and Software Engineering 2(5) (2012) 493–499.

[92] Quelli B, Elhadadi H, Aissaoui H, Bouikhalene B, "AR modelling for cardiac arrhythmia classification using MLP neural networks," International Journal of Computer Applications 47(24) (2012) 44–51.

[93] Acharya UR, Sankaranarayanan M, Nayak J, Xiang C, Tamura T, "Automatic identification of cardiac health using modeling techniques: A comparative study," Information Sciences 178 (2008) 4571–4582.

[94] Neeraj K, Imteyaz A, Pankaj R, "Signal processing of ECG using Matlab," International Journal of Scientific and Research Publications, 2(10) (2012) 1–6.

[95] Louridas P, Ebert C, "Machine learning," IEEE Software 33(5) (2016) 110–115.

[96] "Types of machine learning algorithms | en.proft.me", En.proft.me, 2018. Online. Available: http://en.proft.me/2015/12/24/types-machine-learning-algorithms/. Accessed: 13-Mar-2018.

[97] "Viblo | Free service for technical knowledge sharing", Viblo, 2018. Online. Available: https://viblo.asia/p/intro-to-deep-learning-3P0lPkmPZox. Accessed: 13-Mar-2018.

Chapter 12

Blind source separation for OSAS: data extraction

Tung Ren Sin[1] and Leong Wai Yie[1]

In this research, the electroencephalogram (EEG) signals for sleep apnea were extracted and processed using Blind Source Separation approach. To identify the EEG features, 13 Independent Component Analysis methods were adopted to analyse the data extraction performance. All the EEG signals on Obstructive Sleep Apnea Syndrome (OSAS) were recorded using 10–20 international electrode placement system. The experiment was conducted based on a 20-min sleep recording during rapid eye movement sleep characterized by rapid saccadic movements of the eyes and non-rapid eye movement sleep. Seven electrode positions were identified to record the EEG signals, with a sampling time of 100 Hz. The result was investigated using the proposed 13 ICA algorithms to understand the important EEG signals and features for every process. The wavelets denoising results were obtained to evaluate the robustness of the proposed wavelets denoising algorithms. According to the performance analysis, the proposed wavelets denoising technique could be used to investigate the recorded EEG signals with lower signal amplitude.

12.1 Introduction

Human brain is the most important centre of control for the human nervous system and receives input from the sensory organs. The brain uses exert centralized control for neural activity to communicate with each other. The brain is the most complex organ in a vertebrate's body, usually close to the sensory organs for senses such as vision. The brain cell generates the action potentials: the electrodes are placed on the scalp to record all spontaneous electrical activity in EEG form.

The technology to capture and measure brain's electrical activity using multiple EEG electrodes has greatly been improved. The EEG recording technology is affordable and accurate to measure brain wave activity on the scalp. The electrodes are attached on the scalp of a human and the EEG signals are recorded in frequency domain.

[1]Faculty of Engineering and Information Technology, MAHSA University, Malaysia

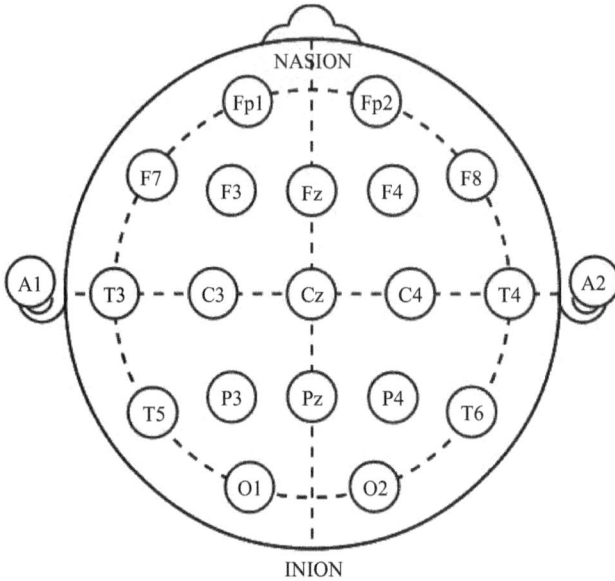

Figure 12.1   A 10–20 international EEG electrode placement system

The depolarization signals from the brain cells are attenuated while passing through the connective tissues in the brain structures. Actually, the brain fluid and the scalp have very complex impedances. In order to prevent collecting noisy signals from the scalp, the skull needs to be prepared for a quality contact with the reason of overcoming the impedance mismatch due to hair and dead skin on the head [1].

During the EEG signals recording, the International electrode 10/20 placement system is adopted to determine the position of the electrodes placement, as shown in Figure 12.1. The EEG recording system is an internationally recognized method on the location identification of scalp electrodes. Therefore, the multiple EEG electrodes tend to record lots of overlapped brain activities and artifacts in frequency domain. These recordings are transmitted by large volume electric conduction and seizure activity from different dynamic neocortical processes (Figure 12.2).

The EEG system is used to record significant brain waves for study purposes. The recording would also consist of abnormities, noise or artifacts. The noise signals or artifacts might overlap with neurotic events. The overlapping leads to difficulties in EEG signals interpretation. One common hypothesis is that the artifacts should be independent from brain activities, in either normal or pathologic conditions. With this assumption, the signals can be considered non-Gaussian. A frequently used method to remove the noise signal is blind source separation (BSS). However, independent component analysis (ICA), which is a special class of BSS, has proven capable of separating the artifacts from the brain sources. There are many ICA algorithms available, which can process the EEG data efficiently [2,3].

In general, the ICA is a statistical and computational approach to separate artifacts and noise from the recorded EEG brain signals. The ICA is recommended

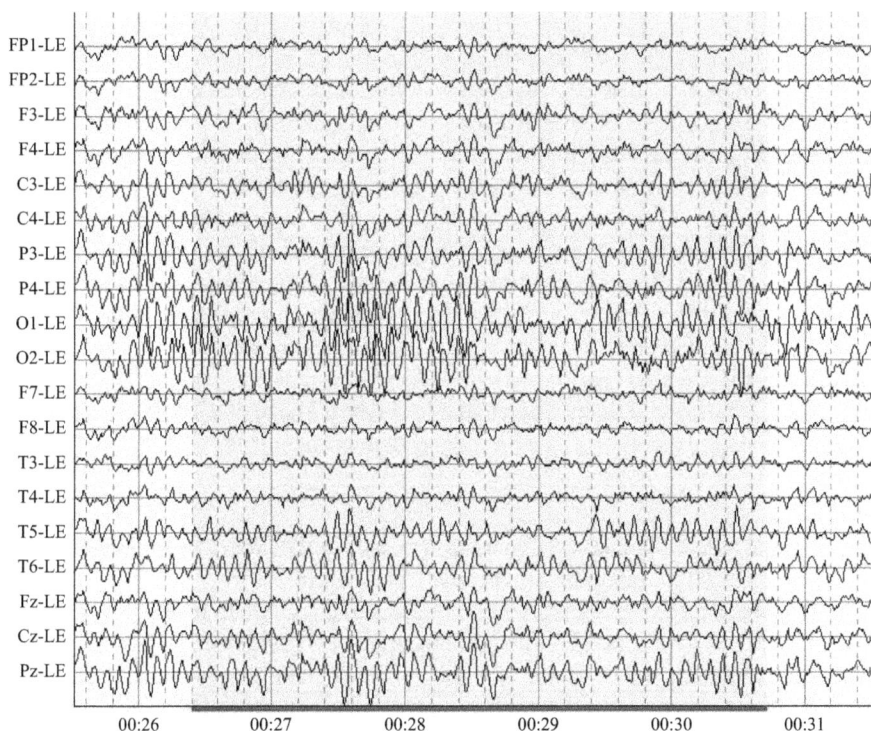

Figure 12.2   The EEG signals recording of alpha activity at multiple electrode locations, namely P3, P4, O1 and O2, for a male adult with both eyes closed

to isolate the brain activities, features and abnormalities from non-brain activities; this technique can be used to understand the brain's spontaneous electric activities by EEG researchers to classify and understand the feature of the brain disorders. ICA could be used blindly to separate the artifacts and overlapping EEG signals into independent source signals. This method is able to remove unwanted signals such as redundancies, noise and artifacts. The ICA will then be used to reconstruct the EEG recording to benefit the brain disorder diagnosis [2].

12.2   Methodology

Noninvasive evaluation in biomedical signal analysis is important to analyse the physiological changes of the body. Having the recorded biomedical signals, the status of various physiological systems is able to be modelled and measured. In general, the biomedical signals are weak, nonstationary and distorted by artifacts, signal processing techniques have played an important role to analyse the recorded EEG signals.

Besides the classical signal analysis tools (e.g. adaptive supervised filtering) used to process the superimposed biomedical source signals, Intelligent Blind Signal Processing techniques such as BSS are used with the aim to recover independent sources given only sensor observations (linear mixture of independent source signals). The BSS can be formulated as the problems of separating or estimating the waveform of the original sources without knowing the parameters of mixing [4].

In particular, ICA is a computational method to separate multivariate signals into several additive subcomponents. The fundamental criterion of adopting ICA approach is that all sources should be zero mean and independent. ICA is a common application for "cocktail party problem" and also for BSS. Generally, ICA has found many applications in image and signal processing, to blindly separate the mixed signals.

ICA can also be defined as statistical "latent variables" model. Consider the linear mixed signals, $x_1, \ldots, x_n$ of n independent components:

$$X_j = a_{j1}s_1 + a_{j2}s_2 + a_{j3}s_3 + \cdots + a_{jn}s_n, \text{ for all } j \tag{12.1}$$

At time index t, the mixed signals are given as x_j. The independent components s_n are assumed to be random variables with zero mean.

To simplify the representation, the vector–matrix notation has always been used instead of having (12.1). The random vector of $\mathbf{x}$ is denoted by the mixtures $x_1, \ldots, x_n$ and the random vector of $\mathbf{s}$ is denoted by the elements $s_1, \ldots, s_n$. Let us then denote $\mathbf{A}$ matrix with the elements of a_{ij} whereby the bold lower case letter indicates vector and bold upper case letter denote matrices. By using the vector–matrix notation, the above mixing model is written as

$$\mathbf{x} = \mathbf{As} \tag{12.2}$$

The statistical model in (12.2) is known as independent component analysis or ICA model. The ICA model is a generative model whereby it describes how the observed data are generated by a process of mixing the components s_i. In this ICA model, the independents are latent variables, meaning they cannot be observed and the mixing matrix is assumed to be unknown. Random vector $\mathbf{x}$ is observable and this is done under general assumptions.

For a random noisy vector $\mathbf{x}(k)$, the mixing ICA model can be represented as:

$$\mathbf{x}(k) = \mathbf{Hs}(k) + \mathbf{v}(k) \tag{12.3}$$

where $\mathbf{H}$ is an (m × n) mixing matrix, $\mathbf{s}(k) = [s_1(k), s_2(k), \ldots, s_n(k)]^T$ is a source vector of statistically independent signals (unknown nonsingular mixing matrix), and $\mathbf{v}(k) = [v_1(k), v_2(k), \ldots, v_m(k)]^T$ is a vector of uncorrelated noise (addictive noise).

The purpose of the ICA is to formulate a linear transformation $\mathbf{W}$ of the dependent sensor signals $\mathbf{x}$ that make the output as independent as possible,

$$\mathbf{y}(k) = \mathbf{Wx}(k) = \mathbf{WAs}(k) \tag{12.4}$$

where $\mathbf{y}$ is an estimate of the sources (independent components) and the sources are exactly recovered when $\mathbf{W}$ is the inverse of $\mathbf{A}$.

From (12.2), there is an ambiguity present in the ICA model. The ambiguity that is present in (12.2) is that we cannot determine the variances (energies) of the independent components. The reason for the ambiguity is that both $\mathbf{s}$ and $\mathbf{A}$ being unknown. Any scalar multiplier in one of the sources s_i could always be cancelled by dividing the corresponding column a_i of $\mathbf{A}$ by the same scalar. However, this ambiguity is, fortunately, insignificant in most application. Besides that, obtaining an exact inverse of the $\mathbf{A}$ matrix in most cases is impossible. Thus, the source separation algorithms aim to find a $\mathbf{W}$ matrix such as the product of $\mathbf{WA}$ in order to permute the diagonal and scalar matrix [4–13].

In the last 20 years, different types of algorithms were proposed and most of the algorithms proposed that the sources are stationary and are based implicitly on high-order statistic (HOS) algorithms. With the application of HOS algorithms, Gaussian sources cannot be separated as they do not have higher than two statistic moments, while the second-order statistic (SOS) does not have such constraint. On the other hand, SOS algorithm uses non-stationary structure of the signals (time or frequency structure) for the separation purpose.

Temporal, spatial and spatio-temporal decorrelations play important roles in the EEG signal analysis and these techniques are based on the SOS algorithm. Furthermore, they are the basis for the modern subspace methods of array processing and frequently used to eliminate redundancy or to reduce noise. In the spatial decorrelation (pre-whitening) technique, the ICA tasks will usually become easier and well-posed (less ill-conditioned) as the unmixing system is described by an orthogonal matrix for real-valued signals and a unitary matrix for complex-valued signals and weights. With the same SOS, one can compute different whitening transformation for nonstationary signals. Moreover, the spatio-temporal and time-delayed decorrelation can be used to identify the mixing matrix and to perform BSS, which mainly on coloured source [2]. In contrast to the correlation-based transformation such as principal component analysis, ICA is not only able to decorrelate the signals (second-order statistic), but it can also reduce higher order statistical dependencies in order to generate signals as independent as possible [3,4,14].

12.2.1   *Second-order blind identification algorithm*

One of the well-known second order-based technique that used to compute the separating matrix is called second-order blind identification (SOBI) algorithm. In the SOBI algorithm, the separation of the matrix is achieved in two steps. The first step is the whitening of the observed signal vector by linear transformation, which is also known as whitening matrix. The second step is applied joint approximate diagonalization (JAD) on a set of different time–delay correlation matrices of the whitened signal vector. As the whitening matrix is estimated based on the noisy observed data, it highly suffers from bias if the SNR is relatively low, especially if the noise correlation matrix is unknown. Besides that, the JAD also suffers from highly time-correlated noise. In such cases, the correlation matrices of the observed signals at nonzero time–delay are still biased by unknown noise correlation matrices. In order to overcome the bias of the whitening matrix in white noise cases, robust SOBI algorithm has been developed to overcome the weakness of SOBI algorithm [15,16].

12.2.2 *Robust SOBI algorithm*

The robust SOBI (SOBI-RO) algorithm formulates a new correlation matrix as a weighted linear combination of a set of time-delayed correlation matrices of the observed signal vector. The weight linear combination is computed in an iterative procedure that makes the formulated correlation matrix in positive define. The positive define correlation matrix is used for computing the whitening matrix and thereby whitening the observed signal vector. In the robust SOBI algorithm, it combines robust whitening and time-delayed decorrelation with the purpose of improving the classical SOBI algorithm. By integration the robust whitening instead of simple whitening, the main objective of using robust whitening is to eliminate the influence of white noise [16].

Recall the equation introduced in (12.3), the source signals s are assumed to be mutually uncorrelated and temporally correlated (instead of independents) in a second-order statistic framework. Computation on this model can be difficult as the presence of noise will influence the correlation between signals. Hence its covariance matrix at lag 0, $\mathbf{R_n}(0) = \mathbf{E}[\mathbf{n}(\mathbf{k})\mathbf{n}(\mathbf{k})^\mathbf{T}]$, can be a full matrix which is unknown and the time-delayed correlation matrix $\mathbf{R_n}(\mathbf{i}) = \mathbf{E}\ [\mathbf{n}(\mathbf{k})\mathbf{n}(\mathbf{k}-\mathbf{i})^\mathbf{T}]$ will become null. With the above assumption, the correlation matrices of the observation have:

$$\mathbf{R_x}(0) = \mathbf{E}\left[\mathbf{x}(\mathbf{k})\mathbf{x}(\mathbf{k})^\mathbf{T}\right] = \mathbf{AR_s}(0)\mathbf{A}^\mathbf{T} + \mathbf{R_n} \tag{12.5}$$

$$\mathbf{R_x}(\mathbf{i}) = \mathbf{E}\left[\mathbf{x}(\mathbf{k})\mathbf{x}(\mathbf{k}-\mathbf{i})^\mathbf{T}\right] = \mathbf{AR_s}(\mathbf{i})\mathbf{A}^\mathbf{T} + \mathbf{R_n} \tag{12.6}$$

The first step (robust whitening) consists of finding a matrix $\mathbf{Q}$ that correlates the signals in x for small time lags. With the helping of ICALAB implementation, which exploits (12.6) for a single time lag $i = 1$. The matrix $\mathbf{R_x}$ (1) is then diagonalized by an eigen-decomposition:

$$\mathbf{R_x}(1) = \mathbf{U_e}\text{diag}\left[\lambda_1{}^2 \dots \lambda_N{}^2\right]\mathbf{U_e}{}^\mathbf{T} \tag{12.7}$$

The pre-whitening matrix $\mathbf{Q}$ can be investigated via the eigenvector matrix $\mathbf{U_e}$ and diagonal eigenvalues matrix

$$\mathbf{Q} = \text{diag}[\lambda_1 \dots \lambda_n]\mathbf{U_e}{}^\mathbf{T} \tag{12.8}$$

With the formation of $\mathbf{Q}$ matrix, the whitened signal z (k-i) = Qx (k − i) for different time lags can be calculated (the default option in ICALAB is 100 time lags).

The second step of robust SOBI is the same as the classical SOBI, namely approximate joint diagonalization of different $\mathbf{R_z}$ (i) matrices, computed with (12.6). Finally, the separation matrix $\mathbf{W}$ is given by

$$\mathbf{W} = \mathbf{A}^\mathbf{T}\mathbf{Q} \tag{12.9}$$

where the matrix **Q** has been computed in the previous whitening or orthogonalization step. Based on the fact that **A** is an orthogonal matrix and the sources are spatially uncorrelated [4,14–17].

12.2.3 Wavelet denoising

During the EEG recording, the recorded signals are not only contaminated with ocular or muscular artifacts; it is also contaminated with noises that come from different sources. Currently, in order to remove the noise from the non-stationary signals, wavelet denoising (WD) is usually adopted on the signals to investigate the separation results. In WD, the recorded signals are decomposed on wavelet basis. After that, we are able to obtain a representation of the signal that concentrates most of its energy in a few wavelet coefficients, which have large absolute values. In the WD process, the noise energy distribution does not change, which means that its energy will not be held by a large value of coefficients. By using large coefficients for denoising, it will lead to an almost noise-free signal. The main problem is the computation of the threshold, which means responding to where to fix the boundary between the small and large wavelet coefficient.

There are a few algorithms that have been proposed in the past years and the most well-known algorithm is known as Donoho's universal thresholding. The Donoho's universal thresholding will compute a threshold level whereby no Gaussian noise will be left in the denoised signal. However, Donoho's universal thresholding is able to provide us an almost noise-free signal, but the important drawback of using this thresholding algorithm is the elimination of possibly informative parts of the signal.

In the EEG signal analysis, it is important not to loose potentially useful information during the diagnosis. Moreover, EEG informative signals often have small amplitude. Therefore, high thresholding algorithm is not appropriate for denoising the EEG signal.

On the other hand, SURE denoising (Stein Unbiased Risk Estimator) and Minimax methods seem adapted to the EEG signal denoising. This is due to two of the algorithms offering low threshold and thus preserving most of the informative signal while eliminating less noise.

For the SURE denoising method, the value of the threshold is computed considering a Gaussian noise hypothesis for which a robust estimation of variance is made. Besides that, SURE denoising method has an important property whereby it can adapt itself to the signal. In simple words, the SURE denoising method threshold depends on the signal but not only depend on the estimated noise.

For the Minimax denoising algorithm, it is used a fixed threshold chosen to yield minimax performance for mean square error against an ideal procedure. The minimax principle is used in statistics in order to design an estimator. As the denoised signal can be assimilated to the estimator of the unknown regression function, the minimax estimator is the one that realizes the minimum of the maximum mean square error.

12.3   The evaluation criteria

In order to validate the ICA separation methods [17], the Index of Separability (IS) is chosen to validate the ICA separation methods. The IS is calculated from the $N \times N$ transfer matrix $\mathbf{G}$ between the original sources and the estimated sources after the ICA separation.

$$\mathbf{G} = \mathbf{WA} \tag{12.10}$$

In order to obtain the IS, it is required to take the absolute value of elements $\mathbf{G}$ and normalize the lines $\mathbf{g_i}$ by dividing each element with the maximum absolute value of the line. As the result, the lines of the resulting matrix $\mathbf{G}'$ will be

$$\mathbf{gi} = \frac{|\mathbf{gi}|}{\mathbf{max}|\mathbf{gi}|} \tag{12.11}$$

The IS is obtained by

$$IS = \frac{\sum_{j=1}^{N} \left(\sum_{i=1}^{N} \mathbf{G}'(i,j) - 1 \right)}{[N(N-1)]} \tag{12.12}$$

For perfect source separation, the IS is equal to zero $(IS = 0)$ [17].

Besides using the IS to validate the proper ICA algorithms to process the EEG signals, the performance index of signal-to-interference ratio (SIR) for mixing matrix $\mathbf{A}$ and the signal $\mathbf{S}$ is chosen as evaluation criteria.

The performance index of SIR for mixing matrix $\mathbf{A}$ can be viewed as follows:

$$y_i = w_i^T X = \left(w_i^T A \right) \mathbf{S} = g_i S = g_{ij} S_j \tag{12.13}$$

where y_i and s_j are estimated components and the j-th source, respectively, w_i^T represents a row vector of demixing matrix and the g_i is a normalized row vector $[0 \ 0 \ g_{ij} \ 0 \ 0]$. As y_i is the estimation of s_j, the ideal normalized vector g_i is the unit vector of $U_j = [0 \ 0 \ \ldots \ 1 \ \ldots \ 0]$. Therefore, one analysis is successful if and only if its vector g_i is similar to unit vector u_j.

For the performance index of SIR for the signal $\mathbf{S}$, each pair of signal (y_i, s_j) is denoted:

$$SIR \ S_{ij} = -10 \log 10 \left(\frac{\|y_i - s_j\|_2^2}{\|s_j\|_2^2} \right) \tag{12.14}$$

12.4   The experimental results

In this study, the ICA algorithm was adopted to process the EEG signal: the signals are generated and compared with the known reference. The five sources are simulated at sampling frequency of 256 Hz. The original sources were mixed randomly, as shown in Figure 12.3.

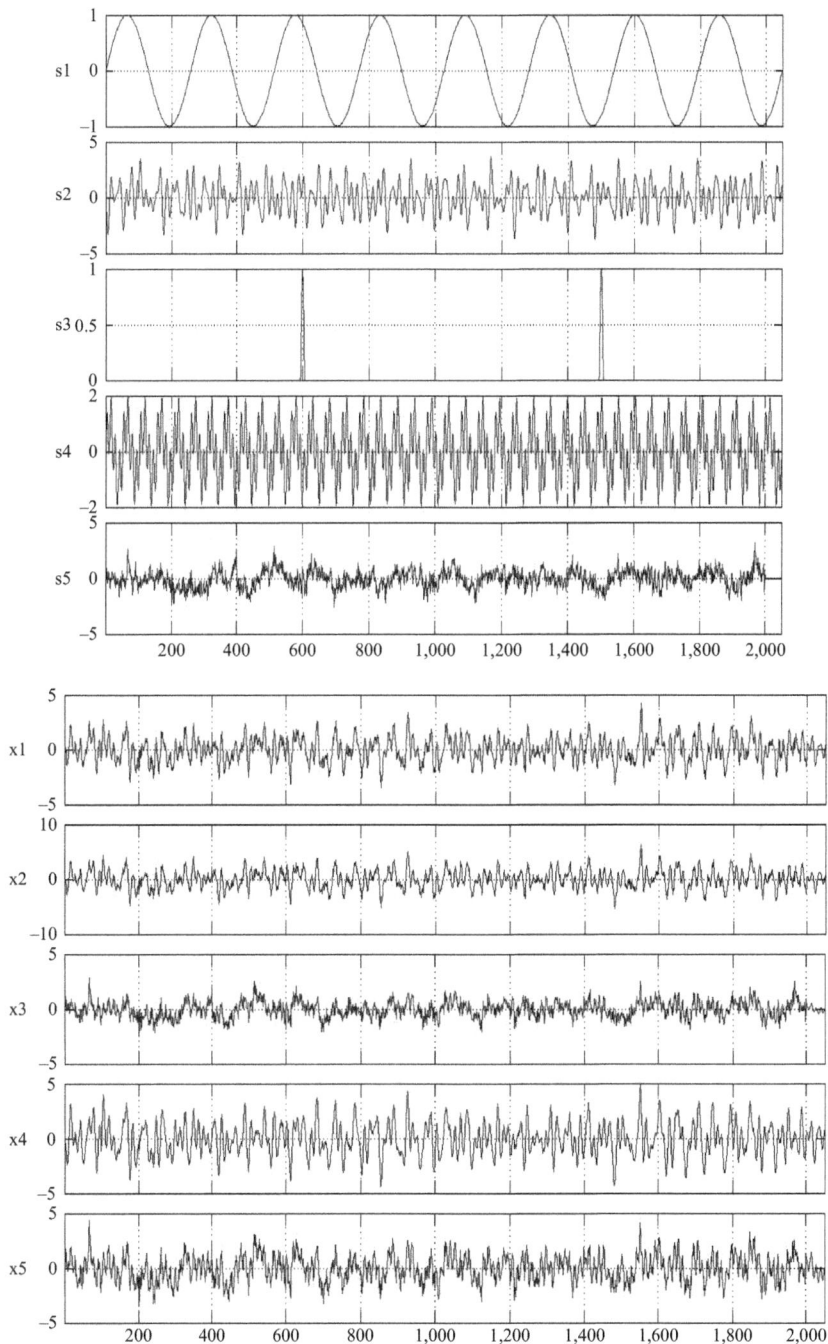

Figure 12.3   (Top) Simulated original noiseless brain sources, (bottom) simulated EEG (mixture)

Three experiments have been conducted to determine the ICA algorithms for EEG signals separation.

(a)   The EEG signals (Figure 12.1) were generated without additional noise to the mixture, in an ideal condition. A total of 13 ICA algorithms were adopted in noiseless condition. The performance results are shown in Table 12.1.

The separability analysis versus ICA was illustrated in Figure 12.4. Both Table 12.1 and Figure 12.4 have shown that the ICA-based robust SOBI (SOBI-RO) algorithm has separated the EEG signals with the separability of 0.0700. When the IS is approaching zero, the signals would have been separated into independent components. These results have shown that the ICA-based second-order statistic algorithms have better separation performance over non-stationary EEG signals.

(b)   To simulate the real EEG signals, the mixtures were added with Gaussian and Uniform noise. Based on our observation, the acquired EEG signals not only

Table 12.1   Comparison of the performance of various ICA algorithms

ICA algorithms	IS	IO
AMUSE	0.0739	0.3126
Evd 2	0.0850	0.2985
SOBI	0.0900	0.2973
SOBI-RO	0.0700	0.1924
SOBI-BPF	0.0904	0.2817
SONS	0.1768	0.5328
FJADE	0.2585	0.4612
JADE TD	0.1950	0.3149
FPICA	0.1226	0.2642
EFICA	0.1099	0.2463
SANG	0.0787	0.3890
ThinICA	0.1199	0.2661
ERICA	0.1742	0.3063

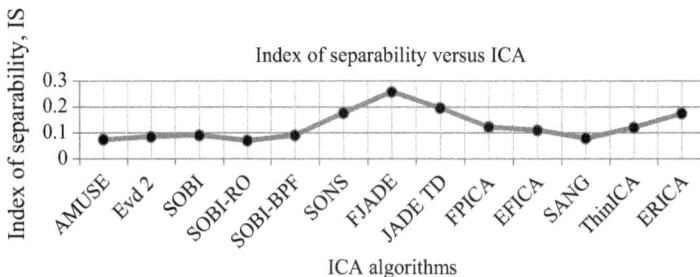

Figure 12.4   The performance analysis of separability versus 13 ICA algorithms

consist of brain activities but also contain non-brain activities. Therefore, by adding different types of noise range from 20 dB to 0 dB, the approximation on the ICA algorithms can then be improved. Thirteen ICA algorithms were investigated with different types of noise (Gaussian and Uniform noise); the result for the additional Gaussian noise and Uniform noise is shown in Tables 12.2 and 12.3, respectively.

Table 12.2 The 13 ICA algorithms are adopted to separate noisy signals (Gaussian noise)

ICA algorithms	20	15	10	5	0	Average of IS
AMUSE	0.1620	0.2557	0.2698	0.3255	0.3194	0.2665
Evd 2	0.1567	0.2321	0.2883	0.3515	0.3360	0.2729
SOBI	0.1340	0.2432	0.3090	0.2923	0.4543	0.2866
SOBI-RO	0.1428	0.1293	0.1731	0.1243	0.1961	0.1531
SOBI-BPF	0.0963	0.1507	0.2421	0.2136	0.2810	0.1967
SONS	0.1588	0.1252	0.1629	0.2822	0.2655	0.1989
FJADE	0.3071	0.2766	0.2813	0.2328	0.3401	0.2876
JEDE TD	0.1972	0.2544	0.3291	0.2473	0.3051	0.2666
FPICA	0.2592	0.2904	0.3160	0.4301	0.3125	0.3216
EFICA	0.2263	0.2021	0.2649	0.3406	0.2829	0.2633
SANG	0.1762	0.2342	0.2623	0.3589	0.3909	0.2845
ThinICA	0.2559	0.2520	0.2989	0.3411	0.3835	0.3063
ERICA	0.2956	0.1801	0.2231	0.3223	0.3332	0.2709

Table 12.3 The 13 noise algorithms were adopted to separate noisy signals (Uniform noise)

Proposed ICA algorithms	20	15	10	5	0	Average index separability, IS
AMUSE	0.1660	0.2582	0.2669	0.3199	0.3366	0.2695
Evd 2	0.1561	0.2609	0.2797	0.2870	0.3538	0.2675
SOBI	0.1359	0.2400	0.2679	0.2860	0.3617	0.2583
SOBI-RO	0.1414	0.1465	0.1349	0.1470	0.1739	0.1487
SOBI-BPF	0.1363	0.1588	0.1410	0.2076	0.2355	0.1759
SONS	0.1180	0.2016	0.1401	0.1823	0.2715	0.1827
FJADE	0.2159	0.1883	0.2576	0.3198	0.3426	0.2648
JEDE TD	0.2405	0.2192	0.2523	0.3520	0.3943	0.2916
FPICA	0.2237	0.2140	0.2780	0.3316	0.3130	0.2721
EFICA	0.2534	0.2480	0.3017	0.3641	0.3544	0.3043
SANG	0.1936	0.2474	0.3146	0.3563	0.3576	0.2939
ThinICA	0.2074	0.2556	0.2432	0.2765	0.3023	0.2570
ERICA	0.3071	0.2333	0.2399	0.3969	0.3801	0.3114

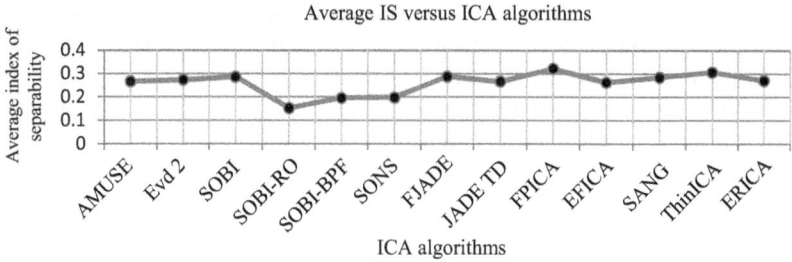

Figure 12.5   The performance analysis of separability versus ICA with Gaussian noise signals

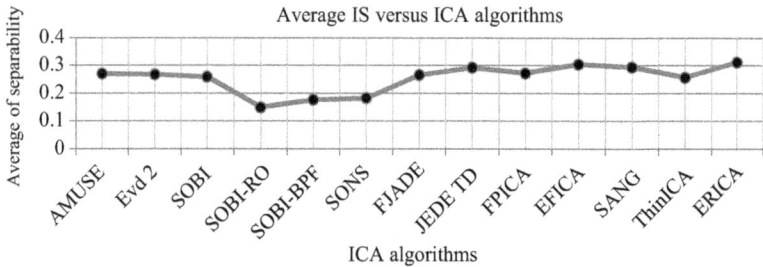

Figure 12.6   The performance results of average separability, IS_{avg}, versus the 13 selected ICA methods with uniform noise

Using the results in Tables 12.2 and 12.3, the performance for IS_{avg} versus ICA algorithms in the presence of Gaussian noise and Uniform noise is shown in Figures 12.5 and 12.6, respectively. From the results of index separability IS_{avg} versus ICA algorithms in the presence of noise (Gaussian or Uniform), the robust SOBI (SOBI-RO) algorithm appears to be a better algorithm in separating the simulated EEG signals.

(c)   Finally, Monte Carlo analysis is used to adopt to ICA algorithms and to verify the robustness of the robust-SOBI (SOBI-RO) algorithm. The mean value of SIR for the mixing matrix, $\mathbf{A} = \mathbf{H}$ and source signal, $\mathbf{S}$, can be calculated. The main purpose of using Monte Carlo analysis is to compare the performance, robustness and consistency of different ICA algorithms for the same mixing conditions.

For the evaluation of ICA algorithms under Monte Carlo analysis, four ICA algorithms have been selected, which are AMUSE, SOBI, SOBI-RO and EFICA. The result for mean values of SIR for mixing matrix $\mathbf{A} = \mathbf{H}$ and mean values for source signal, $\mathbf{S}$, are shown in Figures 12.7 and 12.8, respectively.

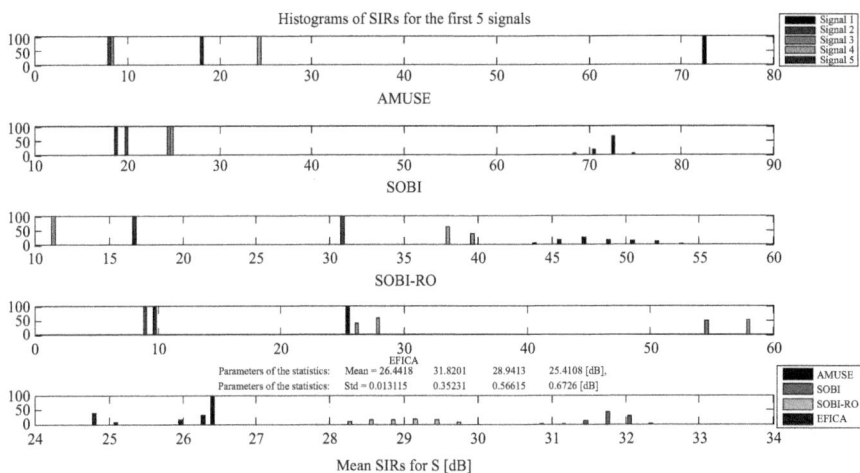

Figure 12.7   The analysis of SIR versus source signals

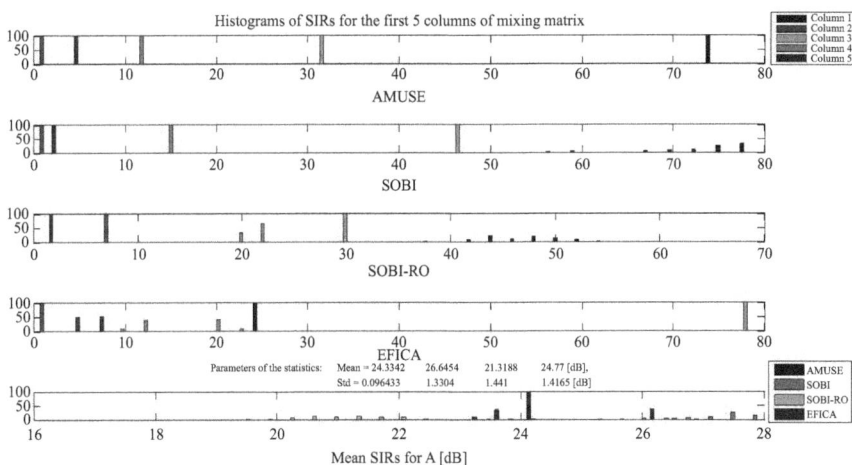

Figure 12.8   The performance analysis of SIR versus ICA algorithms for mixed signals

Based on Figures 12.7 and 12.8, ICA algorithms (AMUSE, SOBI, SOBI-RO and EFICA) could separate the signals successfully with prior knowledge and no additional noise was added to the mixtures. For successful signals separation, the SIR for matrix of **A** and **S** must be greater than 16 dB. The tested algorithms were able to fulfil the criteria for signal (>16 dB) separation.

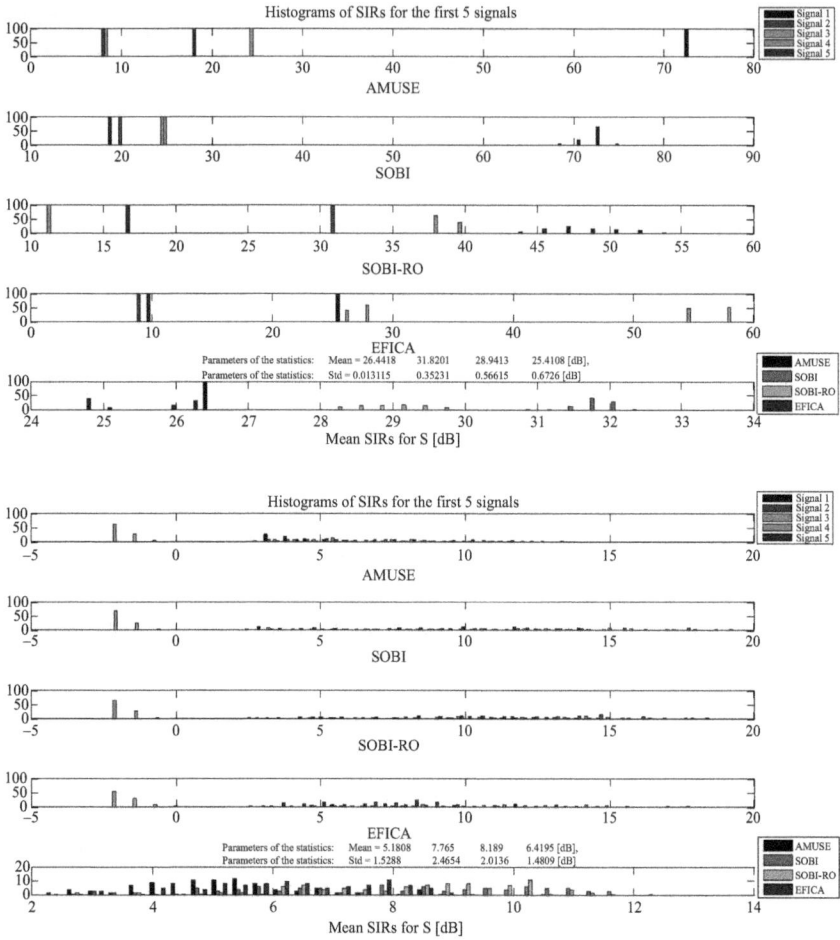

Figure 12.9   The performance analysis for ICA algorithms on noiseless and noisy (20 dB) signals

The ICA algorithms were simulated on signals with 20 dB Gaussian noise. The noisy mixture was simulated using Monte Carlo analysis. The simulation results in Figure 12.9 have shown the mean SIR for the original signals. The noiseless signal was displayed in Figure 12.9 (top); all ICA algorithms have consistently and successfully separated the noisy signals. From Figure 12.9 (bottom), the data were added with 20 dB Gaussian noise. The histogram generated has shown that the ICA-based SOBI-RO and SOBI methods could separate the noisy signals better than the other two algorithms.

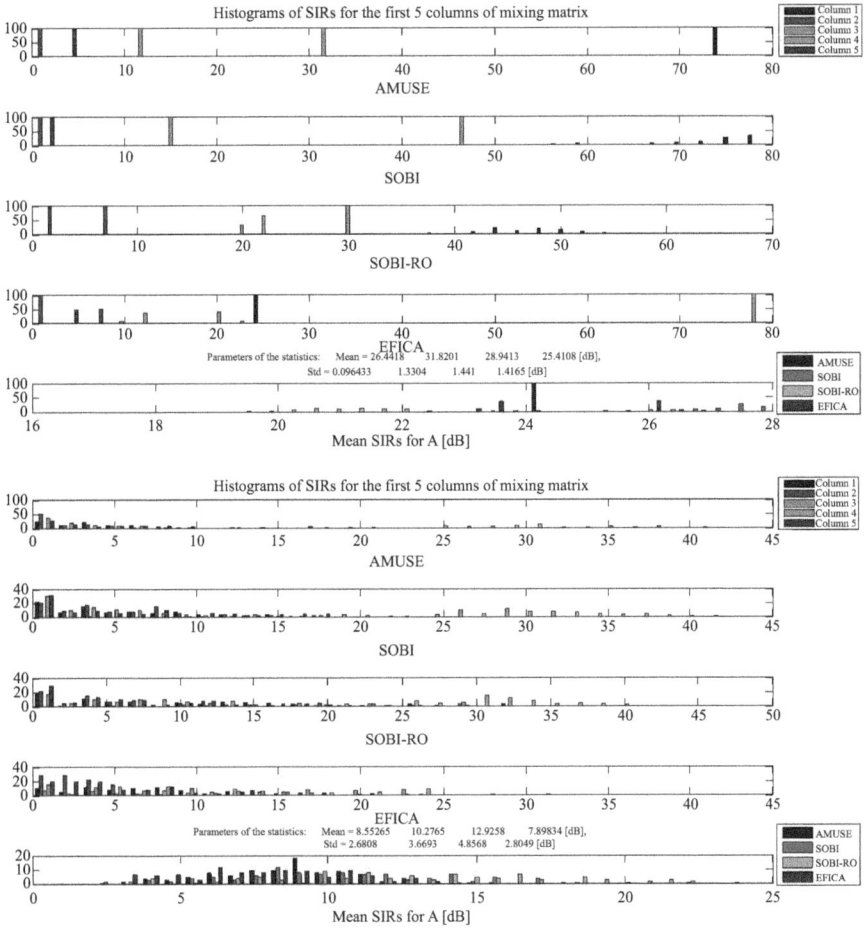

Figure 12.10   The performance comparison of noiseless and noisy signals (20 dB)

In Figure 12.10, the performance results of SIR for source signals and matrix with additional noise give reliable measurement. The noiseless signals (bottom) were successfully separated by all ICA algorithms. As shown in Figure 12.10 (top row), the additional noise (20 dB) has affected the performance of the algorithms.

Figure 12.11 has shown the results of SIR with additional noise signals; the mean value for SIR has decreased. The result has proven that noisy signals always posed an issue for the ICA in separating and reconstructing the signals.

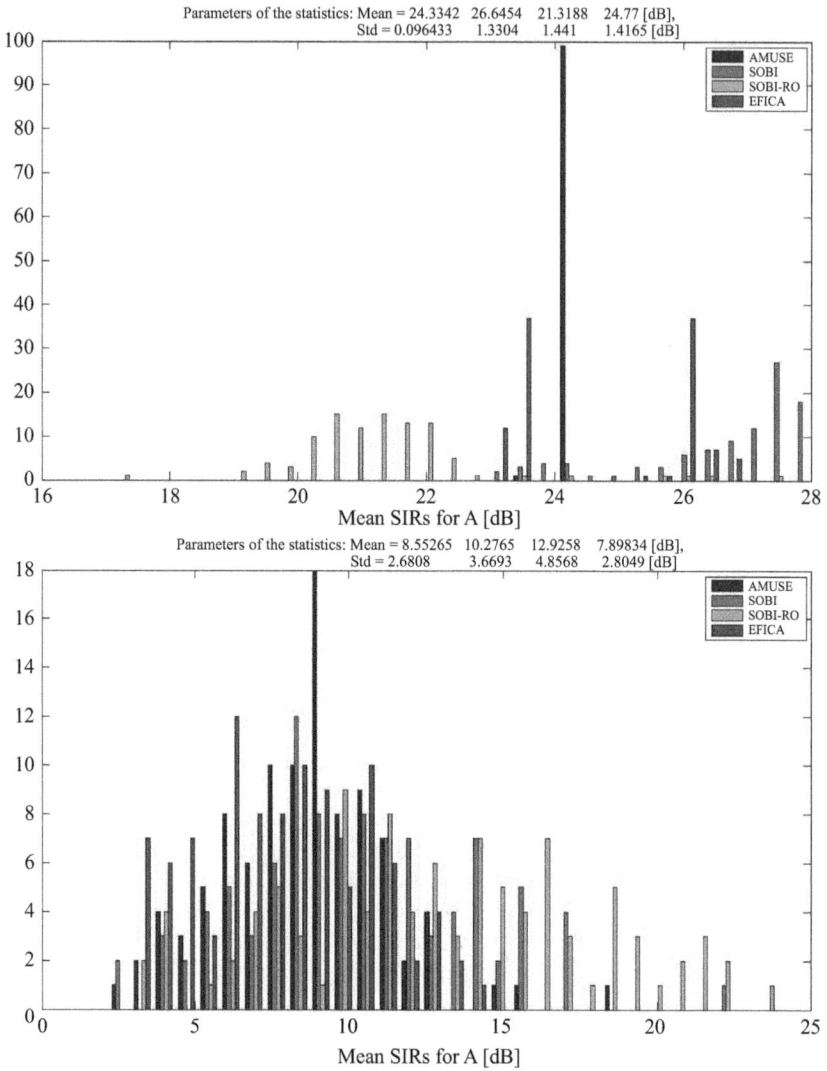

Figure 12.11   Performance results of SIRs versus mean values (top: Original signals; bottom: Noisy signals with 20 dB)

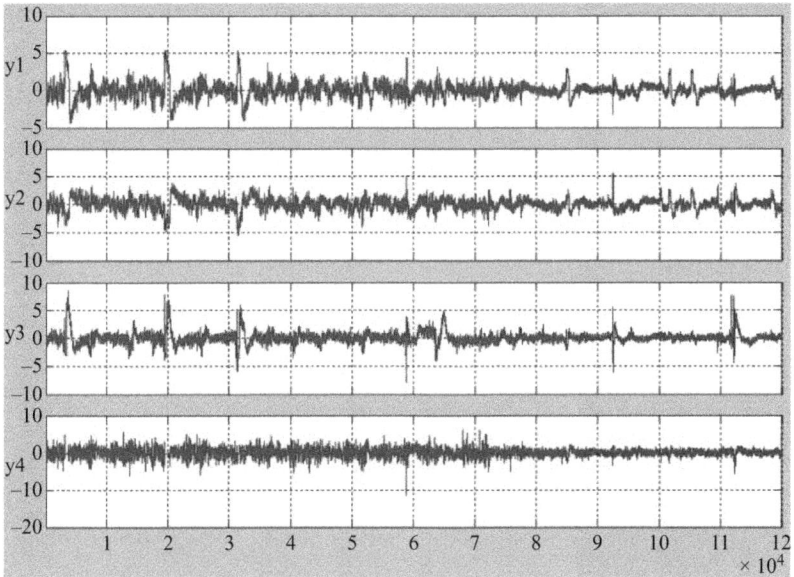

*Figure 12.12   Independent component without denoising (y1 = C3, y2 = O1,
y3 C4 and y4 = O2) running with SOBI-RO algorithms*

12.5   The ICA approach on real EEG signals

The EEG brain signals were captured using a 10/20 international electrode placement system. The 13 proposed ICA separation algorithms and the WD approaches were applied to the signals. The experiment consists of 20 min recording of NREM sleep and REM sleep stages. The EEG electrodes were applied to record the EEG at 100 Hz per sampling. The ICA-based SOBI-RO algorithm was adopted on channel O1, C3, C4 and O2 (Figure 12.12). These four channels were selected due to the electrode placement on the brain scalp.

The WD approach with Heuristic SURE has performed better compared with the fundamental Minimax denoising algorithm (Figures 12.12–12.16). From our observation, the Minimax denoising algorithm tends to remove the important EEG signals that will cause the loss of information and features. The wavelets denoising results were used and magnified to investigate the robustness of the denoising algorithms. The wavelets denoising method has shown better performance to analyse the lower amplitude signals.

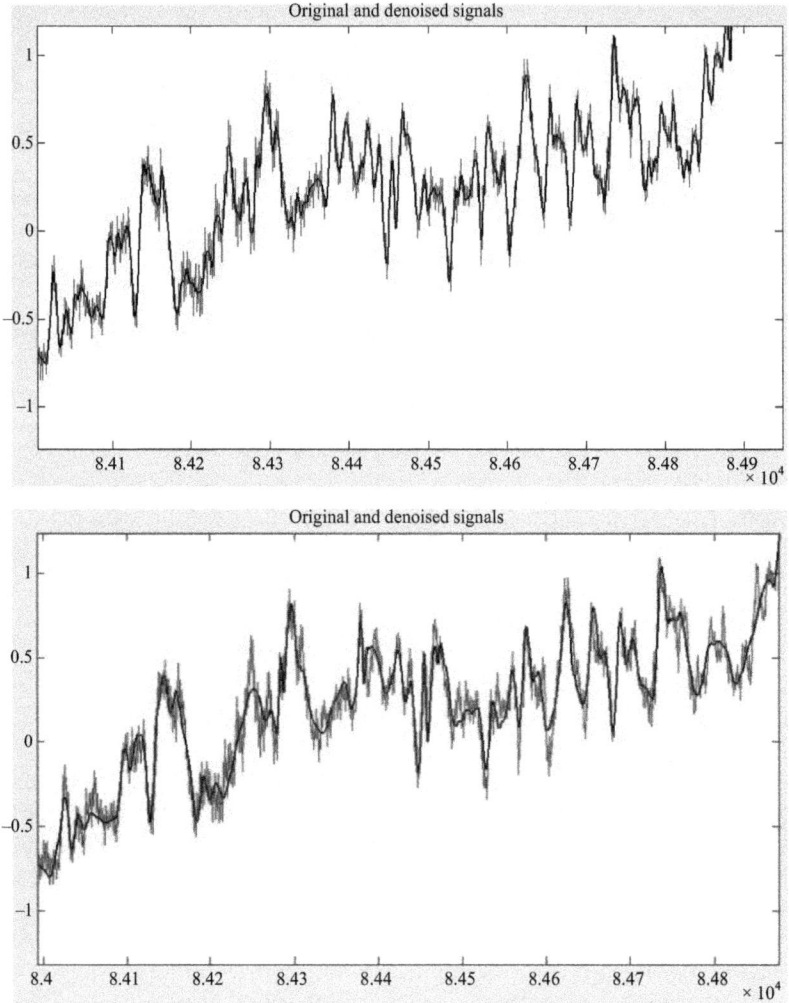

Figure 12.13   Wavelet denoising with Heuristic SURE and Minimax on y1 = C3
channel (top: Heuristic SURE, bottom: Minimax)

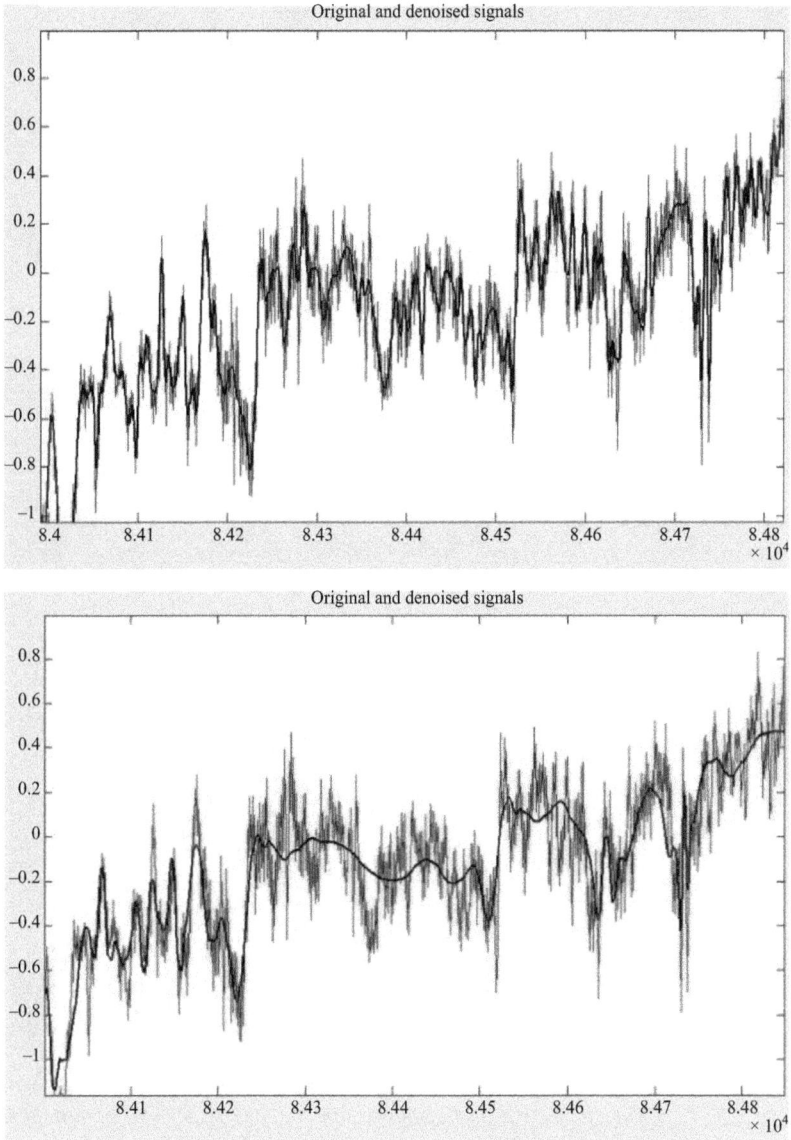

Figure 12.14   Wavelet denoising with Heuristic SURE and Minimax on y2 = O1 channel (top: Heuristic SURE, bottom: Minimax)

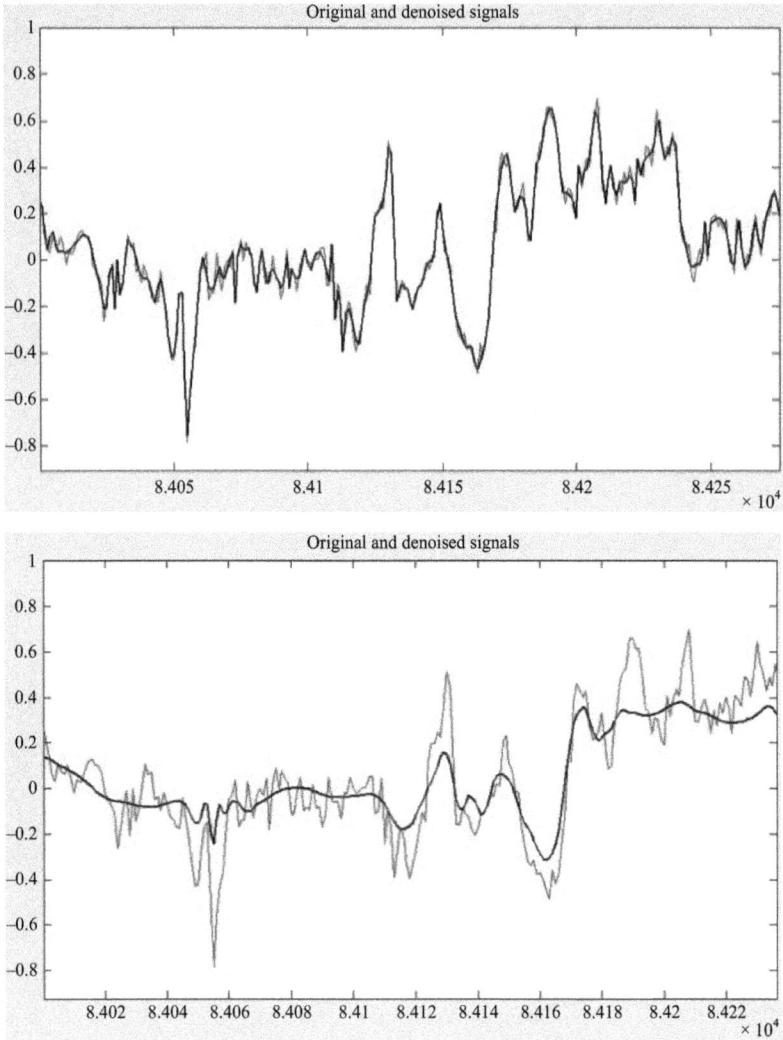

Figure 12.15   The performance results using wavelet denoising algorithm with Heuristic SURE and Minimax approaches on y3 = C4 channel (top: Heuristic SURE approach, bottom: Minimax)

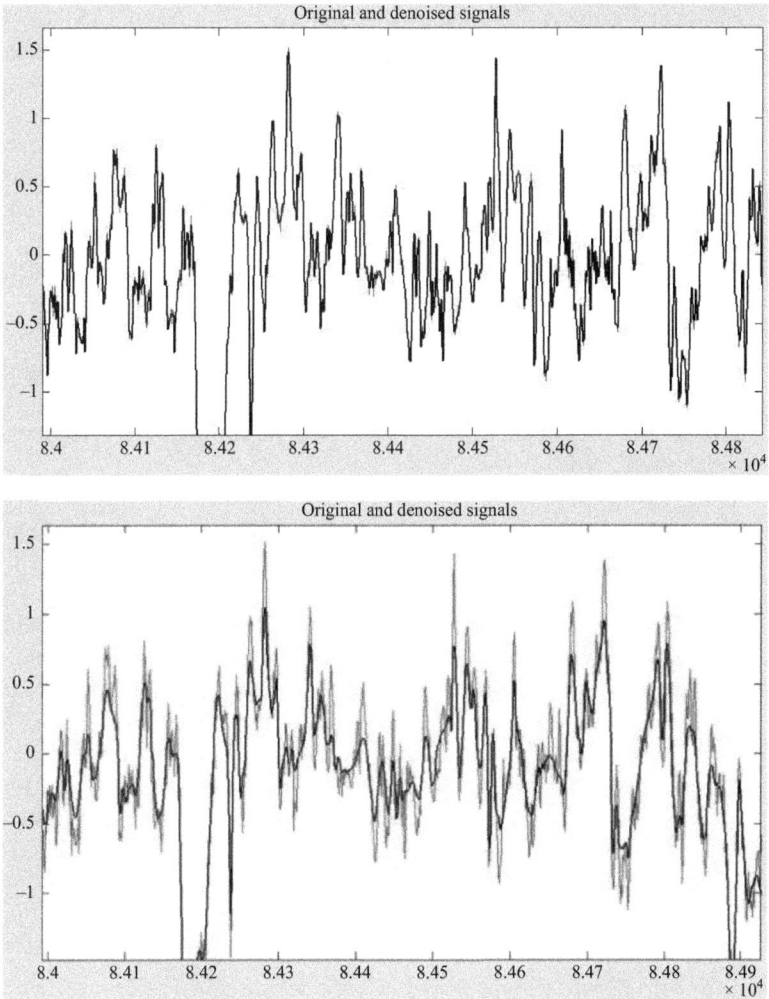

Figure 12.16 *Performance analysis on wavelet denoising with Heuristic SURE and Minimax on y4 = O2 channel (top: Heuristic SURE, bottom: Minimax)*

References

[1] K. Najarian and R. Splinter. Biomedical Signal and Image Processing. CRC Press Taylor & Francis Group. 2006.

[2] A. Delorme, J. Plamer, R. Oostenveld, J. Onton, and S. Makeig. Comparing Results of Algorithms Implementing Blind Source Separation of EEG Data. Swartz Foundation and NIH grant. 4 Apr 2007.

[3]   R. Romo-Vazquez, R. Ranta, V. Luis-Dorr, and D. Maquin. Ocular Artifacts Removal in Scalp EEG: Combining ICA and Wavelet Denoising. *5th International Conference on Physics in Signal and Image Processing*, Mulhouse: France. 2007.

[4]   A. Chichoki and S. Amari. Adaptive Blind Signal and Image Processing. Definition of Blind Signal Extraction. John Wiley Sons, Ltd, England 2002.

[5]   A. Hyvärinen and E. Oja. Independent component analysis: Algorithms and applications. Neural Network, 13 (4–5): 411–430, 2000.

[6]   R. Romo-Vazquez, R. Ranta, V. Luis-Dorr, and D. Maquin. EEG Ocular Artefacts and Noise Removal. 2 Apr 2007.

[7]   K. Ullah, M.A.U. Khan, and R.U. Kundi. What ICA Provides for ECG Signal Extraction from Contaminated ECG Observations without Using Differential Amplifiers. *IEEE* 2010.

[8]   J.V. Stone. Independent Component Analysis. John Wiley & Sons, Ltd, Chichester, 2005.

[9]   W.Y. Leong and D.P. Mandic. Blind Sequential Extraction of Post-Nonlinearly Mixed Sources Using Kalman Filtering. *Nonlinear Statistical Signal Processing Workshop (NSSPW 2006)*, pp. 47–50, 13–15 Sep 2006, Corpus Christi College, Cambridge, United Kingdom.

[10] W.Y. Leong and D.P. Mandic. Towards Blind Separation of Post-Nonlinearly Mixed Sources: Existence and Uniqueness Analysis. *The 7th International Conference on Mathematics in Signal Processing*, pp. 178–181, 17–20 Dec 2006, The Royal Agricultural College, Cirencester, United Kingdom.

[11] W.Y. Leong and J. Homer. An Adaptive Learning Algorithm for Blind Multiuser Detection System in Rician Fading Channel. *2006 IEEE International Workshop on Machine Learning for Signal Processing. Formerly the IEEE Workshop on Neural Networks for Signal Processing*, 6–8 Sep 2006, Maynooth, Ireland.

[12] W.Y. Leong and C. M. Than. Features of sleep apnea recognition and analysis. *International Journal on Smart Sensing and Intelligent Systems*. 7(2): 481–497, 2014.

[13] W.Y. Leong. Implementing blind source separation in signal processing and telecommunications, The University of Queensland, PhD Thesis, 2006.

[14] T.-W. Lee. Independent Component Analysis Theory and Applications. Kluwer Academic Publishers, Boston, 1998.

[15] S.J. Choi, A. Chichoki, and A. Beloucharrne. Second Order Nonstationary Source Separation. Journal of VLSI Signal Processing, Kluwer Academic Publishers, Boston, 2001.

[16] R.R. Gharieb and A. Cichocki. Second order statistic based blind source separation using a bank of subband filters. *Digital Signal Processing* 13 (2003) 252–274.

[17] A. Cichocki, S. Amari, K. Siwek, *et al.* ICALAB Toolboxes. http://www.bsp.brain.riken.jp/ICALAB. 2007.

Index